MW01407912

The Science of

SCENAR

Self Controlled Energic
Neuroadaptive Regulator

Using Modern Electromedicine to Stop Pain, Repair Injuries, and Regenerate Spinal Cords

By

Peter H. Lathrop, Ph. D.

Neurophysiologist

Copyright © 2015 Peter H. Lathrop

All Rights Reserved. No part of this book may be reproduced, scanned, or distributed in any printed or electronic form without prior written permission of both the author and the publisher. Please purchase only authorized electronic editions, and do not participate in or encourage electronic piracy of copyrighted materials. Your support of the author's rights is appreciated.

Neuroadaptive Institute
4275 Executive Square, Suite 200
La Jolla, CA 92037
www.askthescenarexpert.com
peter@neuroadaptiveinstitute.org

"I was impressed with Peter from the moment he came to work with me at the Salk Institute." -- Dr. Francis Crick, Nobel Laureate "The Double Helix"

"Dr. Lathrop will be my successor in leading the field of Electromedicine in the future." -- Dr. Thomas Wing, DC, LAc, inventor of Microcurrent Therapy

"I am so honored to have Dr. Lathrop with me in our practice." -- Dr. Kelly Gibson, DC

"When I think of Dr. Lathrop, many words come to mind: healer, genius, comedian, friend, musician, I could go on. Beyond those descriptions, he is committed to sharing his practice with others so together we can help as many people as possible. That speaks volumes. I have had the pleasure of being an 'apprentice' under him for several months, and he has gone out of his way to help me grow under his tutelage. I have enjoyed the process immensely, and take great pride in sharing the smidgen of his vast knowledge I possess with as many people as possible. Thank you Dr. Lathrop, I am grateful! Everyone who has the opportunity to learn and/or be healed by Dr. Lathrop needs to grab it and go for it! You will be glad you did. " -- Lisa Beguelin, Personal Trainer

Acknowledgements

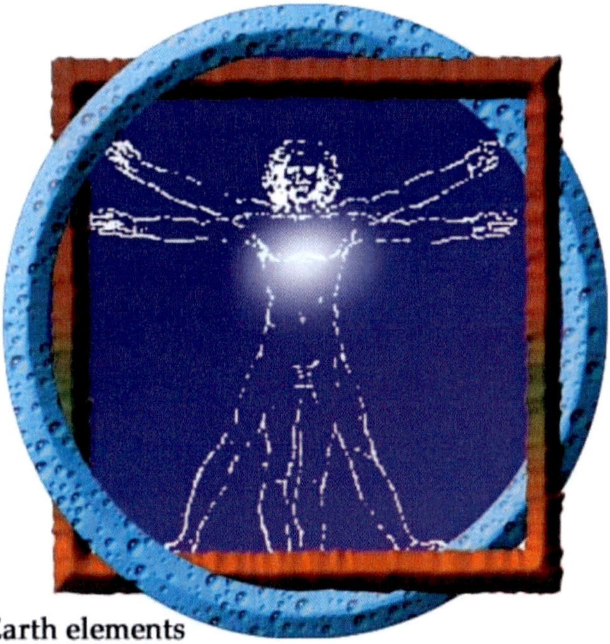

Earth elements

The brown frame represents earth
The blue circle represents water
The white on the man represents the life force

Robert O. Becker, MD, one of my medical school professors who showed me absolutely that I was not alone in my beliefs about the healing properties of electronics.

Thomas Wing, DC LAc, Inventor of Microcurrent Therapy and my mentor for 30 years.

Francis Crick, Ph. D., Nobel Laureate, co-discoverer of DNA and my boss at the Salk Institute. Always positive, my dear friend and never ending source of ideas.

Berny Dohrmann, President of CEO Space, who taught me how to start and run a business even though I am an "out of the box" scientist.

John Choisser, my friend and editor of this book. Without his help, this would never have been written.

Bernie Siegel, MD, author of "Love, Medicine and Miracles" for teaching me visualization techniques.

The Russians, my friends and joint venture partners in Scenar research and American business.

Irena Kossavskaia, MD, my first Russian Scenar instructor and friend for ten years.

Ed Japngie, my fellow out of the box scientist, who started me on the Scenar path ten years ago.

Earl Bakken, founder of Medtronic Inc. who gave me my first job in the field of Electromedicine and his belief in my possibilities.

The many hospitals, clinics, medical device companies, fellow engineers and scientists who have invested in and supported my work in Electromedicine for 35 years.

To Kay, my wife, fellow Medtronic graduate and best friend, who has supported me in my work for 10 years.

Preface

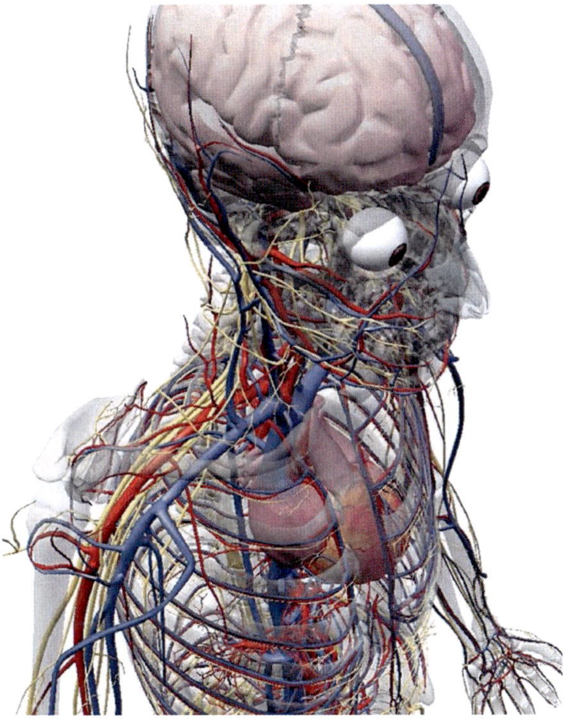

The currently held American belief regarding pain is that it should be managed instead of obliterated. This "pain management" philosophy prevalent among the current allopathic medical establishment promotes reducing pain through drugs and surgery. The question that comes to my mind after saying this is: "Why would one want to manage anything that is so alien to a normal happy life"? It was my understanding all along that we manage only those things that are necessary for our ongoing existence and lifestyle. So where is the paradox here? And how do we solve it?

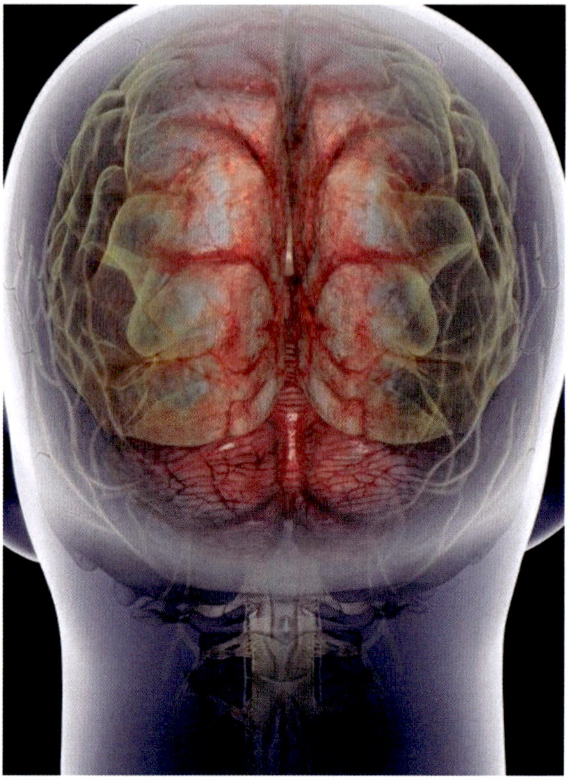

Maybe it is that, as I have found so often in my career, current medical science is not all that it is cracked up to be, if "pain management" is all they have to offer. So, if we are suffering from a chronic and debilitating pain problem, do we want to mask it with a drug that will cause us to lead a limited life both mentally and physically and more importantly become addicted to the very process?

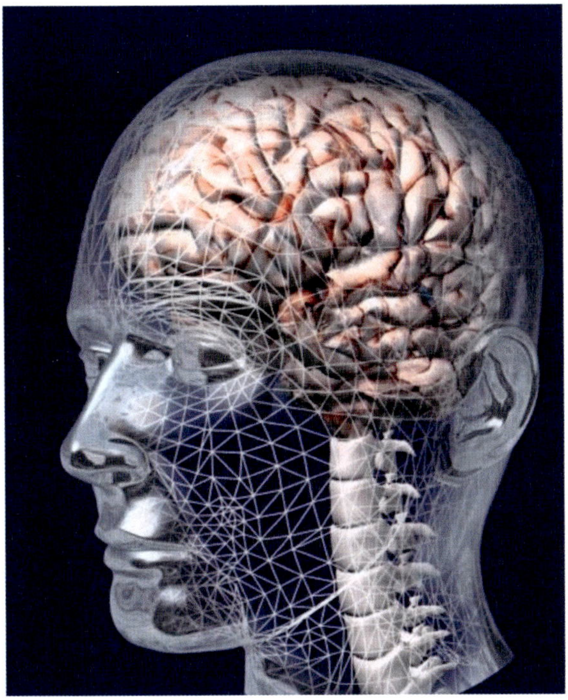

I have spent a great deal of time in my practice over the years, treating people for pain resulting from failed surgeries or their painful after effects. Surgery is not a simple, precise, laser beam treatment which efficiently corrects a problem leading no collateral damage behind. Surgery is an invasive, traumatic, and destructive assault on the body, especially when nerves and spinal columns are involved. There are lasting effects of this in many cases including scar tissue, and other collateral damage such as reduced neuromuscular function.

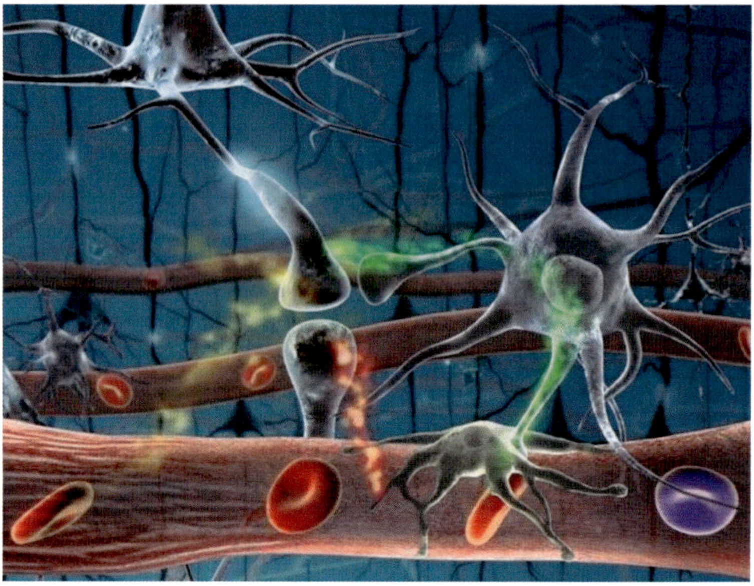

So, how do we solve the previously stated paradox? It might be through technology which has been developed for over 35 years in Russia and in America at the same parallel time and rate. This is called Electromedicine. In America this discovery was made by myself, my colleagues and other scientists working together to develop electrotherapy technology to not only stop pain but speed the healing process of neuromuscular injuries. In Russia it was discovered by two neuroscientists Alexander Karasev and Alexander Revenko. Most physicians in Russia use this technology on a daily basis.

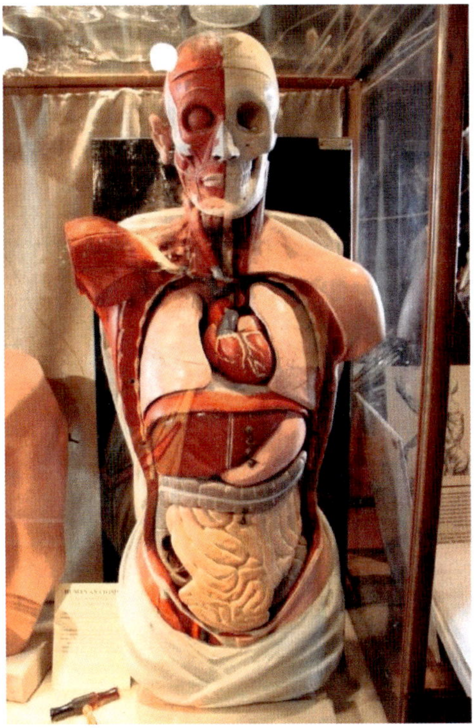

The paradox is solved by the application of an electronic signal to a pain site and the involved tissue. This process accomplishes two things at once. It stops the pain immediately and it rapidly speeds the healing process of the offending cause of the pain.

This form of therapy eliminates the need for narcotics and their debilitating effects, surgery in many cases, and facing life as an invalid. From a fresh injury perspective it stops the growth process of the injury and releases the body's abilities to repair the damage at a cellular level.

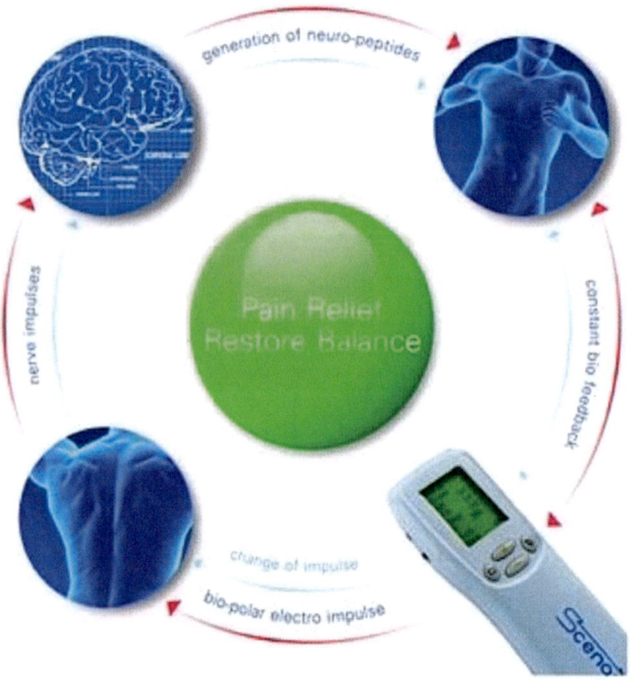
generation of neuro-peptides
constant bio feedback
bio-polar electro impulse
change of impulse
nerve impulses
Pain Relief
Restore Balance

This book is about the SCENAR, its basic principles, function, and application. For a more thorough discussion of the electrochemical, biochemical, and biological basis of the SCENAR as a tool in the practice of Electromedicine, the reader is referred to my two-volume work “Modern Electromedicine”.

About the Author

Peter Lathrop, Ph.D is a neuroscientist, inventor, engineer, educator, and in day-to-day practice a Clinical Neurophysiologist. Every day he helps people suffering with acute and chronic pain and related soft tissue and musculoskeletal injuries to gain sustained pain relief and accelerated healing of their injuries.

When it comes to soft tissue injury (muscles, ligaments, tendons, and nerves) and pain, you name it, he has seen and treated it from the head to the toes and everything in between. Some of the more common conditions include whiplash, neck/cervical strain and pain, shoulder injuries including rotator cuff tears and frozen shoulders, thoracic outlet syndrome, epicondylitis, carpal tunnel syndrome, herniated discs, sciatica, low back pain, knee and ankle sprains, strains, and ligament tears, plantar fasciitis, etc.

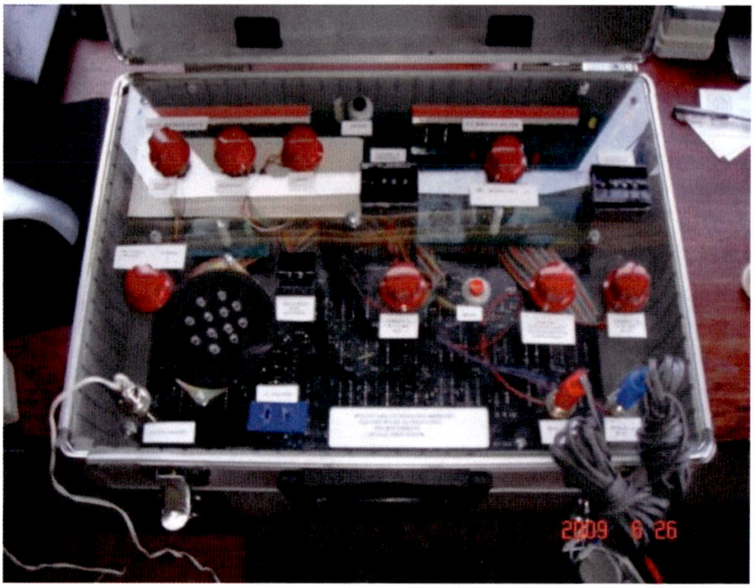
2009 6 26

Throughout his career Dr. Lathrop has spent over 30+ years in clinical practice in San Diego with the San Diego Pain Treatment and Injury Repair Center, the Dynamic Health Institute, Industrial Medical Centers (now US Healthworks), Don Perry & Co - Physical Therapy and Rehabilitation Centers, Blott Chiropractic, Harbor View Medical Center, Paradise Valley Hospital, and San Diego Pain Treatment Center, to name a few.

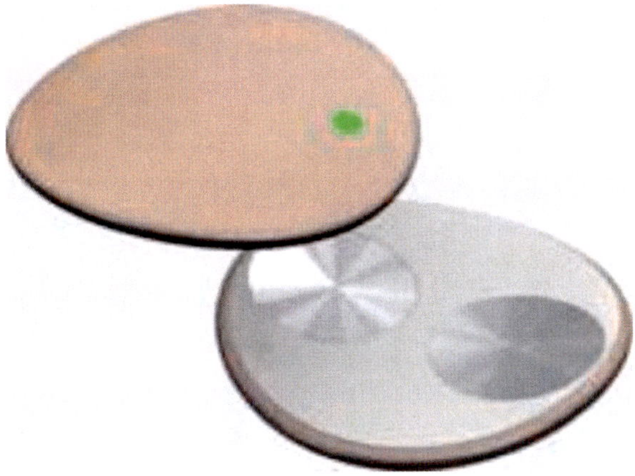

He specializes in the use of therapeutic, regenerative electrotherapy devices to generate healing, including **SCENAR** and microcurrent bioelectric signaling devices. Through the course of his career he has co-developed electrotherapy devices with and for manufacturers, many of which are in wide use today. He worked collaboratively at Medtronic, Inc. in the late 1970s to co-develop the first commercially available **TENS unit**. He partnered with the late **Dr. Thomas Wing** in the development and commercialization of Microcurrent technology. He has received patents for his work in device design for treatment of injuries, viruses, and neurological disorders.

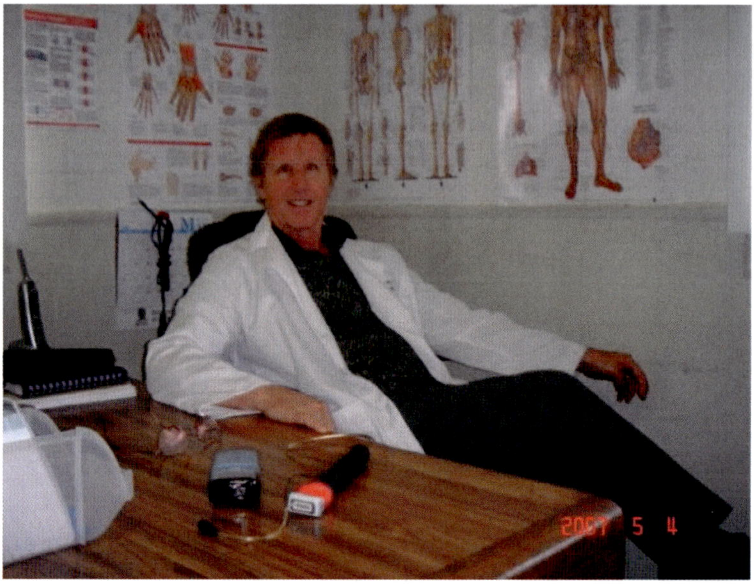

It was in 2006 that Dr. Lathrop was introduced to the SCENAR, long before the FDA clearance was received in the U.S. He has used it now for nine years in clinical practice. He has an excellent rate of success with the device and it has become his "go to" technology for most indications. As an inventor and early adopter of electrotherapy and laser technology he immediately wanted to know more about **SCENAR** and to use it himself. He attended trainings, one which was conducted by a Russian physician and scientist, **Irina Kossovskaia, M.D.** She worked with the original **SCENAR** research team, which included **Dr. Alexander Revenko**, **Dr. Yuri Gorfinkel, Dr. Josef Semikatov**, **Dr. Alexander Karasev** and other top Russian scientists. Given his background in neurophysiology and biochemistry along with most forms of **electrotherapy** Dr. Lathrop rapidly assimilated the information and put the SCENAR to use. **Dr. Lathrop** maintains a significant relationship with the manufacturers in Russia and their representatives.

Always an educator, Dr. Lathrop has trained both patients and practitioners in the use of the SCENAR devices. He is also one of only a few in Southern California to be utilizing the revolutionary Russian SCENAR technology to accelerate healing. He has trained most of them.

Table of Contents

Introduction

Bioelectric Systems

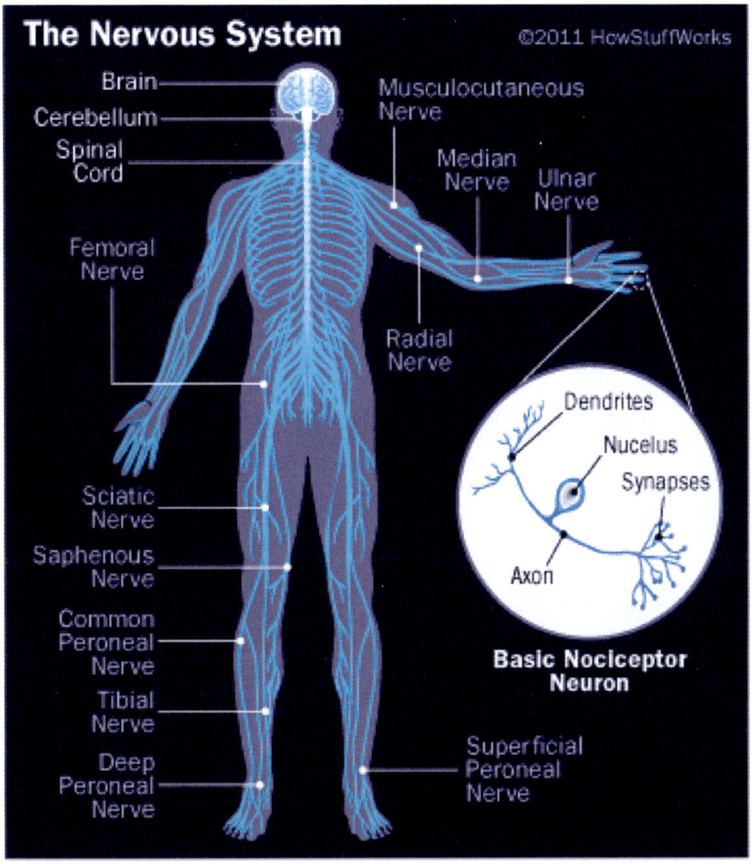

The Nervous System
©2011 HowStuffWorks
Brain
Cerebellum
Spinal Cord
Femoral Nerve
Musculocutaneous Nerve
Median Nerve
Ulnar Nerve
Radial Nerve
Dendrites
Nucelus
Synapses
Axon
Basic Nociceptor Neuron
Sciatic Nerve
Saphenous Nerve
Common Peroneal Nerve
Tibial Nerve
Deep Peroneal Nerve
Superficial Peroneal Nerve

Well what is this about? Most of us think of medicine, the practice of medicine, as needles, drugs, and surgery. Those three things, that's all we need. We need to become addicted to drugs, we need to have marks on our skin from needles and scars from the surgery that is performed to take care of the problems we have. That's pretty much what we're looking at, right? This is called allopathic medicine. It's standard medicine. That's what's practiced in America, unlike Europe, Russia or Canada, where they're a bit more progressive. I'm going to talk about the old/new field of electromedicine. I say old/new because whenever I explain it to people, they say, "Why haven't I heard about this before? It's new, isn't it?"

Yes it's new, since it was invented in 1979 in America and sold worldwide, electromedicine started at **Medtronic** the way it's practiced today in America. At Medtronic, where I worked in 1979, where we invented, designed, and put out to the world the first **TENS unit**. A small electrical device the size of a packet of cigarettes with wires and electrodes which, when attached to the body in an area of pain, stopped the pain signal. I was one of the inventors of this device. Medtronic sold 56 million of them from 1981- 1984.

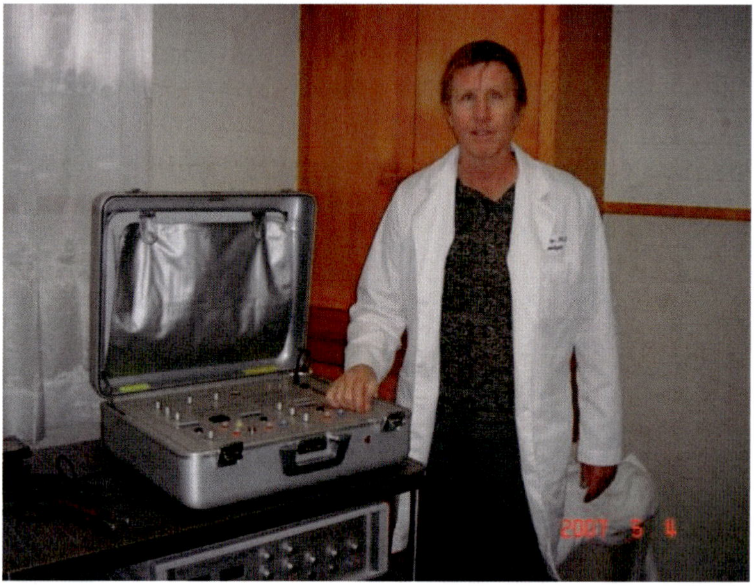

Other companies I've worked for since then have sold millions more, yet I still keep getting asked the question, Why is this so new and why haven't I heard of it before? It's because it's suppressed. There's a better way to do things than needles, drugs, pills, pharmaceuticals, and surgery.

The old/new field of electromedicine kind of goes like this: It is a field of medicine wherein equipment is designed which interacts with the body electronically. The human body is an **electro-chemical** system. It operates on an electric circuit. The body is an electric circuit. These circuits, the nodes of these circuits, are cells. The body is full of billions of cells. Each cell is an electrical piece. It has a positive and a negative charge. They're called ions and they circle the cell. They're in the aqueous fluid around the cell and they're positively charged, negatively charged, neutrally charged, depending on the function of the cell.

Our bodies are made up of billions of them. Inside of each cell is a battery, just like the stuff we plug in our ears and plug everywhere else and use. The battery is called the mitochondria. The **mitochondria** is the cell energy-producing battery of the cell function. They are the activators. Outside of it is the substance that carries the cell and is **charged positively or negatively**. The body is made up of muscles and nerves and other soft tissue. This soft tissue is fed, nourished, and grows by the production of **protein**, which is produced by the transfer of **ions** across the cells, which multiply, producing more protein, converting biochemicals, stimulating the sodium potassium pump in the body. All biochemistry, electrochemistry, this is how the body works. Little tiny engines, the cells, keep reproducing, keep functioning, keep pushing the system and the organs to work. To repair them, to grow them, to replace them constantly.

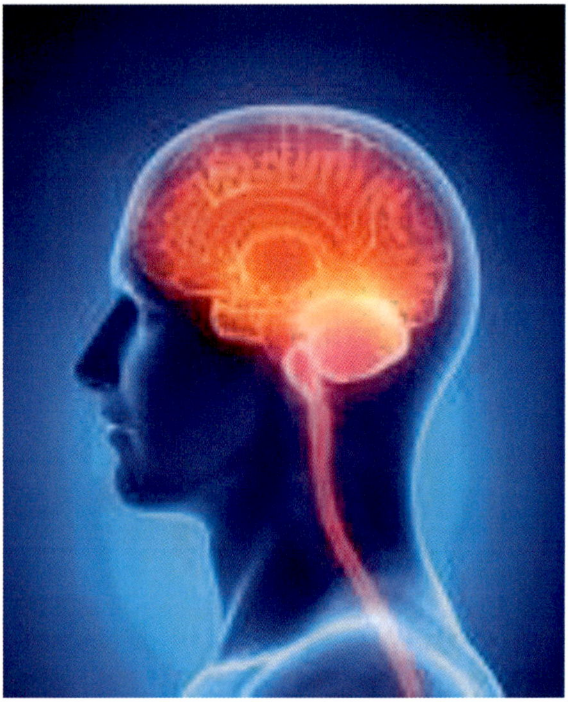

The human body replaces itself in its entirety every six months. What happens is that you have something wrong with your body, if you treat it right, if you reprogram it, the body will repair itself in six months and rid itself of the memory of the old injury or disease. That is pretty much the formula for healthy, functioning cell function. What happens when we have an injury? What happens is that all of this gets changed. The polarity in the cells change, the positive and the negative ions will multiply in one direction or the other, the body becomes out of balance. Electrochemically out of balance. This results in an injury, pain, chronicity, and destruction of the tissue. The injury itself, when it happens and the moment it happens, produces what is called a current of injury.

The current of injury is like a virus. Say you are in a football game and you get hurt, crashed into, your rotator cuff becomes injured, damaged, traumatized, the current of injury immediately starts, and then what once was something the size of your finger, starts growing. If you let it go several hours, overnight, the next day, a few days later, by the time you get to the doctor it's now what started this size at minute one is this size a day or two later because the virus grew, the current of injury grew.

All the cells in the injury then became damaged, malfunctioning, which caused the body's prehistoric method of protection: inflammation, closing the blood supply to the tissue and basically walling off and breaking down the healing process. The healing process needs to occur in order for the injury to get well and go away but what happens is it goes in the reverse to protect itself. So what we do in electromedicine is to put a signal into the body to change that, to correct each and every cell so they're functioning normally and in a healthy manner, to reproduce and to correct themselves, which then will lead to increasing blood supply, reduction of edema, swelling, inflammation. **Returning the body back to its normal state.**

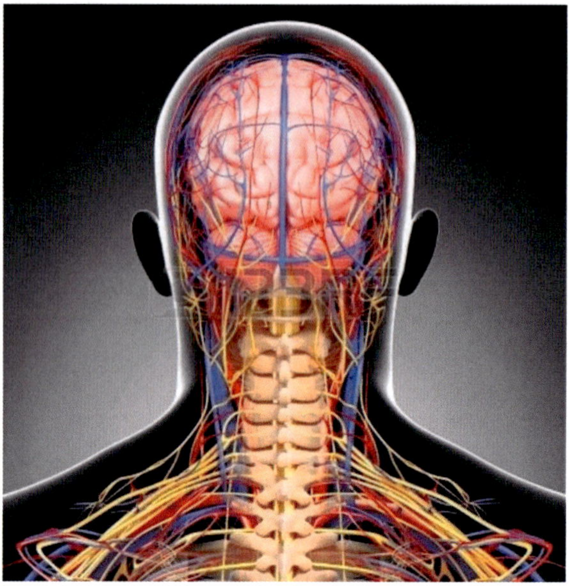

There are two kinds of injuries. There's the acute stage, where it just happened and the current of injury has just occurred and it's growing, and there's the chronic stage where the injury occurred a month or two ago, a few years ago, and the injury stayed with the body, stayed with the memory system of the cell. The cells have a memory. They each remember the way it was so they reproduce the way it was to be the way it will be, which is the way it was. So the cell memory carries forward through the years. This is called a **chronic state of injury.**

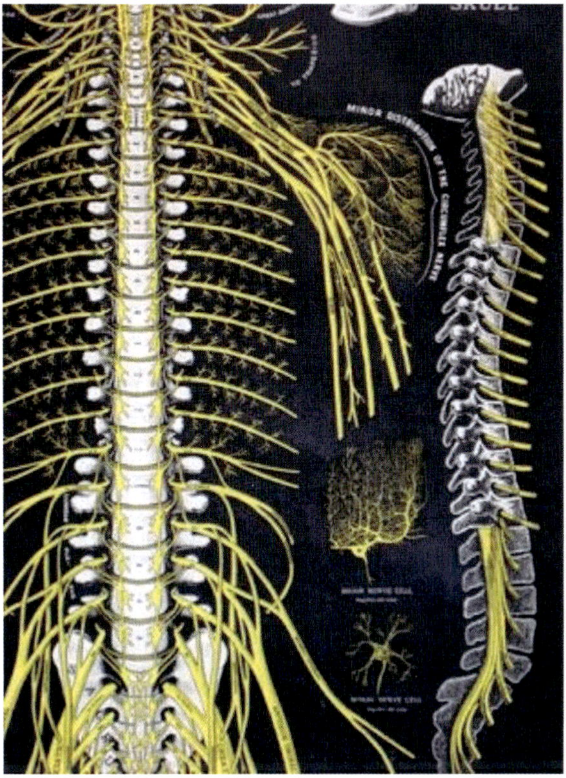

To break the chronic state of injury, the trauma, the memory in the cell, we reprogram the cell with a computer. I have designed computers for 30 years that do this. They are sold worldwide and used in clinical practice. Why haven't I heard of this before? Well, watch. Go somewhere, go to physical therapists, go to chiropractors. Chiropractors, by the way, I have found to be the biggest risk-takers in many ways in the field of electro medicine. The chiropractors have been the ones who primarily took this equipment and used it in their practices because they have the training to do this. They took this and guess what? Their practices improved and they got better and they had better results.

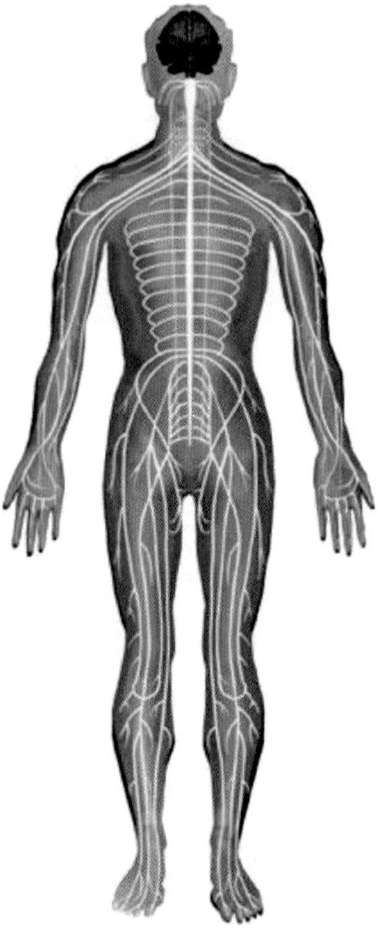

Chiropractors, from a structural point of view and **electrotherapy** from a biochemical/muscle/soft tissue point of view, can pretty well wrap up the problems that people have. Accurately diagnose them and repair them because an injury will cause a structural damage and soft tissue damage, so if we put the spinal column in the right alignment and then we treat the tissue and repair it, and we find we're able to accomplish a great deal this way.

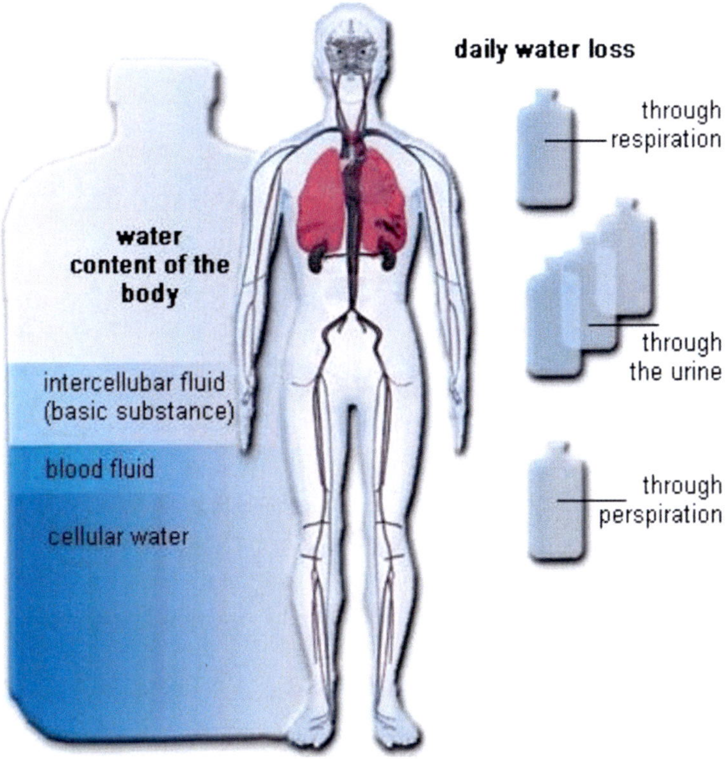
daily water loss
through
respiration
water
content of the
body
through
the urine
intercellubar fluid
(basic substance)
blood fluid
through
perspiration
cellular water

The computers we have designed to do this, interface with the human body in the sense of you hardly feel it, they're hooked up to you, the injury is treated with handheld probes, electrodes, etc., attached to the body, run a few minutes a current into the body, and right at that moment, they are repaired, repaired instantly. A traumatic injury occurring in the moment, can be stopped and repaired. I'm going to give you a live example of that. The injury, in essence, in my work with athletic teams including the Dallas Cowboys and other high school and college teams, we have found that a player that is injured—let's say an offensive lineman is injured, he comes off the field, he's treated, and it only takes five or six minutes to do it, he goes in the next set of downs, uninjured because the injury was erased. That's very possible; we do it all the time. In order to do this, we use different kinds of equipment.

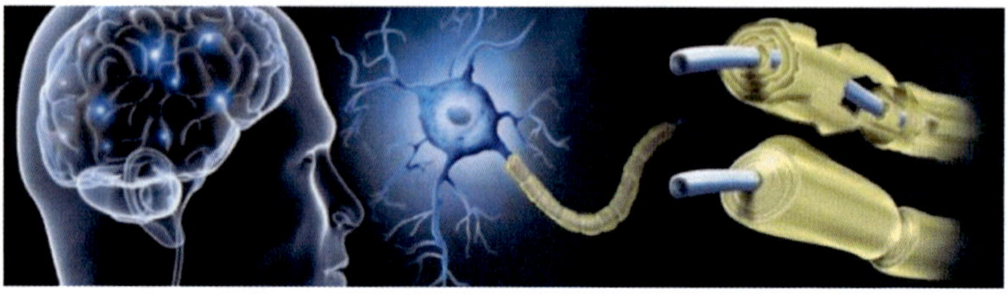

One of the first projects I was involved in was **The Electro-Accuscope**, which is one of the first micro-current devices—micro-current, millionths of an amp, not a car battery, not jumper cables, a millionth of an amp. The average treatment current of the Electro-Accuscope, which reads the tissue, puts back a signal to correct what it reads. It's called a positive feedback loop. The average is somewhere in the neighborhood of half a Hertz and approximately 80-300 micro amps. That's 300 millionths of one amp. Very small. You don't feel it.

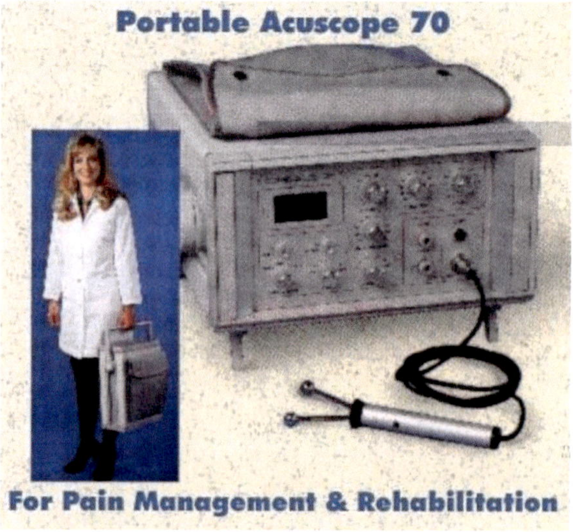
Portable Acuscope 70
For Pain Management & Rehabilitation

I was on the design team for the **Myomatic** in 1980; we developed this device and it's sold and used all over the country. It cost $3,000 and was used in practices all over the country to repair injuries. Basically how it works is that the machine is turned on, the settings are adjusted for the output that you want, what kind of injury you want to repair, what depth you want to go, etc. Then wherever the injury is, it is treated here for 15 seconds, here for 15 seconds, here, here, let's say around the rotator cuff. So you have a treatment time of maybe 10 minutes for an injury. If it's an acute injury that just happened that day or the day before, all you need is maybe one or two treatments and you're done! It's fixed. You didn't have to go to the hospital, go to the doctor, physical therapy, take time off work, whatever, none of it. It's done.

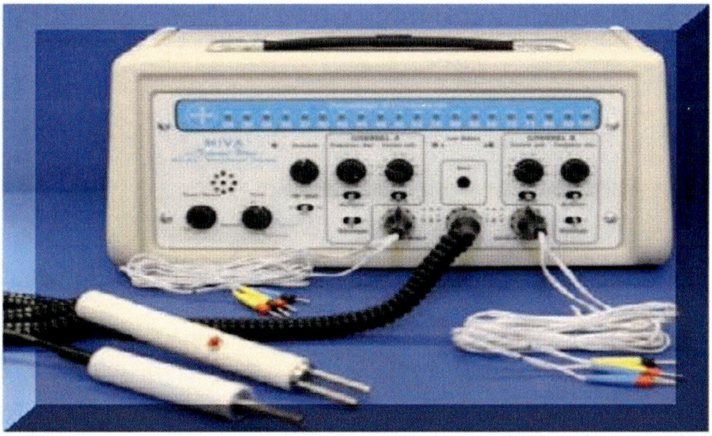

This is how this device works. It goes into the body, it reads the problem, and corrects it automatically. There's a lot of training that goes into teaching somebody how to use this. I have trained people myself, there are trainers that will train therapists how to use it, it's in the protocol where to treat, how to treat, how to have a sense about how to work with the human body. We have two probes; one is held in one hand and has a button on it. And you go here and you read the body until you find the point of injury. The machine will open up and will tell you…(buzzing noise)…that's a perfect circuit there. Now what that says is that there's a full connection so that you would treat and you push the button. Now the Accuscope is the same principle.

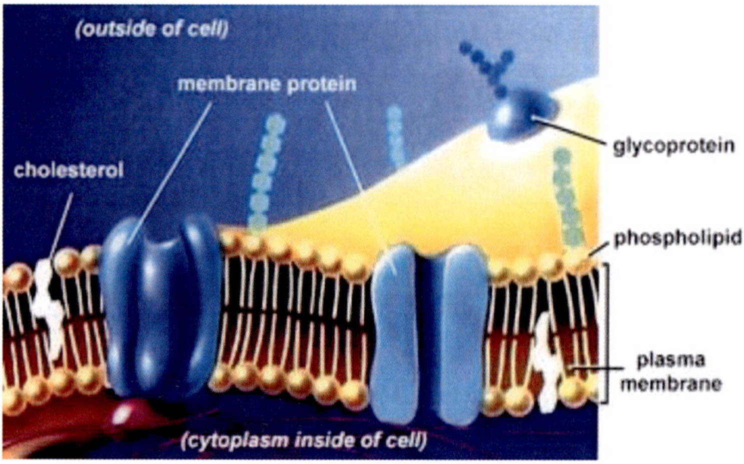
(outside of cell)
membrane protein
glycoprotein
cholesterol
phospholipid
plasma membrane
(cytoplasm inside of cell)

The computers, they are computers, are put in touch with the human body, with the injury, and then they are put to work to repair it and they do it immediately. Now the average is like this—if it's an acute injury, it's done in one, maybe two treatments, if it's a chronic injury, like a year or longer, it may take six, maybe nine treatments, and then the injury is repaired.

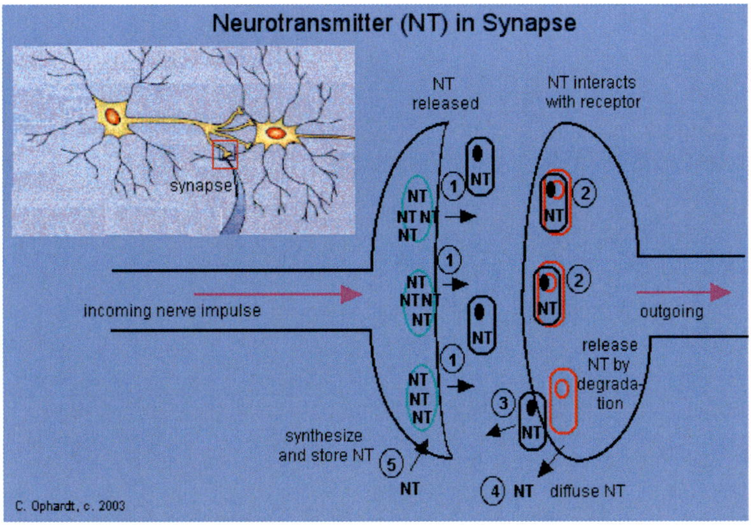
Neurotransmitter (NT) in Synapse
synapse
NT
released
NT interacts
with receptor
incoming nerve impulse
outgoing
release
NT by
degrada-
tion
synthesize
and store NT
NT
diffuse NT
C. Ophardt, c. 2003

The next step in this whole progression is now getting smaller. So we have really big thing here, really big show, we have a smaller big show, and now what we're coming to is a smaller show. Well it's in here now. How does this work? Well, it works this way. We have this little unit and we have this probe, and all we do to treat a patient is I hold this, I find it, this reads the body, finds the injury, and repairs it. That's what we do. We literally find the injury, stop the pain, and return the body back to normal in a few minutes.

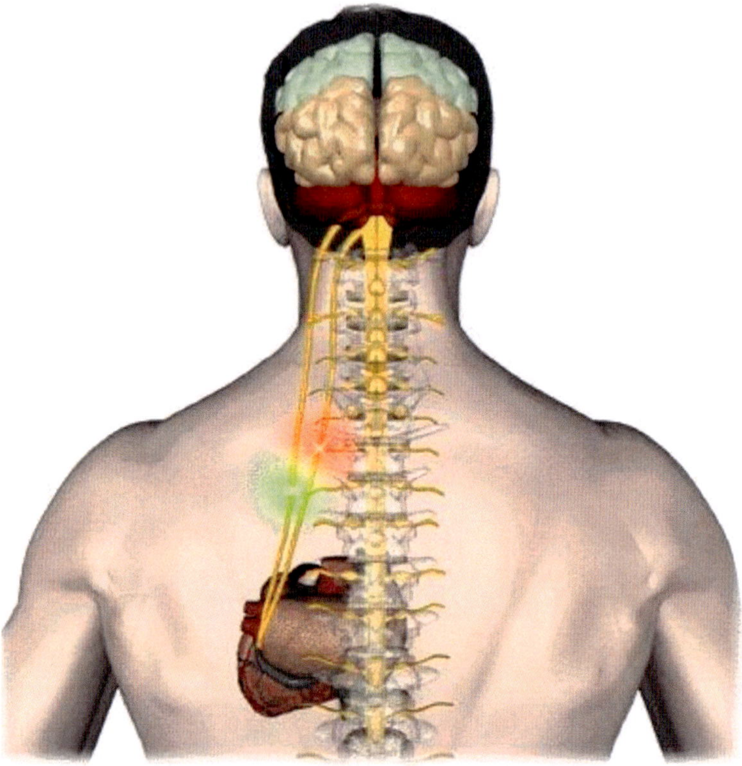

I would like to tell you a couple of things about this kind of technology; some of the patients that I see and some of the injuries and disorders that I treat. They include whiplash injuries, lumbar strains, low back injuries, chronic low back pain, rotator cuff injuries, trigeminal neuralgia which is severe pain of the face.

For example, I had a patient this year that came in with 20 years of trigeminal neuralgia. 18 years of unceasing chronic, severe pain in the right side of his face. When he came in to see me, his face was askew, it was not symmetrical. His eye drooped, his lip drooped, he didn't look right. I treated him, repaired him, stopped the pain, and reconfigured his face so he left with no pain, no trigeminal neuralgia, and his face was symmetrical. That's one thing I do with this equipment.

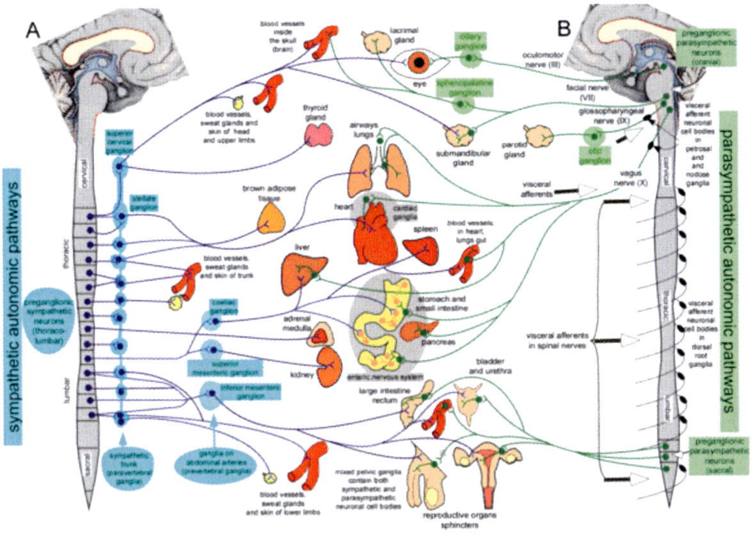
A
B
sympathetic autonomic pathways
parasympathetic autonomic pathways
blood vessels inside the skull (brain)
lacrimal gland
eye
oculomotor nerve (III)
facial nerve (VII)
glossopharyngeal nerve (IX)
vagus nerve (X)
blood vessels, sweat glands and skin of head and upper limbs
thyroid gland
airways lungs
submandibular gland
parotid gland
brown adipose tissue
heart
spleen
blood vessels in heart, lungs gut
visceral afferents
liver
blood vessels, sweat glands and skin of trunk
adrenal medulla
kidney
stomach and small intestine
pancreas
visceral afferents in spinal nerves
bladder and urethra
large intestine rectum
blood vessels, sweat glands and skin of lower limbs
mixed pelvic ganglia contain both sympathetic and parasympathetic neuronal cell bodies
reproductive organs sphincters
cervical
thoracic
lumbar
sacral

Other treatments that we do are athletic injuries, ankles, knees. I tore my medial cruciate ligament a couple of years ago. I heard it tear, I swear I did, it was ugly. I used this equipment to repair myself. I did it in two days. I repaired my leg such that I could walk again. I was badly injured. I played tennis two weeks after the tear. I'm not slow. I'm very fast and aggressive.

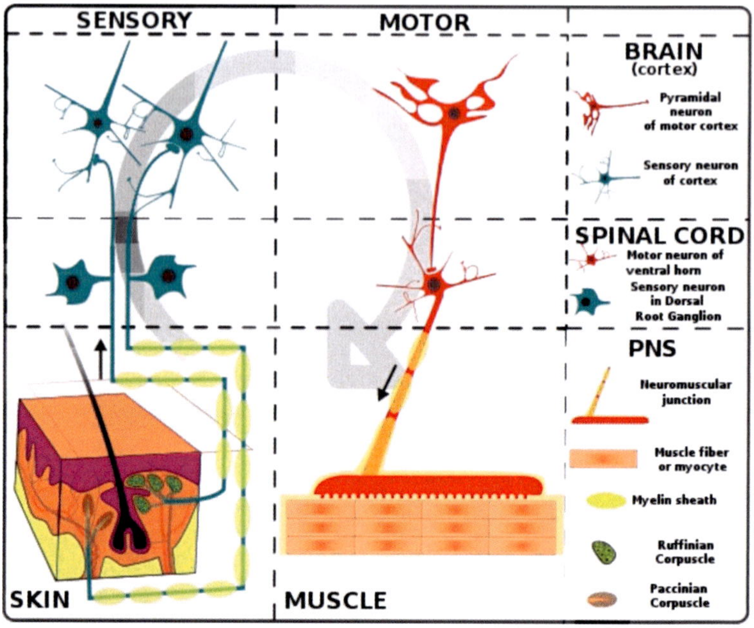
SENSORY
MOTOR
BRAIN
(cortex)
Pyramidal neuron of motor cortex
Sensory neuron of cortex
SPINAL CORD
Motor neuron of ventral horn
Sensory neuron in Dorsal Root Ganglion
PNS
Neuromuscular junction
Muscle fiber or myocyte
Myelin sheath
Ruffinian Corpuscle
Paccinian Corpuscle
SKIN
MUSCLE

The thing is, this stuff works. I'll call it **"new" medicine**. I've only been in it 30 years; I guess it's still new. It does work. We can do pretty much miracle kind of medicine. Some of the kinds of injuries I treat include carpel tunnel syndrome, peripheral neuralgia, paralysis, lack of sensation, parenthetic injuries, strains, sprains, tears, rotator cuff injuries, anterior cruciate ligament tears, strains. I can repair the tissue at the cellular level by reprogramming it with this equipment.

This is pretty much what I do. I call myself a television repair man for the human body. Bring in your set, I'll attach my tools and fix it. What we can do then, is electronically change the signal, so the signal does not say hurt, it says '**NORMAL**'. So we can do this electronically and we've been doing it for years

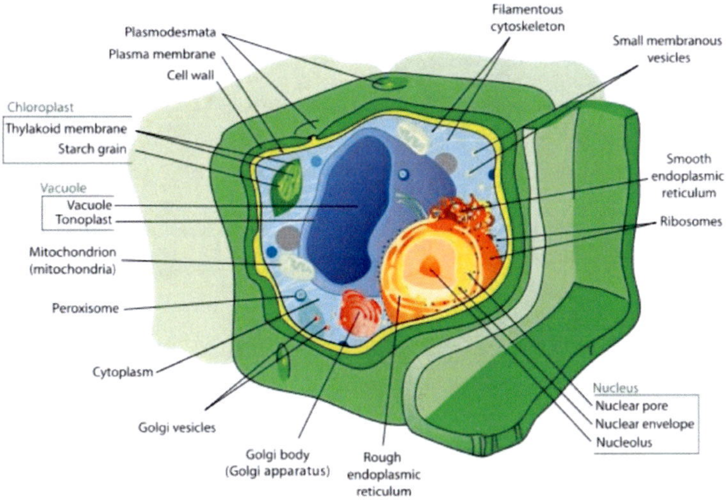
Filamentous cytoskeleton
Plasmodesmata
Plasma membrane
Cell wall
Small membranous vesicles
Chloroplast
Thylakoid membrane
Starch grain
Smooth endoplasmic reticulum
Vacuole
Vacuole
Tonoplast
Ribosomes
Mitochondrion (mitochondria)
Peroxisome
Cytoplasm
Nucleus
Nuclear pore
Nuclear envelope
Nucleolus
Golgi vesicles
Golgi body (Golgi apparatus)
Rough endoplasmic reticulum

I have been thinking about how I explain to clients what is happening in their body when soft tissue is injured. One way I describe a new or fresh soft tissue injury is like a pebble thrown into the middle of a still lake. Think about it - skipping pebbles at the lake. "See" what happens when it "plops". An injury is just like this. It often starts as just a very tiny circle. As the minutes and hours pass an injury grows like the circles in the lake from the initial "plop" of the tossed pebble.

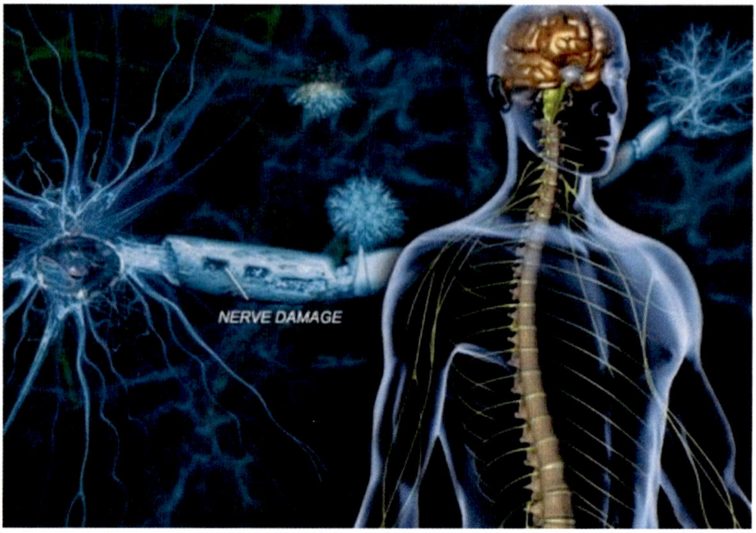
NERVE DAMAGE

Injuries grow immediately through involvement of cell after cell after nerve, muscle, and tendon or ligament fiber. **Biochemicals** gather about the injury to wall it off from the rest of the body, producing swelling and inflammation as a "warning" not to use the injured part. This process is not necessary today as we, unlike the caveman, have no need to keep fighting, surviving, or using the injured appendage. Still the injury grows, involving more and more tissue. It rapidly swells and becomes painful.

What to Do?

If you have a **regenerative electrotherapy** device like a **SCENAR** you would treat yourself immediately. Yes, home units are available. I see the day when we will all have one in our home. They are not complicated to use and they are worth it over your lifetime. Actually my experience is that most people get their return on investment with one, maybe two injuries or issues.

Better a SCENAR in your home than a bottle of pills given their side effect profiles.

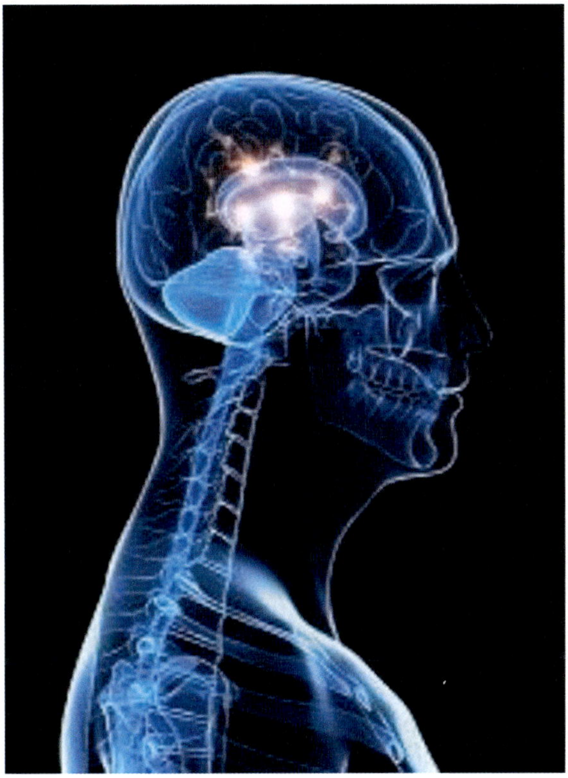

The sooner a regenerative electrotherapy modality like SCENAR is applied the sooner an injury can be repaired. It could be as soon as overnight if applied the same day as the injury. Really.

If you don't have a SCENAR

So you don't have your own SCENAR yet. Well, this is the injury that might make you say "now". What you need to do is immediately, within minutes, sit or lie down and apply ice to try to stop the progression of the injury. Use ice for 20 minutes several times during the day of the injury. Taking an **anti-inflammatory** several times the first couple of days of the injury can also be useful. I suggest fish oil. Rest the injury!

Chapter 1.
What is Scenar?

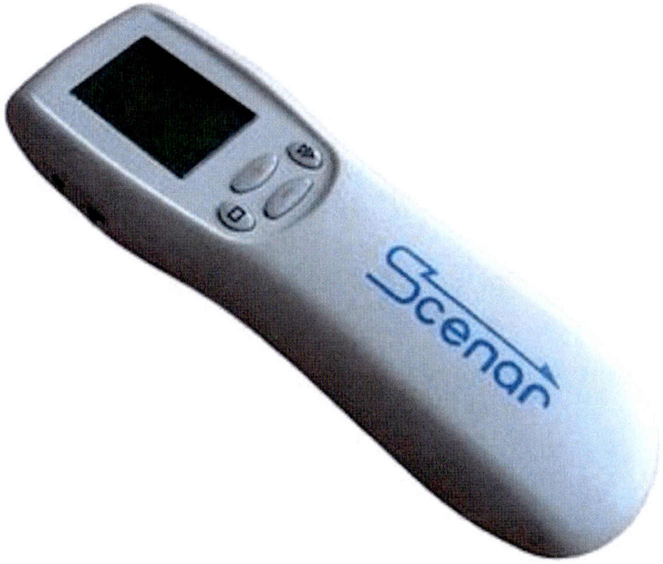
Scenar

SCENAR stands for Self Controlled Energo-Neuro Adaptive Regulator

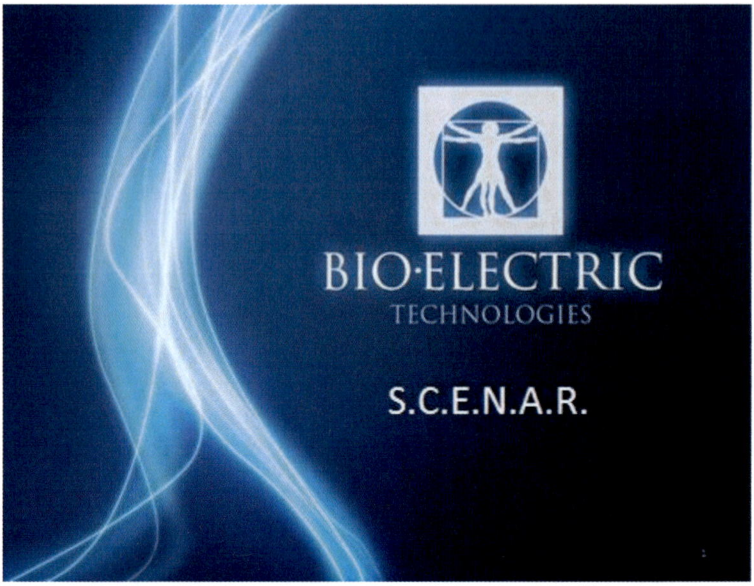
BIO·ELECTRIC
TECHNOLOGIES
S.C.E.N.A.R.

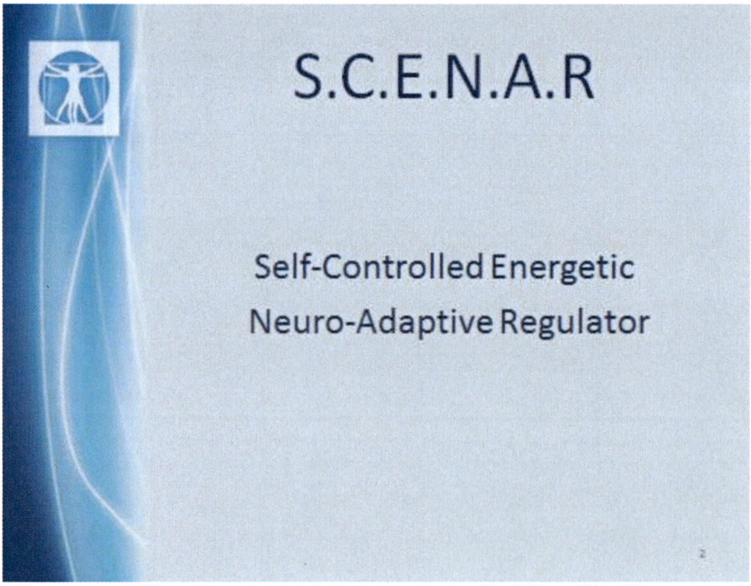
S.C.E.N.A.R
Self-Controlled Energetic
Neuro-Adaptive Regulator

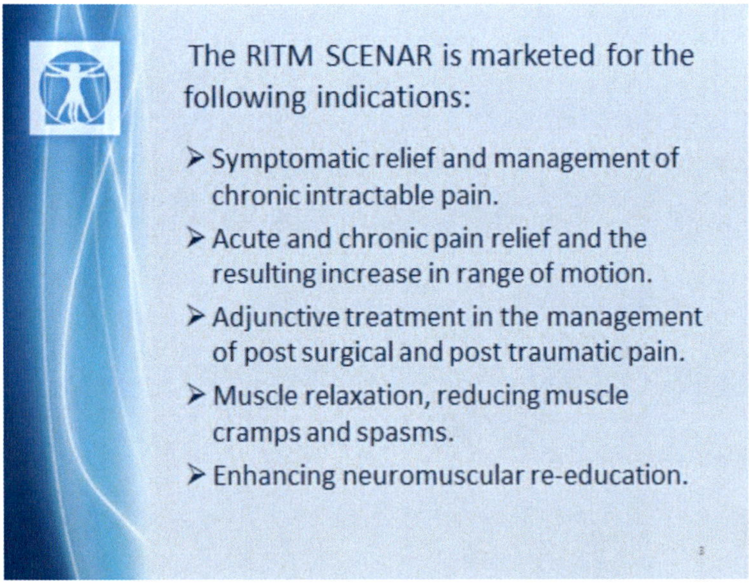
The RITM SCENAR is marketed for the following indications:
➤ Symptomatic relief and management of chronic intractable pain.
➤ Acute and chronic pain relief and the resulting increase in range of motion.
➤ Adjunctive treatment in the management of post surgical and post traumatic pain.
➤ Muscle relaxation, reducing muscle cramps and spasms.
➤ Enhancing neuromuscular re-education.

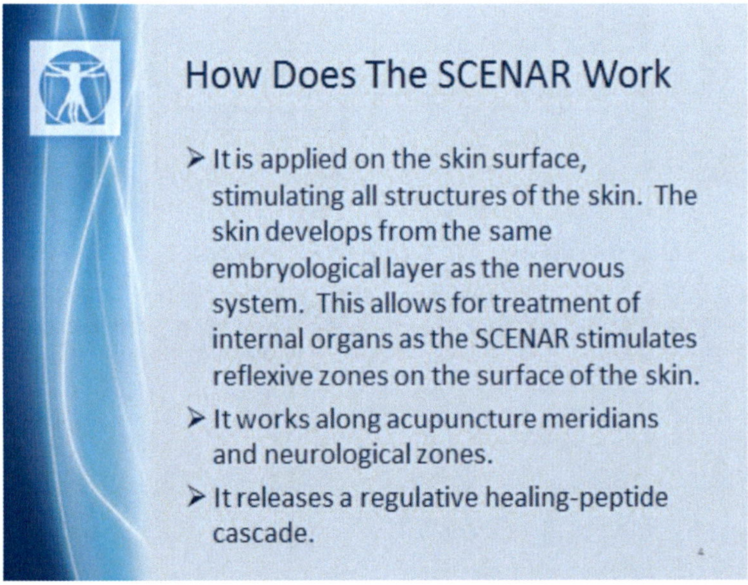
How Does The SCENAR Work
➤ It is applied on the skin surface, stimulating all structures of the skin. The skin develops from the same embryological layer as the nervous system. This allows for treatment of internal organs as the SCENAR stimulates reflexive zones on the surface of the skin.
➤ It works along acupuncture meridians and neurological zones.
➤ It releases a regulative healing-peptide cascade.

- It helps to restore homeostasis.
- It eliminates repetitive contral nervous system patterns.
- It works along ascending pathways in the spinal cord to affect the cortex of the brain. This causes efferent pathways from the cortex to convey impulses, which affect a response in the organs associated with the reflex area on the skin.
- It works directly on local spinal reflexes.
- It re-establishes normal membranous resonance.

Contraindication:

- Pacemakers
- Cardiac Fibrillation
- Intoxication

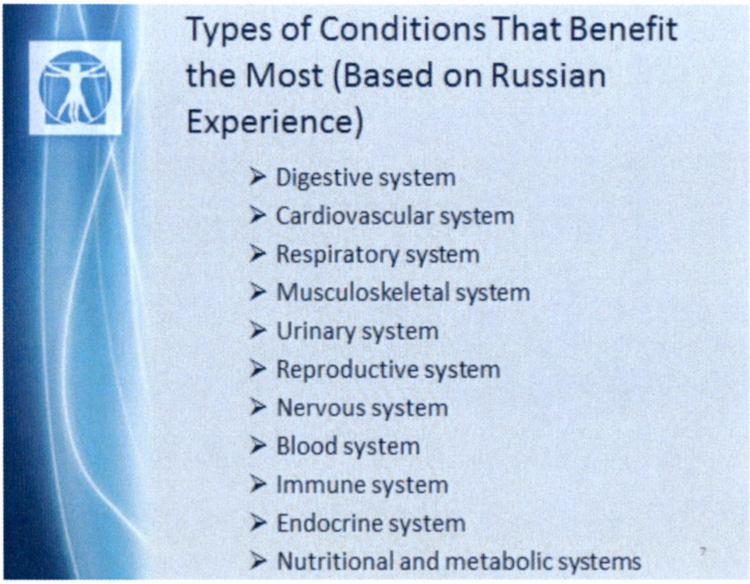
Types of Conditions That Benefit the Most (Based on Russian Experience)
➢ Digestive system
➢ Cardiovascular system
➢ Respiratory system
➢ Musculoskeletal system
➢ Urinary system
➢ Reproductive system
➢ Nervous system
➢ Blood system
➢ Immune system
➢ Endocrine system
➢ Nutritional and metabolic systems

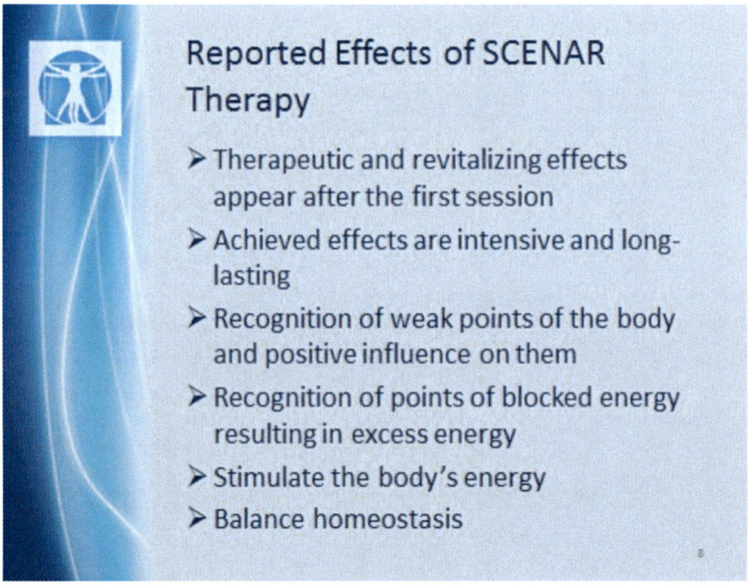
Reported Effects of SCENAR Therapy
➢ Therapeutic and revitalizing effects appear after the first session
➢ Achieved effects are intensive and long-lasting
➢ Recognition of weak points of the body and positive influence on them
➢ Recognition of points of blocked energy resulting in excess energy
➢ Stimulate the body's energy
➢ Balance homeostasis

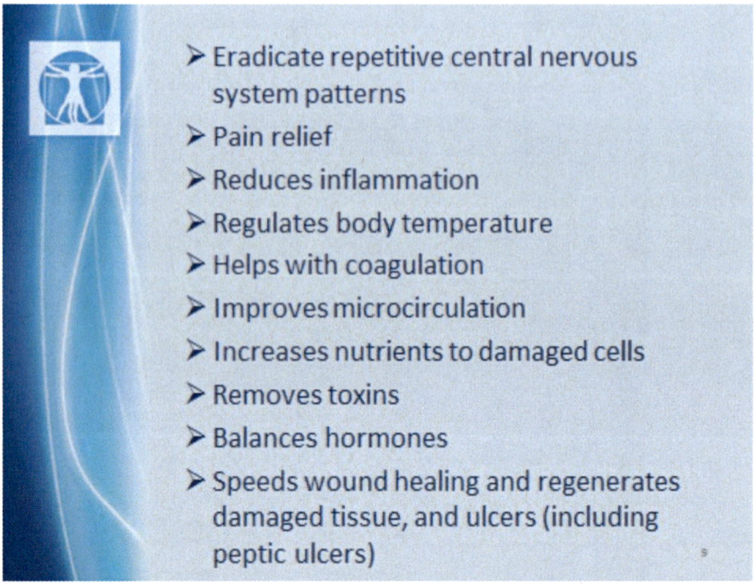
➤ Eradicate repetitive central nervous system patterns
➤ Pain relief
➤ Reduces inflammation
➤ Regulates body temperature
➤ Helps with coagulation
➤ Improves microcirculation
➤ Increases nutrients to damaged cells
➤ Removes toxins
➤ Balances hormones
➤ Speeds wound healing and regenerates damaged tissue, and ulcers (including peptic ulcers)

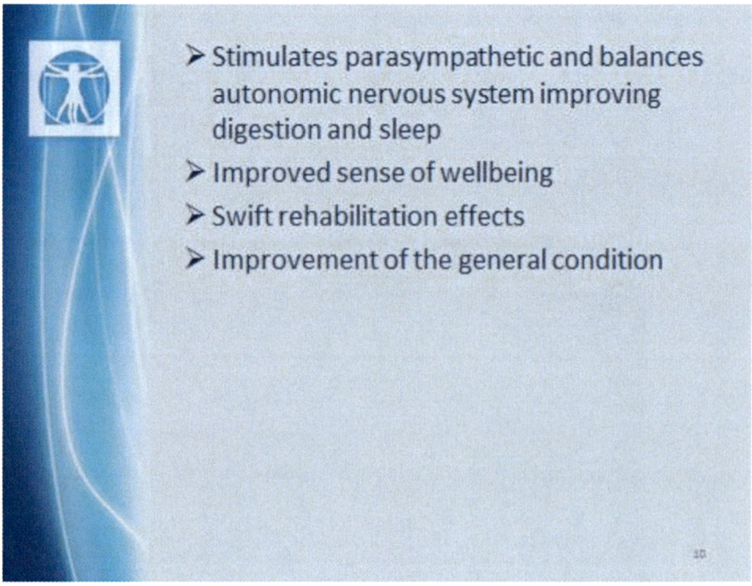
➤ Stimulates parasympathetic and balances autonomic nervous system improving digestion and sleep
➤ Improved sense of wellbeing
➤ Swift rehabilitation effects
➤ Improvement of the general condition

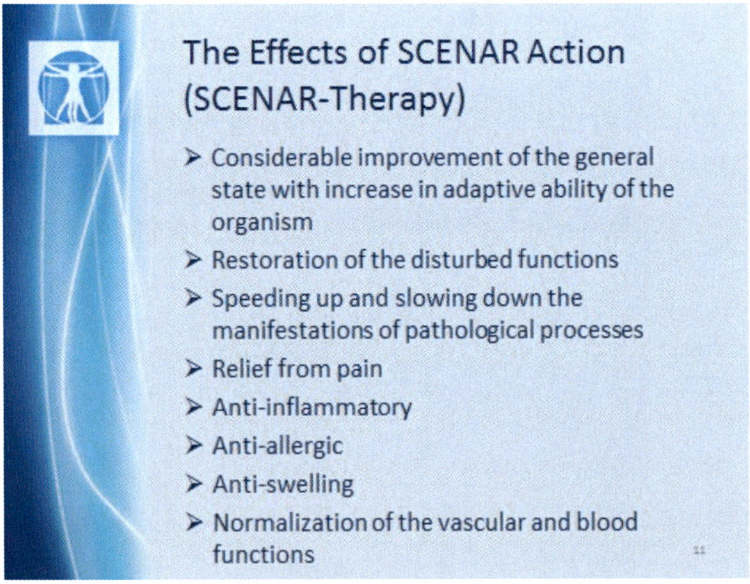
The Effects of SCENAR Action (SCENAR-Therapy)
➢ Considerable improvement of the general state with increase in adaptive ability of the organism
➢ Restoration of the disturbed functions
➢ Speeding up and slowing down the manifestations of pathological processes
➢ Relief from pain
➢ Anti-inflammatory
➢ Anti-allergic
➢ Anti-swelling
➢ Normalization of the vascular and blood functions
11

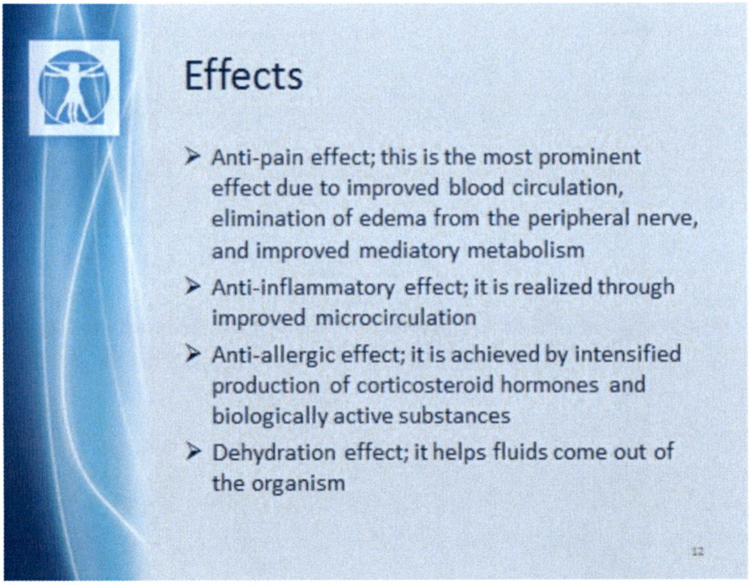
Effects
➢ Anti-pain effect; this is the most prominent effect due to improved blood circulation, elimination of edema from the peripheral nerve, and improved mediatory metabolism
➢ Anti-inflammatory effect; it is realized through improved microcirculation
➢ Anti-allergic effect; it is achieved by intensified production of corticosteroid hormones and biologically active substances
➢ Dehydration effect; it helps fluids come out of the organism
12

- Immunoregulating effect; it occurs due to stimulation of the immune system. If patient has a low immunity, SCENAR application helps increase it. But if there is an autoimmune process in the organism, then the SCENAR application helps reduce the immune response
- Vascular effect; it normalizes vascular tone, improved hemodynamics, and activates microcirculation due to elimination of spasm in vessels
- Vascular effect; it normalizes vascular tone, improves hemodynamics, and activates microcirculation due to elimination of spasm in vessels

13

- Hemostatic effect; it occurs due to activated collateral blood supply and relieved stress in the arterial vessel
- Improved collateral blood circulation effect; it occurs involuntarily due to direct electrical current application to the sensitive and vegetative nerve fibers
- Normalized metabolic (albominous, fatty, carbohydrate, mineral) effect to be due to improved functions of the kidneys, skin, sweat glands, lungs, liver, internal secretion glands and central nervous system
- Anti-shock effect; it becomes apparent under any form of shock: traumatic, pain, anaphylactic, etc.

14

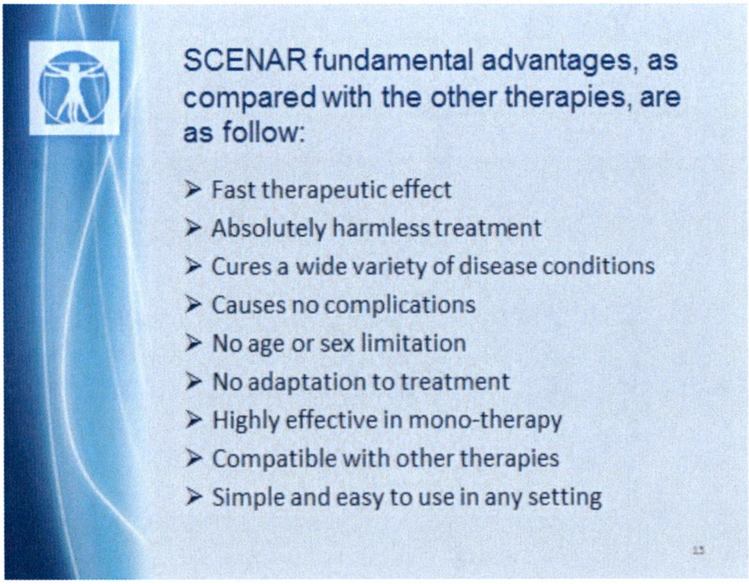
SCENAR fundamental advantages, as compared with the other therapies, are as follow:
➤ Fast therapeutic effect
➤ Absolutely harmless treatment
➤ Cures a wide variety of disease conditions
➤ Causes no complications
➤ No age or sex limitation
➤ No adaptation to treatment
➤ Highly effective in mono-therapy
➤ Compatible with other therapies
➤ Simple and easy to use in any setting

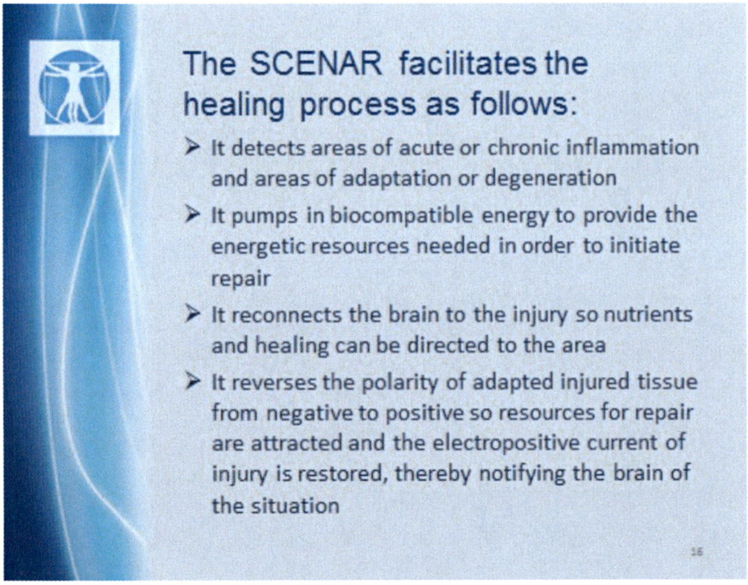
The SCENAR facilitates the healing process as follows:
➤ It detects areas of acute or chronic inflammation and areas of adaptation or degeneration
➤ It pumps in biocompatible energy to provide the energetic resources needed in order to initiate repair
➤ It reconnects the brain to the injury so nutrients and healing can be directed to the area
➤ It reverses the polarity of adapted injured tissue from negative to positive so resources for repair are attracted and the electropositive current of injury is restored, thereby notifying the brain of the situation

- It provides a signal that stimulates the release of neuropeptides from the pharmacy of chemicals in the skin to augment the ingredients needed for repair
- It tones down the sympathetic nervous system and tunes up the parasympathetic nervous system
- It provides a sequenced series of nerve-like impulses alternating with pauses to prevent adaptation/habituation to the signals
- It dynamically changes the signal characteristics in accordance with the bio-feedback from the body

17

SCENAR application is indicated at any stage in treatment of the following diseases

- Nervous system (various diseases of the vertebral column with secondary disorders of the nervous activity, static and dynamic's disorders of the vertebral column, deformation of the spinal column, radiculitis, neuritis, strokes and their consequences, diseases of the vegetative nervous system etc.)
- Musculo-skeletal system (myositis, arthritis, arthrosis, bruising of the soft tissue, at the fractures at different stages of the process)

18

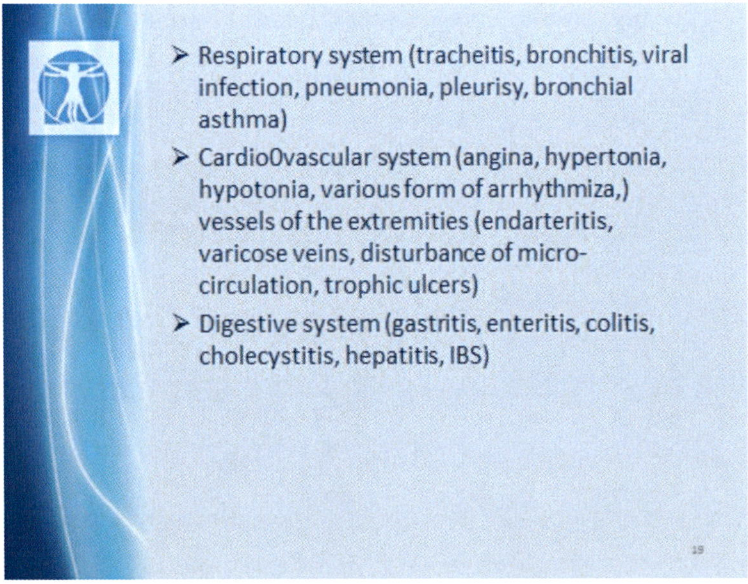
➢ Respiratory system (tracheitis, bronchitis, viral infection, pneumonia, pleurisy, bronchial asthma)
➢ CardioOvascular system (angina, hypertonia, hypotonia, various form of arrhythmiza,) vessels of the extremities (endarteritis, varicose veins, disturbance of micro-circulation, trophic ulcers)
➢ Digestive system (gastritis, enteritis, colitis, cholecystitis, hepatitis, IBS)

Nerve endings on the skin continually inform the brain of any changes in the body, both inside and outside. **Any changes on the skin surface can characterize the body's condition**. SCENAR devices activate practically all the organs and systems of the body.

SC - Self-Controlled The RITM SCENAR® device establishes a biofeedback link with the body when in use, constantly changing the properties of the applied electric impulses, depending on the measured reaction from the body.

EN - Energo-Neuro The effect of RITM SCENAR® is based on electric impulses of a specific shape; patterned after the natural nervous discharges of the human body.

AR - Adaptive Regulator The RITM SCENAR® device not only provides direct therapeutic effect but also activates the natural defenses of the body. The effect is achieved through the stimulation of reflective zones and acupuncture points on the skin surface.

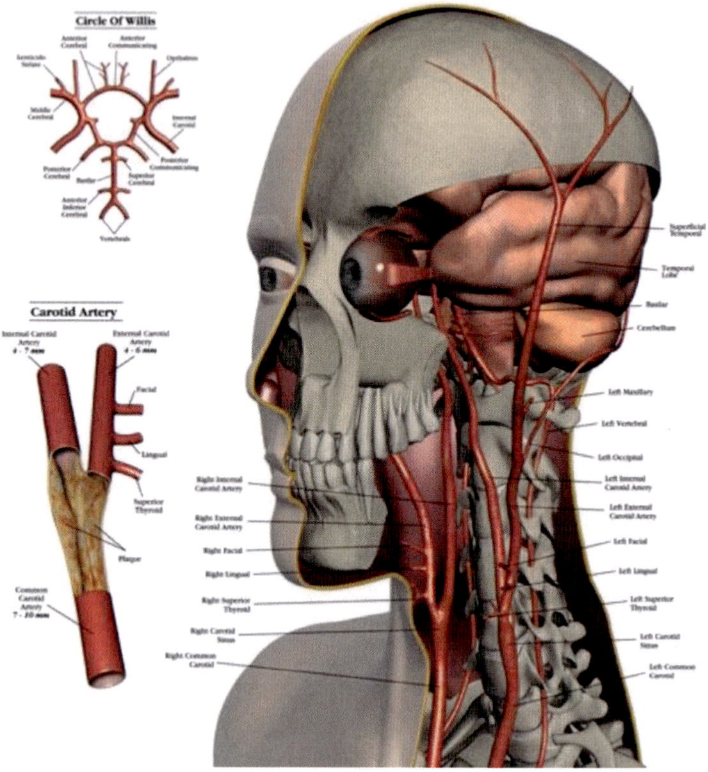
Circle Of Willis
Carotid Artery
Internal Carotid Artery 4 - 7 mm
External Carotid Artery 4 - 6 mm
Facial
Lingual
Superior Thyroid
Plaque
Common Carotid Artery 7 - 10 mm
Superficial Temporal
Temporal Lobe
Basilar
Cerebellum
Left Maxillary
Left Vertebral
Left Occipital
Left Internal Carotid Artery
Left External Carotid Artery
Left Facial
Left Lingual
Left Superior Thyroid
Left Carotid Sinus
Left Common Carotid
Right Internal Carotid Artery
Right External Carotid Artery
Right Facial
Right Lingual
Right Superior Thyroid
Right Carotid Sinus
Right Common Carotid

The first **RITM SCENAR®** prototype was manufactured in 1976. The FDA cleared RITM SCENAR in May 2011 for the treatment of acute, chronic and post operative pain. The FDA and Health Canada have cleared RITM SCENAR® Devices for treatment of chronic and acute pain.

Device Operation and Information to the Brain

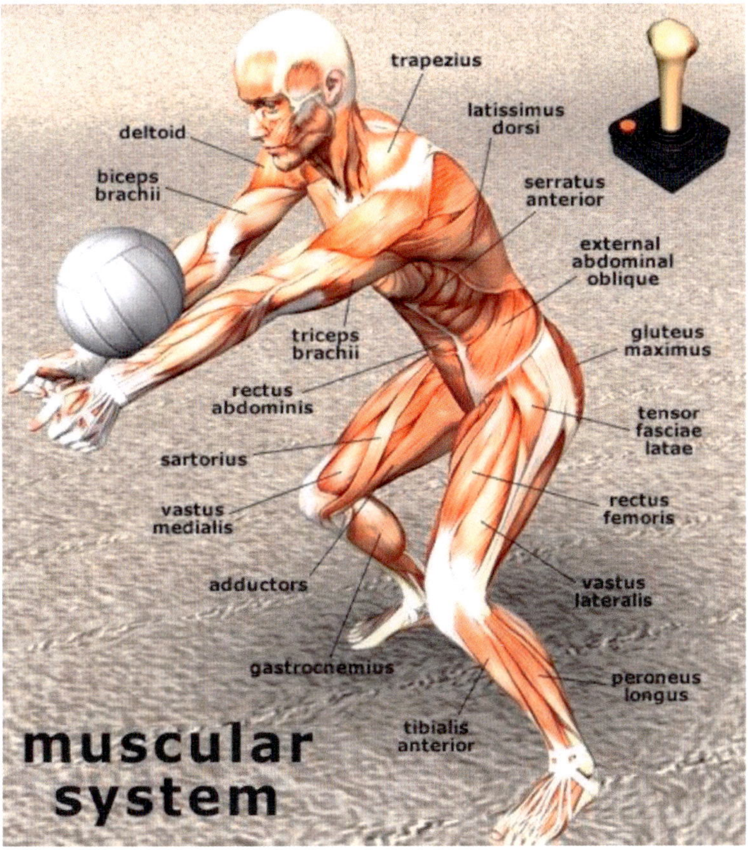
trapezius
latissimus dorsi
deltoid
biceps brachii
serratus anterior
external abdominal oblique
triceps brachii
gluteus maximus
rectus abdominis
tensor fasciae latae
sartorius
rectus femoris
vastus medialis
adductors
vastus lateralis
gastrocnemius
peroneus longus
tibialis anterior
muscular system

Spinal cord (segment), Skin, Blood vessels, Sweat glands, Internal organ interoreceptors Afferent information links (sensory), Efferent information links (motor).

The **command (signal)** that is required for the normalization of the organism's internal media then comes to the executive organs, which produce normalization of the body temperature and improvement of the patient's state. When an impulse is transmitted along nerves and synapses, the conduction is only possible with the help of neurotransmitters such as **adrenaline, acetylcholine**, **glycine** etc. **Neuropeptides** are found in all part of the Central Nervous System and Peripheral Nervous System. Physiological functions are under the control of a whole range of neuropeptides or group of chemical compounds known as **regulative peptides** (RP), which are the "**Programming Package**" for triggering certain complex functions. RP's have a long life span in the organism. In comparison, histamine exists at effective concentrations for only a few seconds; RPs from tens of minutes to tens of hours.

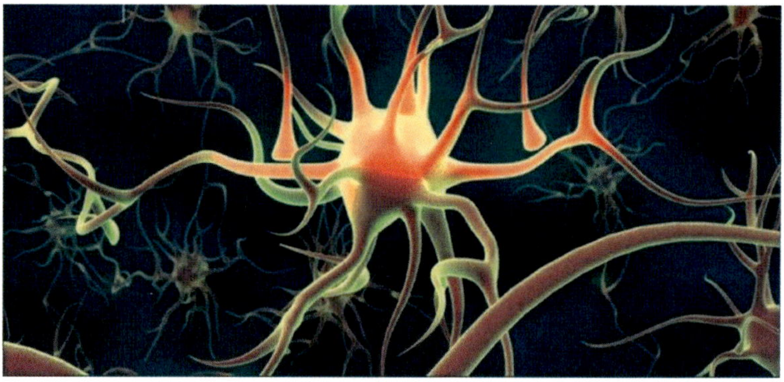

Another peculiarity of RP's is that when they break down it is not just a simple process of decomposition of the regulators, but a reaction resulting in the formation of new **bio-active compounds.** These new compounds have bio-activities which may be fundamentally different from the original RP's functions. The release of the effective dosage of a RP will increase the cascade reactions due to the release of long chains of other RP's. Distant effects of RPs are explained by the presence and action of protein carriers. RP's influence the activity of certain genes and the activity of the **genome.**

Chapter 2.
Mechanisms Involved In Pain Relief

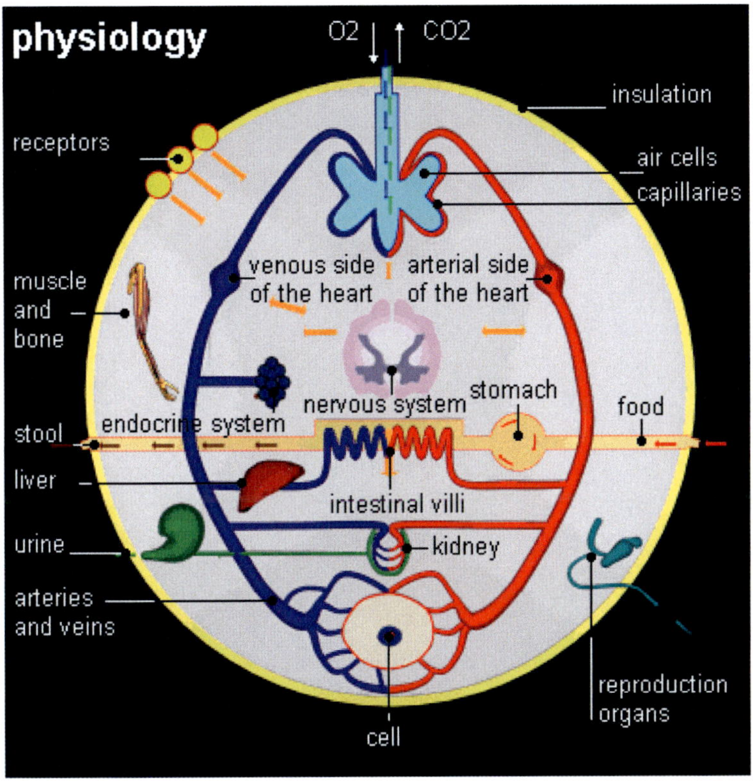
physiology
O2
CO2
insulation
receptors
air cells
capillaries
venous side of the heart
arterial side of the heart
muscle and bone
nervous system
stomach
food
stool
endocrine system
liver
intestinal villi
urine
kidney
arteries and veins
reproduction organs
cell

Neurophysiological:

SCENAR impulse causes impulses in thick and thin nerve fibers and in the brain this prevents the passage of pain impulses. SCENAR impulses act on A fibers which activate the substantia in the spinal cord and in its excited state it depolarizes the pain impulses arriving at this time. This prevents transmission of the pain Impulses from the periphery to the brain, that is, it closes the gate (**gate theory**).

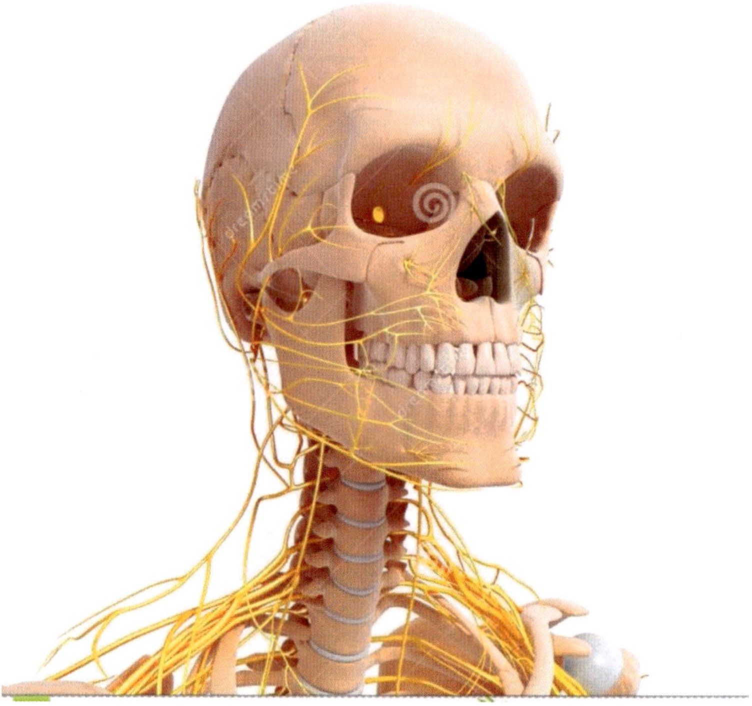

Neurochemical: Nociceptors are pain **receptors** and in the brain there is a nociceptive system, which is counteracted by an antagonistic system, the anti-nociceptive system.

Pain impulses begin in free **nerve endings**. These endings are called nociceptors. Sharp pain is conducted via **A delta fibers** which terminate in lamina I and V of the spinal cord.

Prolonged, often burning pain is conducted via **C fibers**, which terminate in laminae II 'and V of the cord. The **neurotransmitter** of these pain afferent endings is called **substance P**. The neurons of these contribute to the formation of the lateral spino-thalamic tract. This pathway not only projects fibers directly to the thalamus but also provides collaterals at every level of the spinal cord and brain stem.

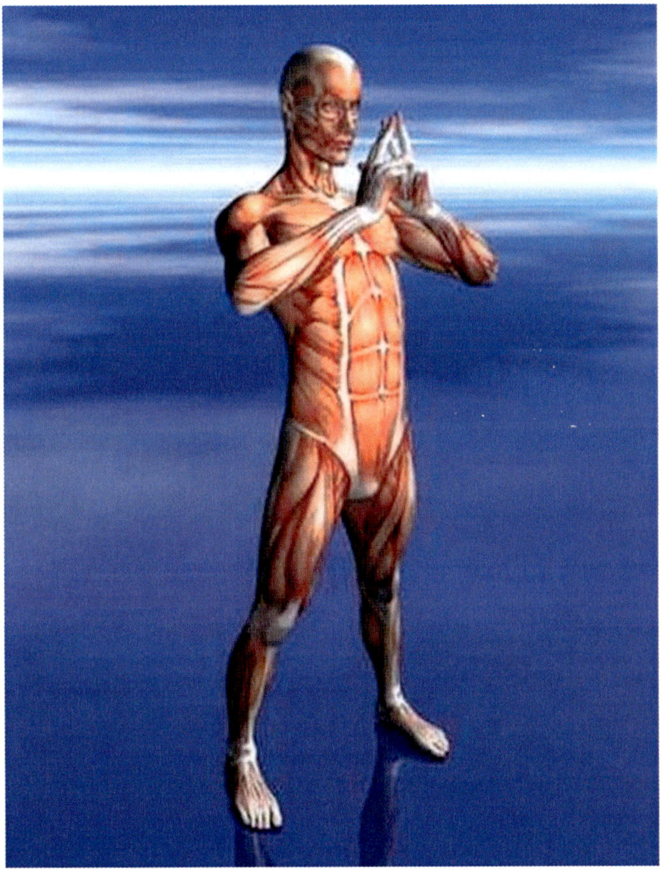

From the **cortex** descending pain inhibitory pathways begin. Fibers follow towards **thalamus,** then to midbrain region and to the reticular formation which allows a mixing of other systems and changes **neurotransmitters** to enhance and refine the degree of inhibition. Descending pathways fibers synapse with inter-neurons with both incoming **primary pain afferents** and cels whose axons form the lateral spinal-thalamic tract, closing the inhibitory arch.

There are three **hormone** systems in the **anti-nociceptive system**, opiate, **serotonin** and **adrenalin** systems, all of which influence each other. Electrical stimulation from the device acting on peripheral nerve fibers influences both nociceptive and anti-nociceptive systems. This releases opiod-like compounds which block release of compound P at the level of the substantia gelatinosa and block transmission of the pain impulses chemically. **The device also releases vasodilators locally**, which enhances oxygen supply and eases pain. There may be cells, which are self-stimulating and have a memory for chronic pain. SCENAR treatment may suppress their memory.

Scenar Physiological Aspects

NERVOUS SYSTEM OF THORAX AND UPPER LIMB (ANTERIOR VIEW)

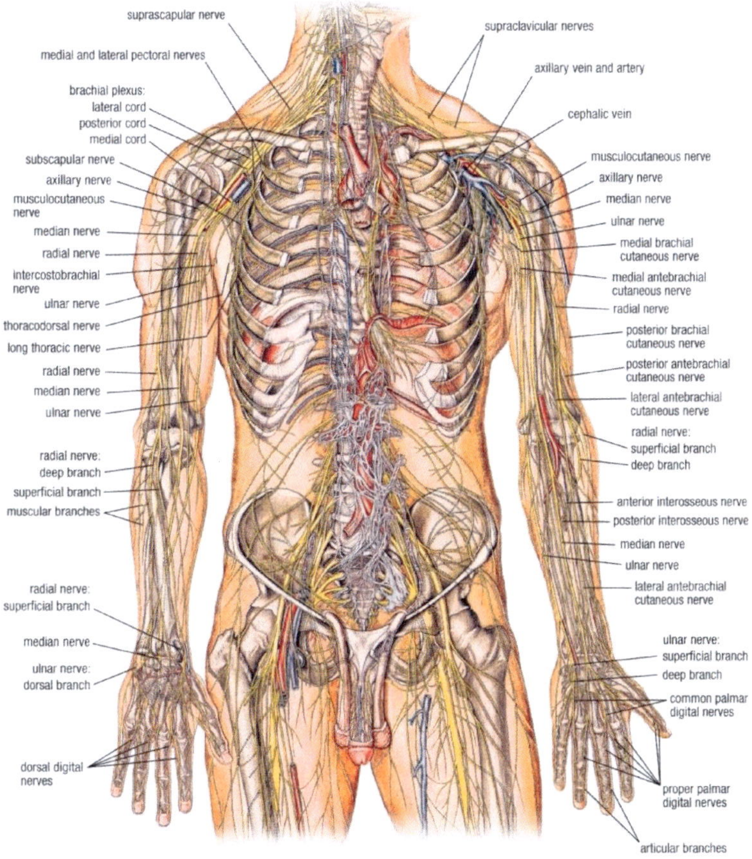
suprascapular nerve
medial and lateral pectoral nerves
brachial plexus:
lateral cord
posterior cord
medial cord
subscapular nerve
axillary nerve
musculocutaneous nerve
median nerve
radial nerve
intercostobrachial nerve
ulnar nerve
thoracodorsal nerve
long thoracic nerve
radial nerve
median nerve
ulnar nerve
radial nerve:
deep branch
superficial branch
muscular branches
radial nerve:
superficial branch
median nerve
ulnar nerve:
dorsal branch
dorsal digital nerves
supraclavicular nerves
axillary vein and artery
cephalic vein
musculocutaneous nerve
axillary nerve
median nerve
ulnar nerve
medial brachial cutaneous nerve
medial antebrachial cutaneous nerve
radial nerve
posterior brachial cutaneous nerve
posterior antebrachial cutaneous nerve
lateral antebrachial cutaneous nerve
radial nerve:
superficial branch
deep branch
anterior interosseous nerve
posterior interosseous nerve
median nerve
ulnar nerve
lateral antebrachial cutaneous nerve
ulnar nerve:
superficial branch
deep branch
common palmar digital nerves
proper palmar digital nerves
articular branches

In response to an adequate irritant with electrical current there will be a release of bioactive compounds, predominantly **neuron-peptides** (regulative peptides), having specific influences on surrounded tissues. SCENAR sends electrical impulses through the skin. The effect of the excitement of the nervous tissue depends on the type of the fibers.

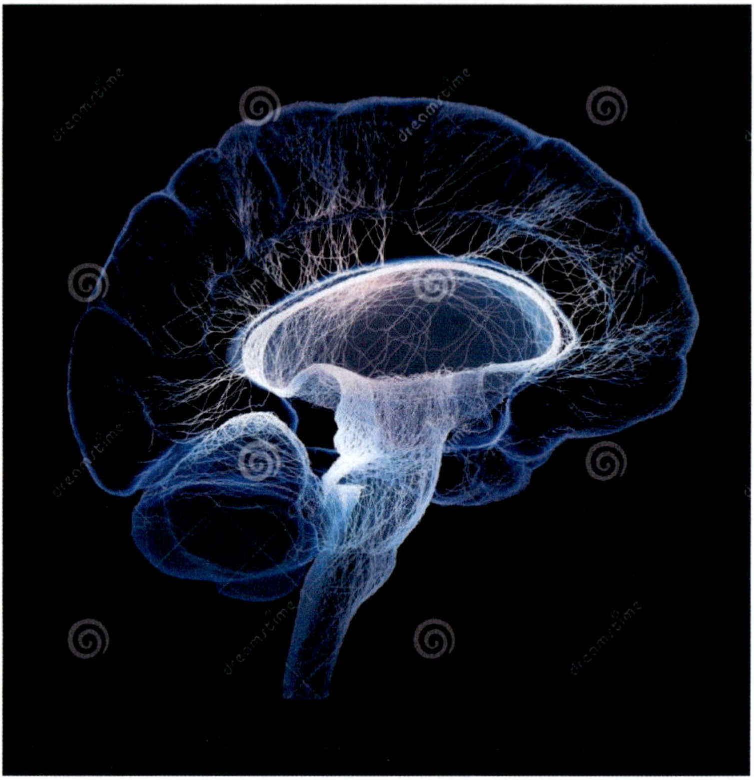

For activation of **C fibers** the force of the current should be 225 – 1600 times higher than for type A and B. C-fibers account for about 85% of all type of nerve fiber. When an impulse is transmitted along nerves and synapses, the conduction is only possible with the help of neurotransmitters such as **adrenaline, acetylcholine, glycine** etc. Neuropeptides are found in all part of the **Central Nervous System and Peripheral Nervous System**. Physiological functions are under the control of a whole range of neuron -peptides or group of chemical compounds known as Regulative Peptides (RP), which are the "**Programming Package**" for triggering certain complex functions. RP's have a long life span in the organism. In comparison, histamine exists at effective concentrations for only a few seconds; RP's from tens of minutes to tens of hours. Another peculiarity of RP's is that when they break down it is not just a simple process of decomposition of the regulators, but a reaction resulting in the formation of new **bio-active compounds**

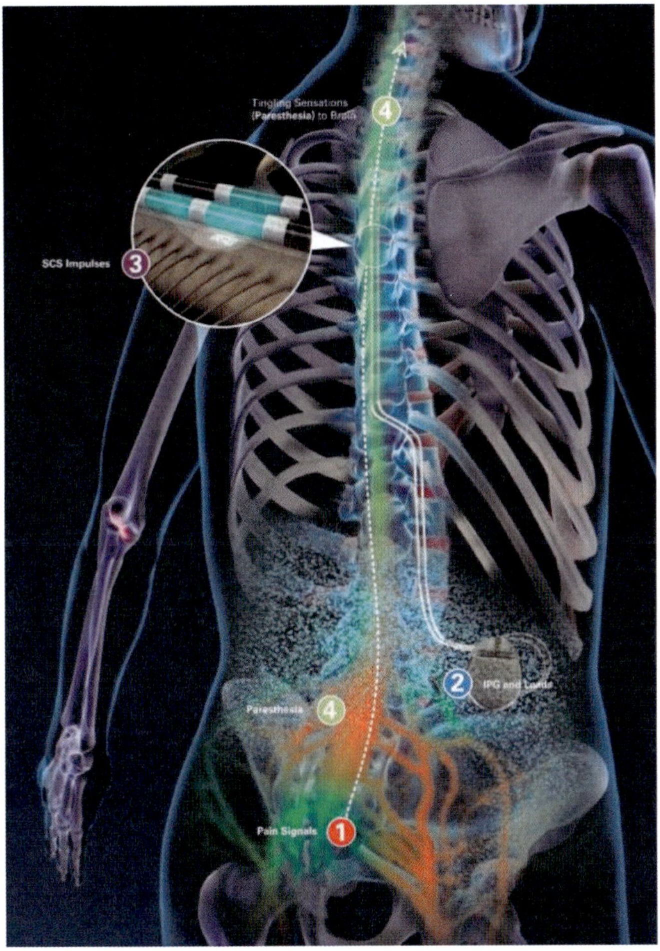
Tingling Sensations
4
SCS Impulses
3
2
Paresthesia
4
Pain Signals
1

The release of the effective dosage of a RP will increase the cascade reactions due to the release of long chains of other RPs. Distant effects of RPs are explained by the presence and action of protein carriers. RPs influences the activity of certain genes and the activity of the genome.

Scenar and the Nervous System

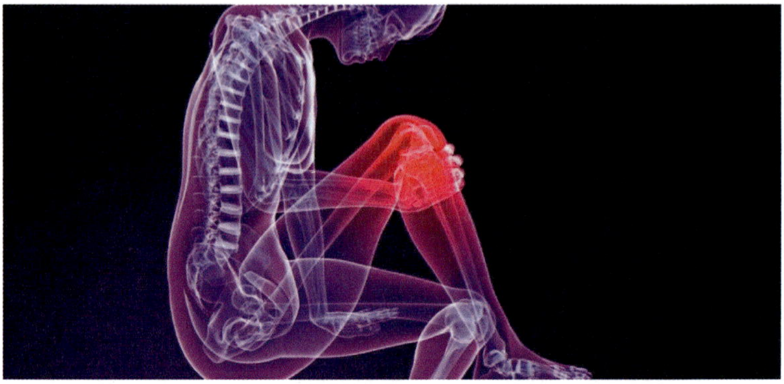

In order to understand the operating mechanism of the device and to set up, on its basic, effective methods of treatment to various diseases of particular patient, as well as to explain high effectiveness of the device to many diseases, it is necessary first to become acquainted (in a general way) with the mechanism of human body life support regulation processes, provided by the nervous system.

The **organism** is an ultra-stable, self-organizing system, which regulates its stable state on its own, keeping fluctuations of its organs' functioning within the proper limits. The organism chooses and maintains itself at a necessary level for its organs and systems function, depending on requirements (work, rest, managing the infection, etc.).

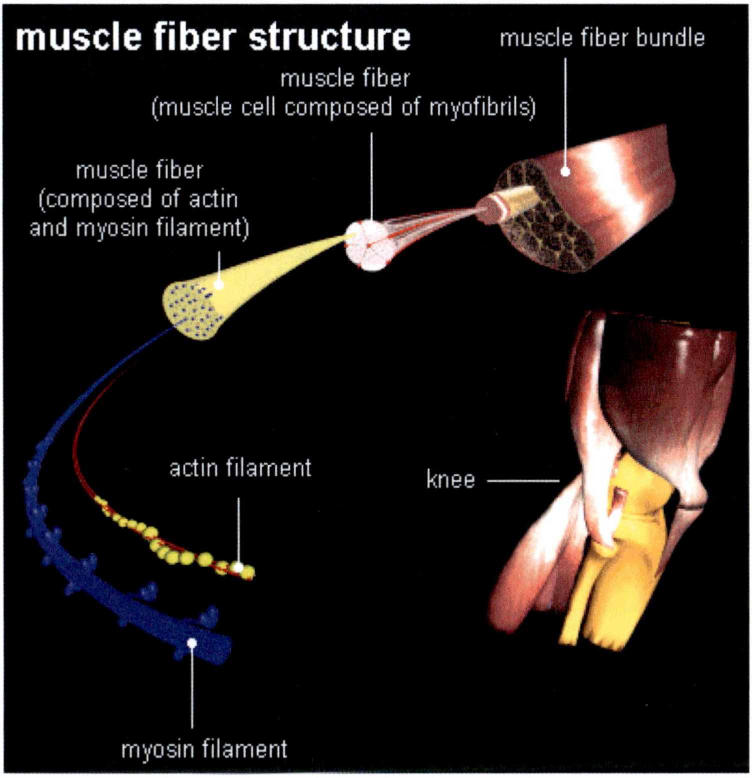
muscle fiber structure
muscle fiber bundle
muscle fiber
(muscle cell composed of myofibrils)
muscle fiber
(composed of actin
and myosin filament)
actin filament
knee
myosin filament

Besides, the organism is an open system to the environment, since it is not able to survive without stable inflow of oxygen from the environment, water, nutrients and discharge into it of carbon dioxide and unnecessary (and sometimes harmful) metabolic products. The environment provides not only efficient, but also harmful effects on men. So the organism should "know" what is happening inside and outside of it. The state of a man will be normal only in the case, when proper interrelations are maintained between internal organs and systems, organism and environment.

Scenar Works on These Principles

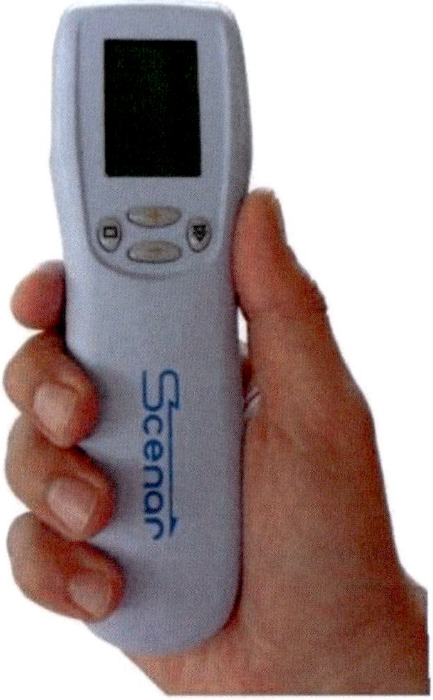
Scenar

The SCENAR is **applied** to the body through an electrode on the back of it. This is what is called a **biofeedback device**. What does that mean? Biofeedback means it reads, computes, and treats. It reads the tissue, it reads the damage, and reads the disease. It pulls that information back into the computer, calculates a cure and puts it back into the body and repairs or fixes the problem. Biofeedback, that's what it means, that what this is registered as, a biofeedback device. This is fairly new. The TENS unit was not a biofeedback device. It simply put a signal in. Later in life as we went on about our research and work both in **Russia** and America, **we developed biofeedback devices and we found this to be the best way to go in order to cure and repair injuries**. So, that's what the SCENAR does, it reads the tissue, finds the injury, finds the disease, finds the problem, computes the problem and puts back a signal to correct it. So what do we do with this?

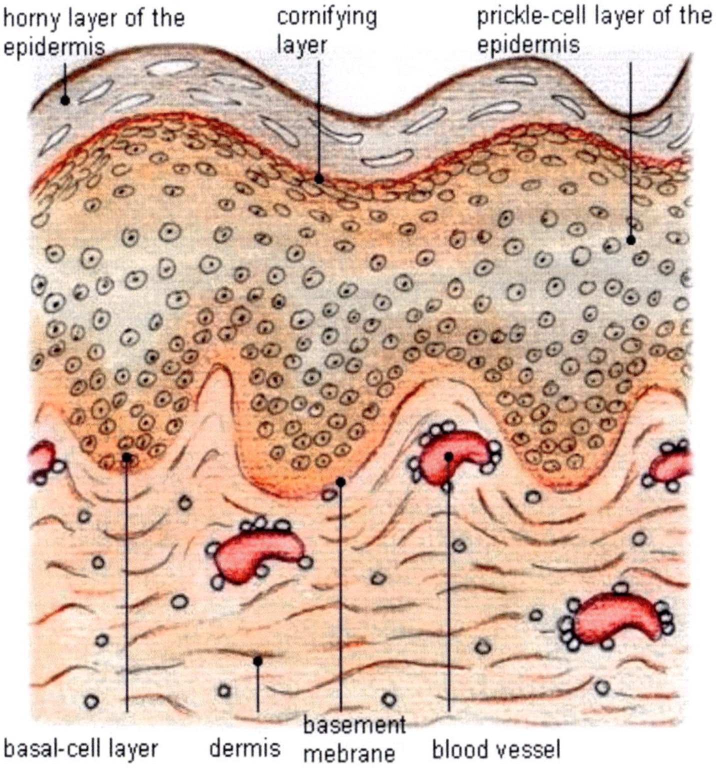
horny layer of the epidermis
cornifying layer
prickle-cell layer of the epidermis
basal-cell layer
dermis
basement mebrane
blood vessel

The **skin** develops from the same embryological layer as the nervous system. Reflexology and acupuncture treat areas on the skin that represent internal organs and **energy pathways**. Using the **SCENAR**, it is possible to influence every system of the body and to balance energy flow in the meridians SCENAR adds energy to the system, a system that may be depleted in its reserves as it attempts to heal itself. Normally the body undergoes adaptive reactions to changes in the environment and often these are suppressed by such things as cough mixtures, anti-inflammatory medicines, etc. **The signal received from the SCENAR, acting on the skin, causes a regulating adaptive reaction within a short period of time**. This may restore lost functions and goes some way to explain how unresolved problems from the past resurface to be dealt with.

How the SCENAR Works

The **SCENAR uses biofeedback,** enabling the body to heal itself. The SCENAR sends out a series of signals through the skin and measures the response. Each signal is only sent out when a change is recorded in the electrical properties of the skin, in response to the previous signal. **Visible reactions include reddening of the skin, numbness, stickiness (the SCENAR will have the feeling of being magnetically dragged), a change in the numerical readout and an increase in the electronic 'clattering' of the device**.

The body can get accustomed to a stable pathological state, which may have been caused by injury, disease or toxicity. The SCENAR initiates the healing process by **stimulating the production of regulatory peptides** for the body to use where necessary, thereby re-establishing the body's natural physiological state. Neuron and other regulatory peptides are produced by C-fibers, which comprise 85% of all nerves in the body. C-fibers react most readily to SCENAR electro-stimulation and the peptides produced last up to several hours, meaning the healing process will continue long after the treatment is over. The large quantity of neuropeptides and C-fibers in the Central Nervous System can also result in the treatment on one area aiding with other chemical imbalances, correcting sleeplessness, appetite and behavioral problems.

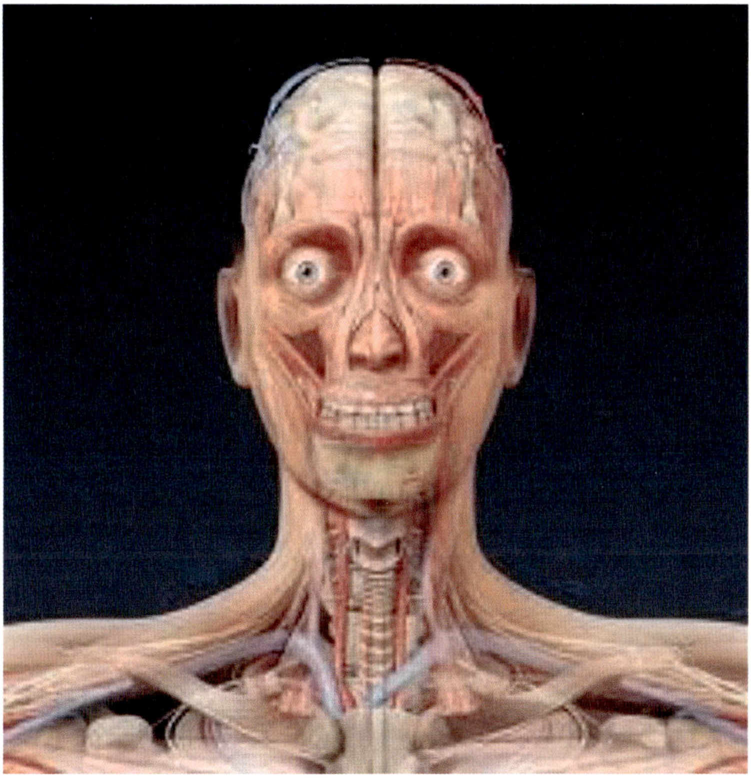

In Russia, some 600 practitioners currently use the SCENAR as their principal treatment instrument, with over 50,000 reported cases of individual use. A vast wealth of information on the SCENAR is available from research papers, clinical reports and training manuals. **The SCENAR can be used on most types of disease or injury: circulatory, sensory, respiratory, neurological, genital-urinary, musculoskeletal,**

gastro-intestinal, endocrine, immune and psychological disorders. The SCENAR is also credited with vastly reducing recovery times. Russian athletes have been known not only to compete after serious injuries, but even to break world-records post SCENAR therapy. In Russian accident and emergency wards the SCENAR is used to aid recovery from cardiac arrest, massive trauma and coma. The SCENAR has recently been shown to aid in improving learning ability, memory, sexual function and improved physical health. Finally trials in Russia have also realized SCENAR's usage for pain management. Both cancer and fracture patients have found more pain relief from the release of natural opioids after SCENAR treatment than from those externally administered.

SCENAR Operation

The SCENAR is run over the spine and abdomen or infected area. The software records the resistive response to its signals and returns a fresh signal, causing a gentle tingling/stroking sensation. The practitioner is looking for anomalies on the skin surface, which may be highlighted by redness, numbness, stickiness or a change in numerical display or sound. Although these areas may not seem to directly relate to the obvious symptoms, by treating these **'asymmetries'** (as the Russians call them) with the SCENAR, the healing process will commence. Experienced SCENAR practitioners state that, though the SCENAR device may be used after the preliminary training, it takes up to four years to master. A chronic problem may require up to 6 weeks SCENAR treatment, with long-lasting effectiveness. Acute problems may just take one or two treatments. It is reported that SCENAR proves effective in 80% of all cases, of which full recovery occurs in 2/3rds of them and significant healing in the remainder.

SCENAR Overview

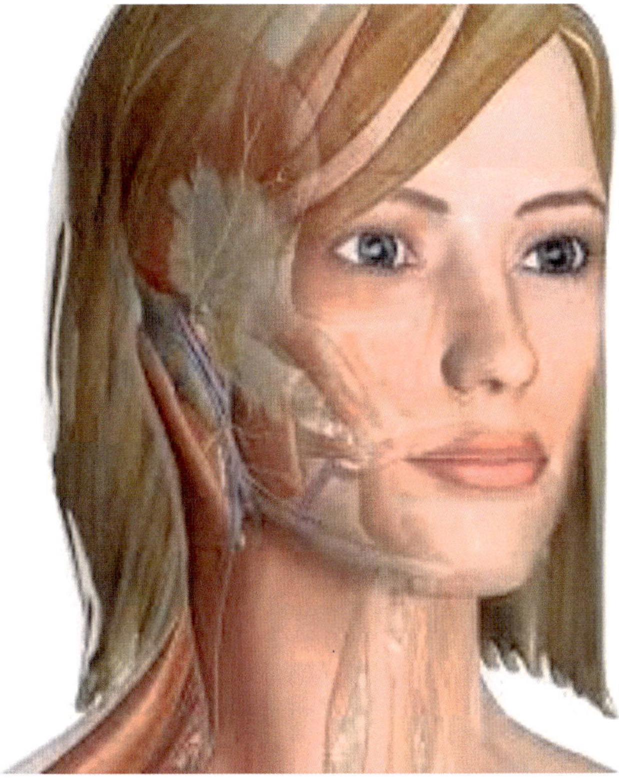

Of all the devices reviewed by the author, few demonstrate the rapid treatment capabilities of the SCENAR. Not only is the SCENAR versatile in its range of treatment, but it also displays an amazing ability to accelerate the healing process. As a stand-alone treatment system, the SCENAR is excellent for alleviation of acute symptoms.

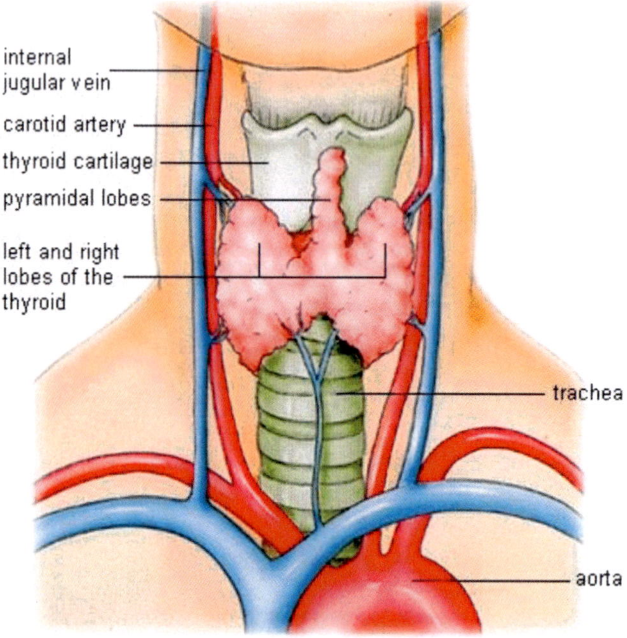
internal
jugular vein
carotid artery
thyroid cartilage
pyramidal lobes
left and right
lobes of the
thyroid
trachea
aorta

SCENAR Therapy is non-drug medical technology, which is directed at activating the self-healing resources of the human organism. These devices are non-invasive energy regulators of the body's systems.

Scenar devices were invented in Russia nearly 20 years ago in order to keep cosmonauts in good health while in space. In 1986 the first SCENAR device, having passed clinical trials, was given permission by USSR Medical Council to be used in hospitals and homes.

These devices are intended to stimulate the body's self-recovery program by using its own "internal pharmacy" of neuropeptides. This enables the body to choose the most appropriate chemical combination for each particular case.

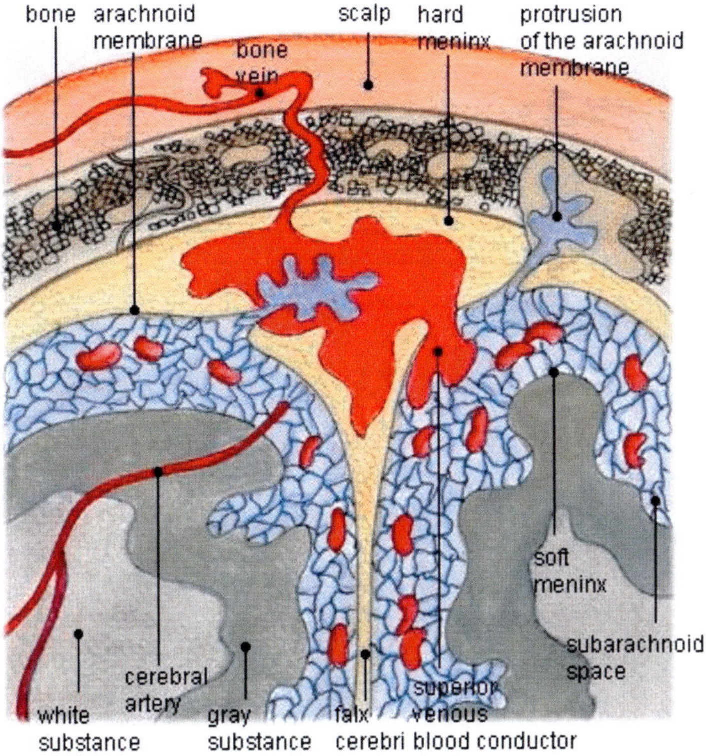
bone
arachnoid membrane
bone vein
scalp
hard meninx
protrusion of the arachnoid membrane
soft meninx
subarachnoid space
cerebral artery
white substance
gray substance
falx cerebri
superior venous blood conductor

Lately, great popularity has been associated with the medicine-free methods of treatment that would help our organism to fight diseases in the most natural way and considerably reduce or even exclude drug taking at all.

The **Scenar stimulates cellular reactions** to help restore respiratory capacity in tissues and organs, lower concentration of hydrogen ions in tissues, restore or improve utilization of free oxygen by the cell and restore metabolic processes in the body.

This is called **homeostasis,** which is the state in which all the processes responsible for energy transformations in the organism are dynamically balanced and stable despite environmental changes.

Since the brain controls the tissues and organs with electric pulses, it is natural that Scenar generated pulses can influence the internal organs and systems through feedback from the body.

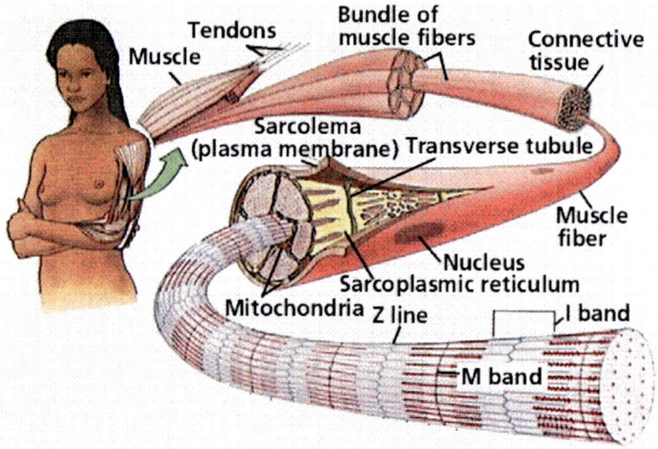

Tendons
Muscle
Bundle of
muscle fibers
Connective
tissue
Sarcolema
(plasma membrane)
Transverse tubule
Muscle
fiber
Nucleus
Sarcoplasmic reticulum
Mitochondria
Z line
I band
M band

The Scenar is effective in managing pain associated with soft tissue dysfunction and in controlling chronic, severe pain.

The outcome of the neuron stimulation is that it affects the area of pathological activity locally through increased blood circulation, neuropeptide release, stimulation of the lymph flow, reduction of acute or chronic inflammation and muscle relaxation.

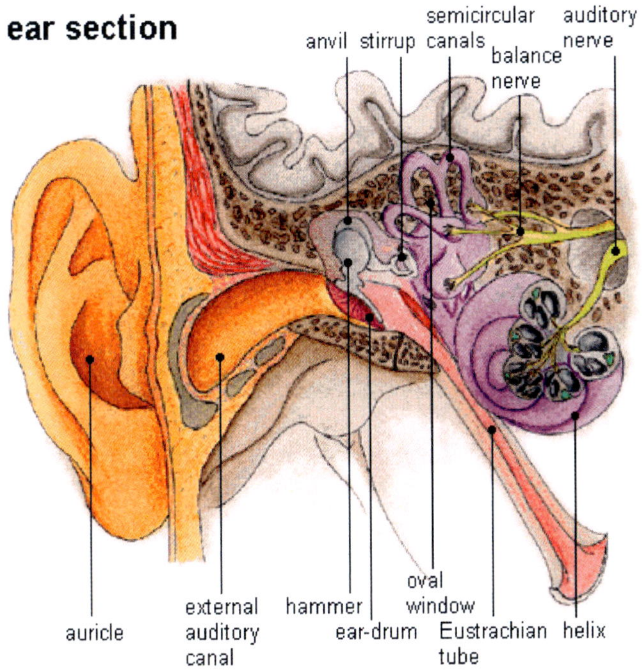
ear section
anvil
stirrup
semicircular canals
balance nerve
auditory nerve
auricle
external auditory canal
hammer
ear-drum
oval window
Eustrachian tube
helix

As the pathological systems are eliminated, there is disappearance of complaints and restoration of function.

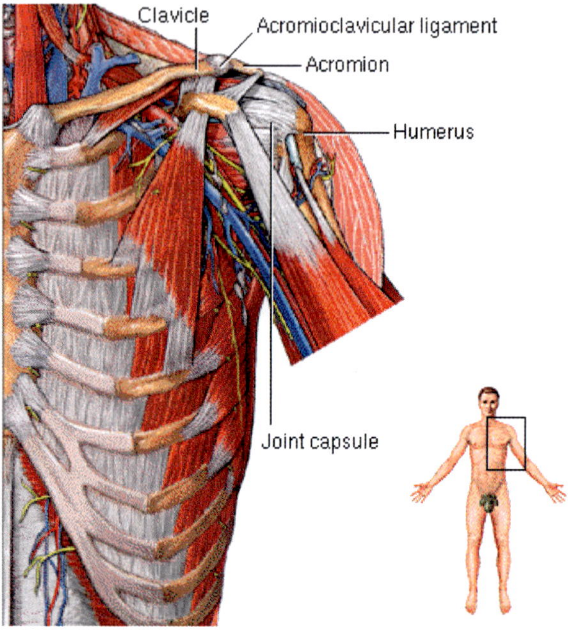
Clavicle
Acromioclavicular ligament
Acromion
Humerus
Joint capsule

It **detects areas of degeneration**. Then it pumps in biocompatible energy to provide the energetic resources needed to initiate repair.

It **reverses the polarity** of adapted injured tissue from negative to positive so resources for repair are attracted and the electropositive current of injury is restored, thereby notifying the brain of the situation.

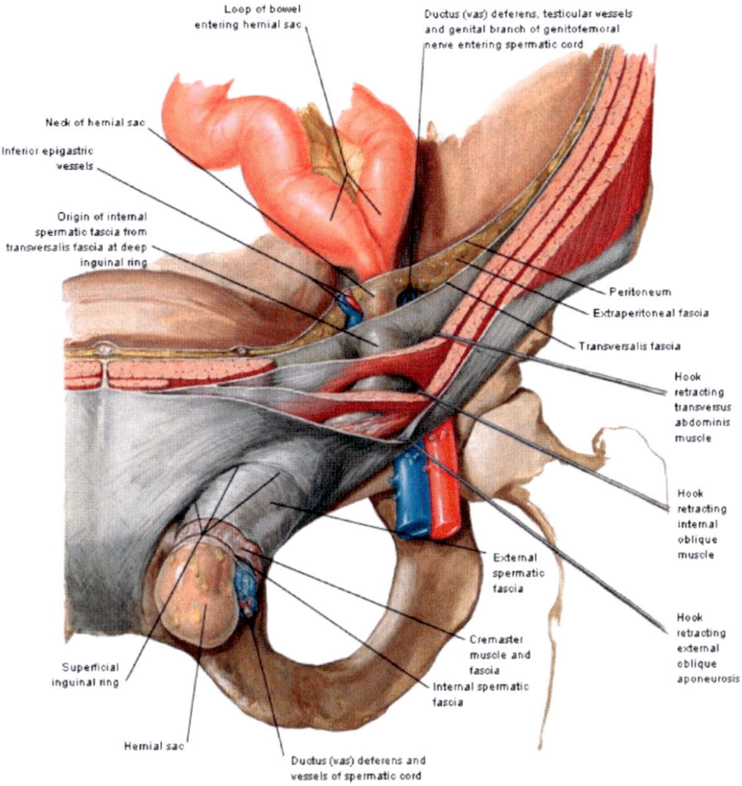
Loop of bowel entering hernial sac
Ductus (vas) deferens, testicular vessels and genital branch of genitofemoral nerve entering spermatic cord
Neck of hernial sac
Inferior epigastric vessels
Origin of internal spermatic fascia from transversalis fascia at deep inguinal ring
Peritoneum
Extraperitoneal fascia
Transversalis fascia
Hook retracting transversus abdominis muscle
Hook retracting internal oblique muscle
External spermatic fascia
Hook retracting external oblique aponeurosis
Cremaster muscle and fascia
Superficial inguinal ring
Internal spermatic fascia
Hernial sac
Ductus (vas) deferens and vessels of spermatic cord

It provides a signal that **stimulates the release of neuropeptides** from the pharmacy of chemicals in the skin to augment the ingredients needed for repair.

The SCENAR is applicable in a wide variety of clinical situations from acute injury to post-operative recovery, and the treatment of chronic pain.

It is portable, small and easy to use as the Scenar is hand held, lightweight and battery operated.

Scenar Works in Three Ways

Central mechanism

It acts via **ascending pathways** in the **spinal cord** on the cortex of the brain. As a result, efferent pathways from the cortex convey impulses, which affect a response in the organ, the organ corresponding to the projection of the area of skin treated. It acts via ascending pathways in the **spinal cord** on the cortex of the brain. As a result, **efferent pathways** from the cortex convey impulses, which affect a response in the organ, the organ corresponding to the projection of the area of skin treated.

Intercostal Nerves and Arteries

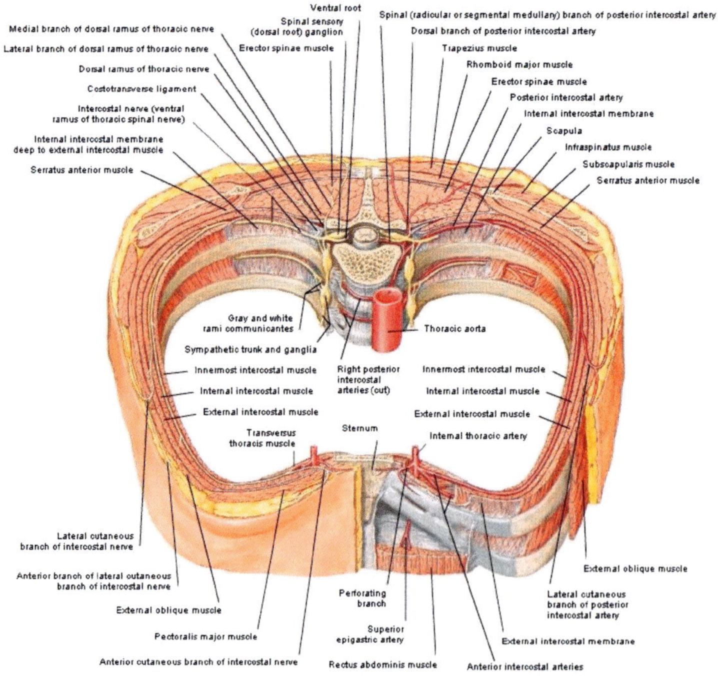

Ventral root
Spinal sensory (dorsal root) ganglion
Erector spinae muscle
Medial branch of dorsal ramus of thoracic nerve
Lateral branch of dorsal ramus of thoracic nerve
Dorsal ramus of thoracic nerve
Costotransverse ligament
Intercostal nerve (ventral ramus of thoracic spinal nerve)
Internal intercostal membrane deep to external intercostal muscle
Serratus anterior muscle
Spinal (radicular or segmental medullary) branch of posterior intercostal artery
Dorsal branch of posterior intercostal artery
Trapezius muscle
Rhomboid major muscle
Erector spinae muscle
Posterior intercostal artery
Internal intercostal membrane
Scapula
Infraspinatus muscle
Subscapularis muscle
Serratus anterior muscle
Gray and white rami communicantes
Sympathetic trunk and ganglia
Thoracic aorta
Innermost intercostal muscle
Internal intercostal muscle
External intercostal muscle
Right posterior intercostal arteries (cut)
Innermost intercostal muscle
Internal intercostal muscle
External intercostal muscle
Transversus thoracis muscle
Sternum
Internal thoracic artery
Lateral cutaneous branch of intercostal nerve
Anterior branch of lateral cutaneous branch of intercostal nerve
External oblique muscle
Pectoralis major muscle
Anterior cutaneous branch of intercostal nerve
Perforating branch
Superior epigastric artery
Rectus abdominis muscle
External oblique muscle
Lateral cutaneous branch of posterior intercostal artery
External intercostal membrane
Anterior intercostal arteries

Segmental mechanism

It acts directly on local spinal reflexes.

Local mechanism

Membranous Resonance.

Each cell in the body vibrates in its own fashion and there is an overall resonance. The action of the SCENAR creates its own resonance and by sending vibrations through the **membranes** it reaches into any pathological focus.

Molecular Polarization

Molecules reposition themselves within an electrical field according to their electrical charge. This is an additional factor in the transmission of impulses in all directions.

Microphoresis

There exists a mini-pharmacy on the surface of the skin and the action of the SCENAR stimulates the selective re-absorption of trace elements and minerals etc. through the skin in minute dosages by microphoresis as required by the body. For this reason it is recommended not to bathe or shower two hours before or after treatment.

Chapter 3.
What is The SCENAR Looking For?

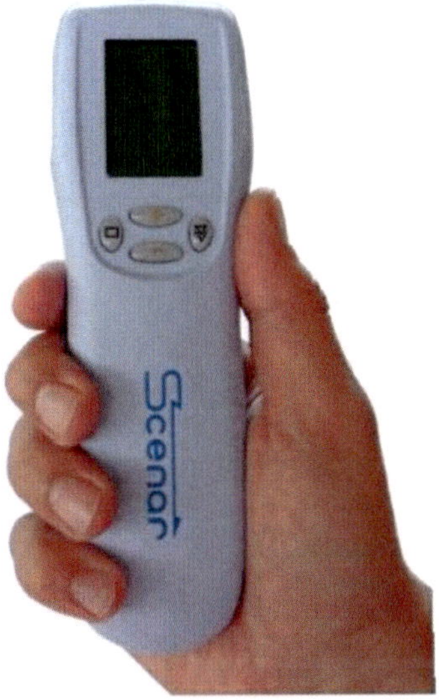
Scenar

The SCENAR is looking for **asymmetries**. **Asymmetries in SCENAR language are what we call diversions from the norm or something that's off, something that's broken, something that's damaged, something that's diseased**. And how do you read asymmetries through the skin? Well what is the skin? The skin is the largest organ in the human body, and what is the skin besides that? **A mirror of everything** underneath it. So if you have electrical signals going on underneath the skin, why wouldn't the skin recognize it and conduct it? Well it does, just like an electrical circuit. If you have a lot of bare wires hanging out under a cable, the signal is going to go through all those bare wires. So if the cable, or if the covering of it is conductive, then it will read everything that's going on in the wires and the flow of electricity through them. That being said, this is what it does. It looks at the galvanic **skin response** and several other factors on the skin that are determinants of disease and injury. It computes them and it comes up with a solution as to how to correct them, and then puts it back into the skin. Then that travels into the cells and corrects them and normalizes the cell function so the cells can operate properly, **produce ATP, produce protein and repair the damage.**

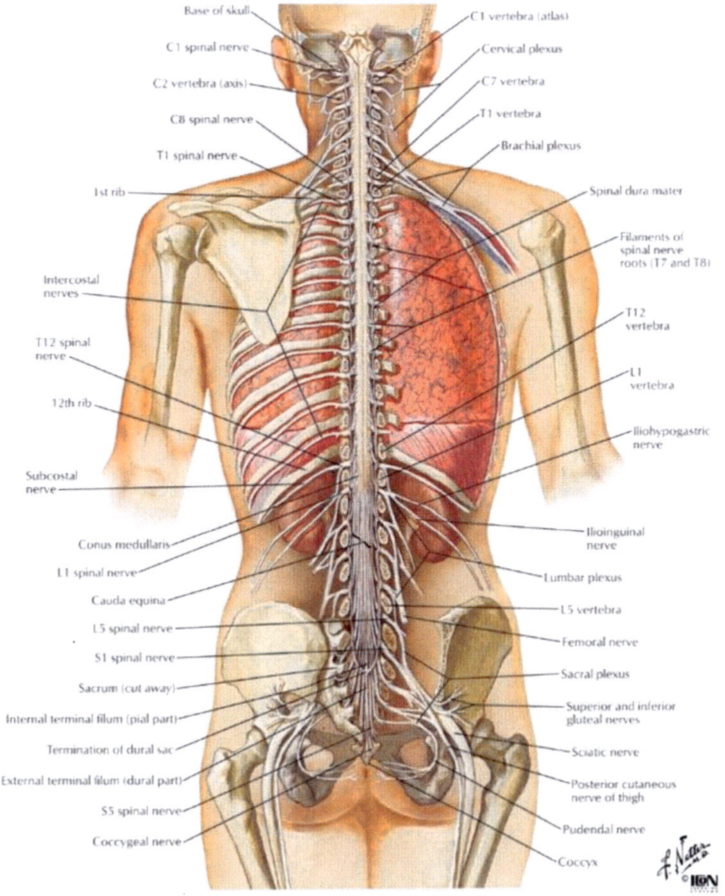
Base of skull
C1 spinal nerve
C2 vertebra (axis)
C8 spinal nerve
T1 spinal nerve
1st rib
Intercostal nerves
T12 spinal nerve
12th rib
Subcostal nerve
Conus medullaris
L1 spinal nerve
Cauda equina
L5 spinal nerve
S1 spinal nerve
Sacrum (cut away)
Internal terminal filum (pial part)
Termination of dural sac
External terminal filum (dural part)
S5 spinal nerve
Coccygeal nerve
C1 vertebra (atlas)
Cervical plexus
C7 vertebra
T1 vertebra
Brachial plexus
Spinal dura mater
Filaments of spinal nerve roots (T7 and T8)
T12 vertebra
L1 vertebra
Iliohypogastric nerve
Ilioinguinal nerve
Lumbar plexus
L5 vertebra
Femoral nerve
Sacral plexus
Superior and inferior gluteal nerves
Sciatic nerve
Posterior cutaneous nerve of thigh
Pudendal nerve
Coccyx

How does it do this? Well there are a whole lot of factors in the SCENAR that do this work. Imagine a graph where you have a line that shoots up, a line that shoots down, up and down, up and down and those are called transmission cycles, and these cycles are what the SCENAR produces, electrical signals that are varied shapes, up and down, slow and fast and sharp and dull and they're paired together many in a group, one in a group, several in a group, two in a group, three in a group, depending on what's wrong with the body. It produces wave forms which change according to the need of the body to be fixed. So this is done by adjusting the SCENAR as to frequency. **What is frequency? Beats per second frequency, called Hertz**, after the inventor and discoverer of the whole concept of beats and electrical systems. So we have frequency. We have amplitude. What is amplitude? Amplitude is the measurement of power. **Amplitude is WHAT is done with the power**, and in the SCENAR case it is milliamps. What's a **milliamp**? One one thousandth of an amp. So if you're putting 70 milliamps into the body you are putting 70 one thousandths of an amp, which is a very small current. And then we have other things that are in the SCENAR which adjust for wave form and adjust amplitude for up and down and fast and slow and strong and weak to as to accommodate the accommodation factor of the human body which will accommodate or not bother to react to an electrical signal if it is too boring.

It changes according to that. So we have many **frequencies**. And what we find is like Royal Rife in 1938, we find that every **disease** and **injury** has a frequency. Cancer has a **frequency**. An injury has a frequency. There are thousands and thousands of frequencies in the human body that make thousands of changes to particular issues and parts. So the frequency is an important thing for the SCENAR to do properly and for example, we have found in SCENAR research that, if we set the SCENAR to 59.6 Hertz, that's beats per second, that is a healing frequency for soft tissue. And we can heal pretty much anything with that.

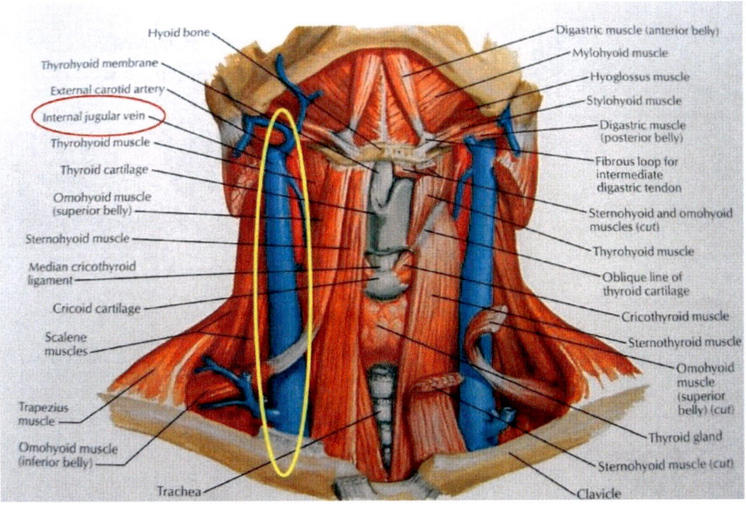
Hyoid bone
Thyrohyoid membrane
External carotid artery
Internal jugular vein
Thyrohyoid muscle
Thyroid cartilage
Omohyoid muscle (superior belly)
Sternohyoid muscle
Median cricothyroid ligament
Cricoid cartilage
Scalene muscles
Trapezius muscle
Omohyoid muscle (inferior belly)
Trachea
Digastric muscle (anterior belly)
Mylohyoid muscle
Hyoglossus muscle
Stylohyoid muscle
Digastric muscle (posterior belly)
Fibrous loop for intermediate digastric tendon
Sternohyoid and omohyoid muscles (cut)
Thyrohyoid muscle
Oblique line of thyroid cartilage
Cricothyroid muscle
Sternothyroid muscle
Omohyoid muscle (superior belly) (cut)
Thyroid gland
Sternohyoid muscle (cut)
Clavicle

If we can't do it with that, then we can use several others instead. So we have whole lot of capabilities to do this. The SCENAR itself put into certain modes, we have one mode called FM, which stands for Frequency Modulation. **Frequency Modulation** means ever changing frequencies in a signal line. So if we turn it on to that, it will find the frequency and do the work because it will review all the **frequencies** that it's used to doing for this kind of work.

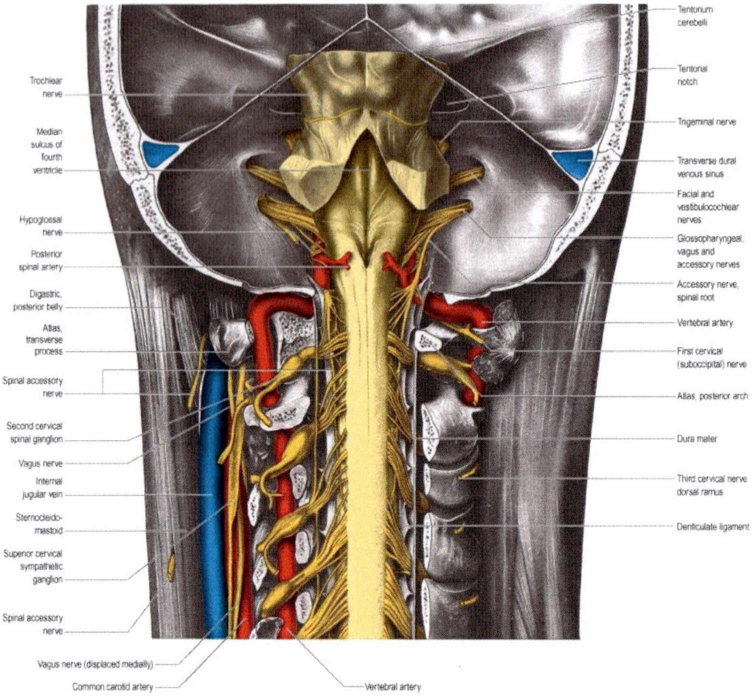
Trochlear nerve
Median sulcus of fourth ventricle
Hypoglossal nerve
Posterior spinal artery
Digastric, posterior belly
Atlas, transverse process
Spinal accessory nerve
Second cervical spinal ganglion
Vagus nerve
Internal jugular vein
Sternocleido-mastoid
Superior cervical sympathetic ganglion
Spinal accessory nerve
Vagus nerve (displaced medially)
Common carotid artery
Vertebral artery
Tentorium cerebelli
Tentorial notch
Trigeminal nerve
Transverse dural venous sinus
Facial and vestibulocochlear nerves
Glossopharyngeal, vagus and accessory nerves
Accessory nerve, spinal root
Vertebral artery
First cervical (suboccipital) nerve
Atlas, posterior arch
Dura mater
Third cervical nerve dorsal ramus
Denticulate ligament

So the **SCENAR has a brain**. It is a biofeedback device. It reads the problem, computes the problem and puts a correction to the problem back into the body. And this is done by placing the SCENAR on the skin for a few seconds, reading the asymmetry, which we call the **'initial response'** or **IR**. The initial response is the immediate read of a problem and it measures the problem. The amount of a problem in a body underneath an electrode is measured and delivered in numerical form so that you can tell whether you have an inflammation, a strain, a tear, a fracture, all different kind of injury or damage. It has this capability. It pretty much is a complete diagnostic and treatment unit for most everything you can think of. So that is in a nutshell, is an introduction to the SCENAR, how it works and the theory behind it.

Pain Factors

Neurophysiological factor, i.e., the pain is provoked by the receptors' or their afferent fibers' irritations. SCENAR application produces additional afflux of neurotype pulse signals, thus impeding transfer of the pain pulses to the brain.

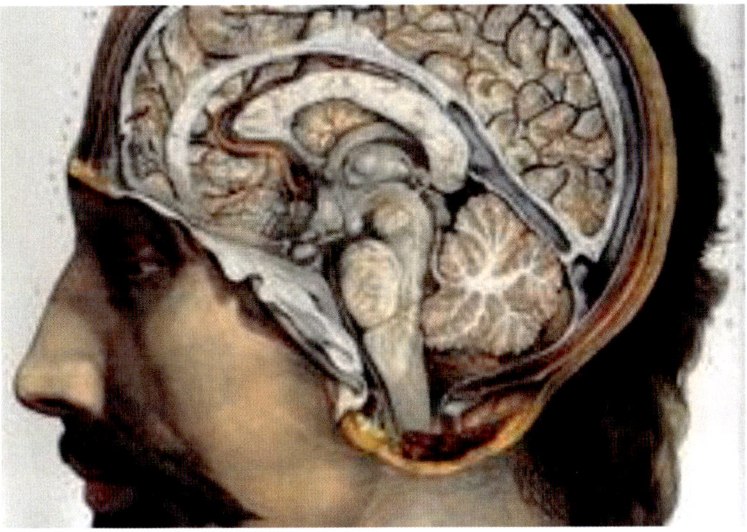

Neurochemical factor - it is produced by **neuropeptides**, SCENAR stimulation of neurons of vegetative ganglia initiates formation of the opiate-like substances which are antagonistic to the pain conductive neuropeptides thus blocking pain stimulation transferring.
Transdermal electrostimulation along with stimulation of the central serotonin secretion brings about on-the-spot secretion of an active vasodilation substance that restores redox processes and eliminates pain.

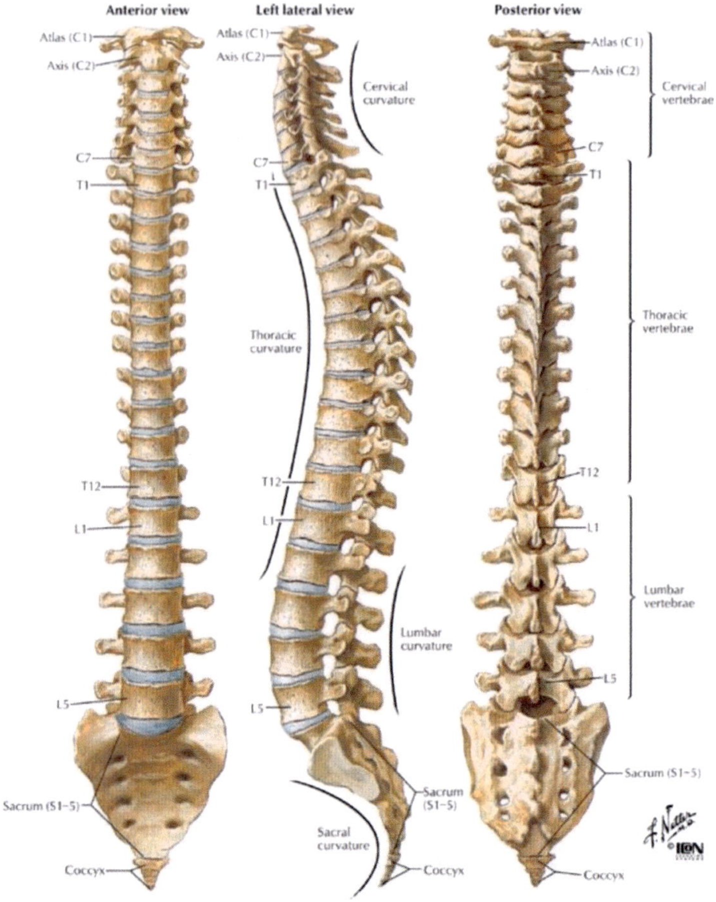

Anterior view
Left lateral view
Posterior view
Atlas (C1)
Axis (C2)
C7
T1
T12
L1
L5
Sacrum (S1–5)
Coccyx
Cervical curvature
Thoracic curvature
Lumbar curvature
Sacral curvature
Cervical vertebrae
Thoracic vertebrae
Lumbar vertebrae

Effects of Scenar Treatment

Pain-killing effect usually lasts for at least four hours and gives a more profound effect than narcotics.

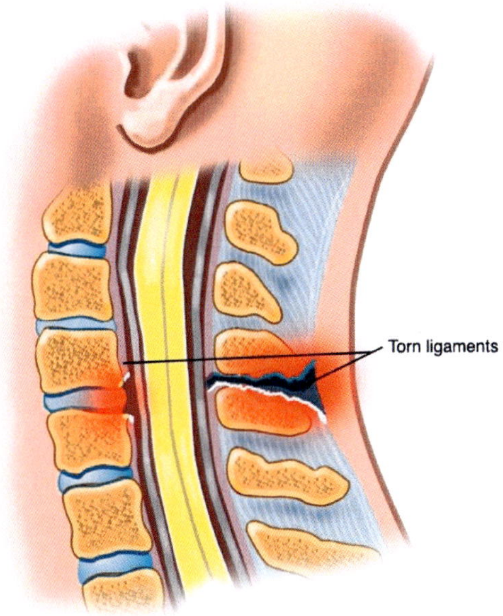
Torn ligaments

Mechanisms:

Refraction in the nerve endings of the peripheral nerve fibers blocks the transmission of the **pain impulse**.

A new dominant focus is established in the cortex of the brain, which suppresses the pain focus.

SCENAR action considerably reduces edema around the nerve fibers and so reduces the pressure on nociceptors.

Three factors are involved.

- Neurophysiological
- Neuro-chemical
- Psycho-emotional

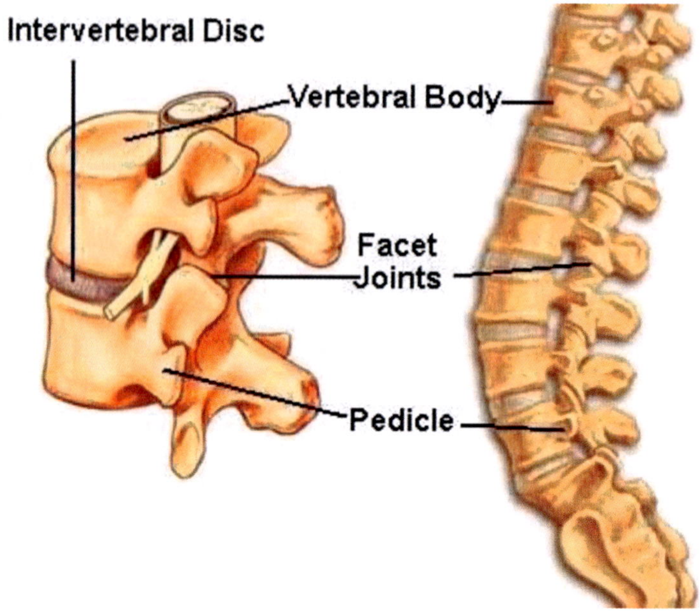
Intervertebral Disc
Vertebral Body
Facet
Joints
Pedicle

Anti-inflammatory Effect

An inflammatory focus is surrounded by a leukocyte cuff in order to prevent the inflammation from spreading to the surrounding tissues. Eventually this cuff will be in the way of reorganization and recovery, as new leucocytes cannot reach the focus of inflammation. The action of the SCENAR reduces the cuff and speeds recovery. **Maximum benefit is obtained if treatment occurs every two hours**.

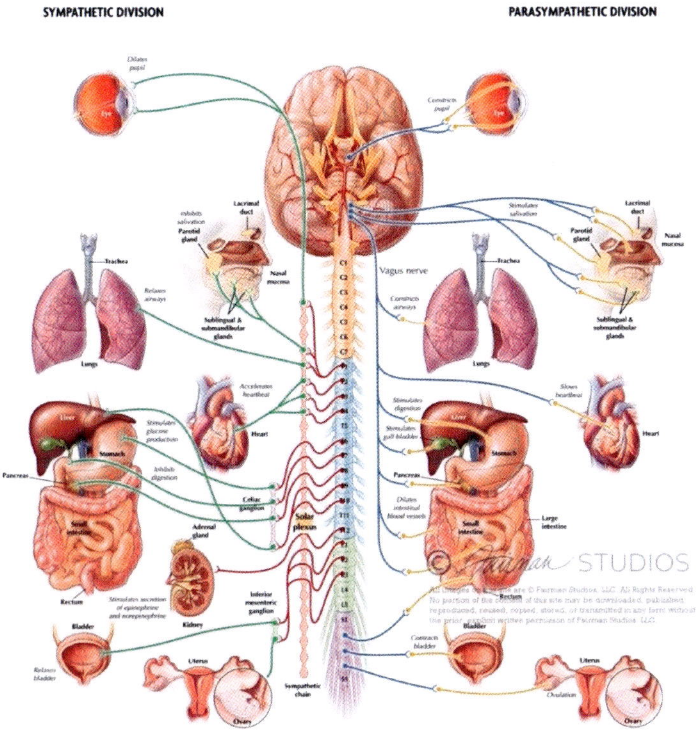
SYMPATHETIC DIVISION
PARASYMPATHETIC DIVISION
Dilates pupil
Eye
Constricts pupil
Lacrimal duct
Inhibits salivation
Parotid gland
Nasal mucosa
Stimulates salivation
Trachea
Relaxes airways
Lungs
Sublingual & submandibular glands
Vagus nerve
Constricts airways
Accelerates heartbeat
Heart
Slows heartbeat
Liver
Stimulates glucose production
Stomach
Stimulates digestion
Stimulates gall bladder
Pancreas
Inhibits digestion
Celiac ganglion
Solar plexus
Dilates intestinal blood vessels
Small intestine
Large intestine
Adrenal gland
Rectum
Stimulates secretion of epinephrine and norepinephrine
Kidney
Inferior mesenteric ganglion
Bladder
Relaxes bladder
Contracts bladder
Uterus
Ovary
Ovulation
Sympathetic chain
STUDIOS

Anti-edema

Helps reduces swelling by redistributing the fluid between the lymphatic and vascular systems. Again, for maximum effect, treat two hourly.

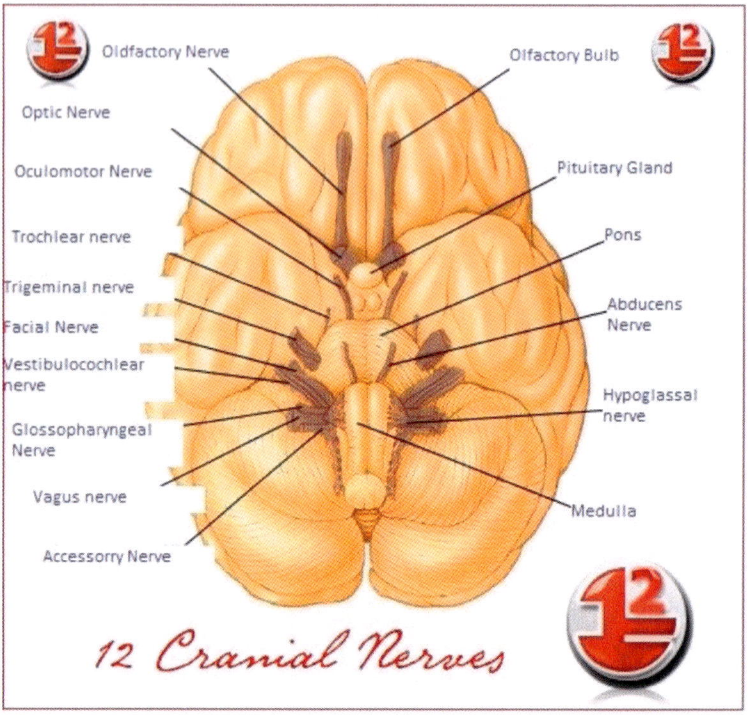
Oldfactory Nerve
Olfactory Bulb
Optic Nerve
Oculomotor Nerve
Pituitary Gland
Trochlear nerve
Pons
Trigeminal nerve
Facial Nerve
Abducens Nerve
Vestibulocochlear nerve
Hypoglassal nerve
Glossopharyngeal Nerve
Vagus nerve
Medulla
Accessorry Nerve
12 Cranial Nerves

Hemostatic Effect

As a result of collateral blood supply and the reduction of pressure in the main vessel, bleeding stops. Bleeding rate may increase before stopping.

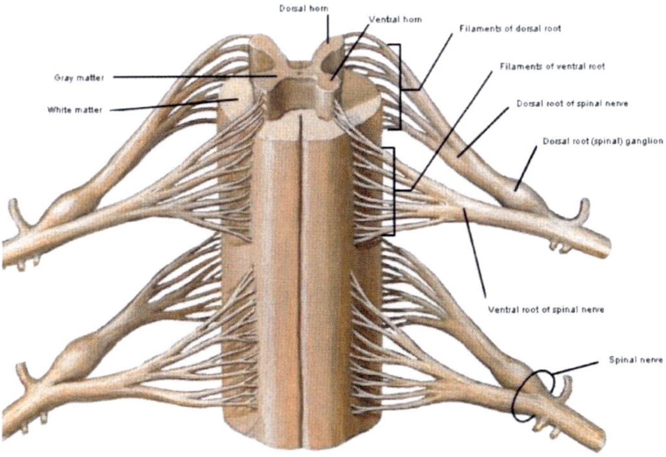
Dorsal horn
Ventral horn
Filaments of dorsal root
Filaments of ventral root
Dorsal root of spinal nerve
Dorsal root (spinal) ganglion
Gray matter
White matter
Ventral root of spinal nerve
Spinal nerve

Hyperemia Effect

Increased blood flow. **Vasodilators** increase the lumen of micro-circulation blood vessels and blood flow to the place of treatment increases. This is maximal 30-60 minutes after treating and is especially observed when treating coronary artery spasm.

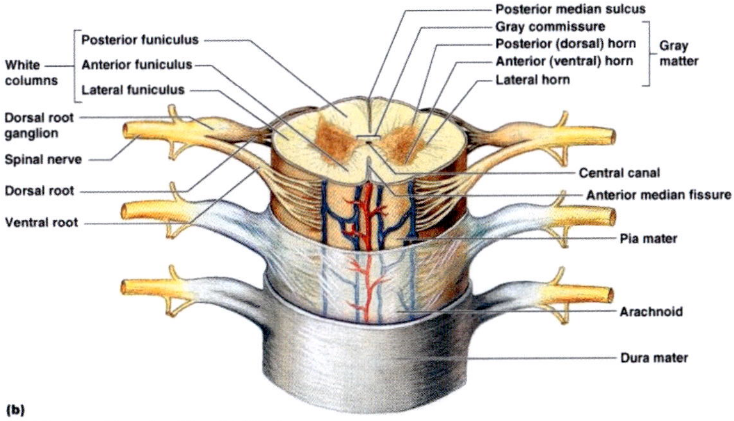
Posterior median sulcus
Gray commissure
Posterior (dorsal) horn
Anterior (ventral) horn
Lateral horn
Gray matter
White columns
Posterior funiculus
Anterior funiculus
Lateral funiculus
Dorsal root ganglion
Spinal nerve
Dorsal root
Ventral root
Central canal
Anterior median fissure
Pia mater
Arachnoid
Dura mater

(b)

Copyright © 2004 Pearson Education, Inc., publishing as Benjamin Cummings.

Anti-shock /Anti-allergic Effects

Local or general reaction can be observed with food allergy, drug reactions and insect bites, and may manifest as urticarial rashes, edema (including that of the larynx), rhinitis, bronchospasm and so on. These symptoms are treated as they occur.

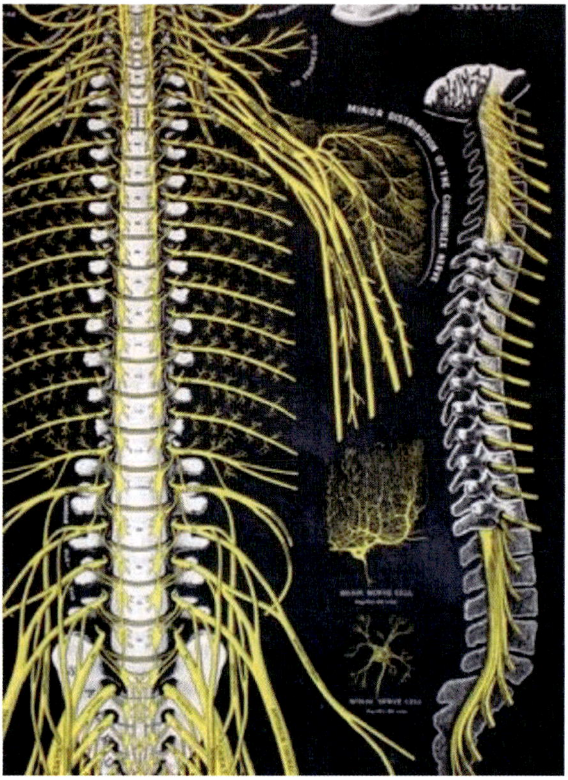

Antipyretic effect

Lowering of high temperatures can be obtained by treating the main blood vessels. It's best to treat only very high temperatures, as mild pyrexias are usually normal adaptive reactions.

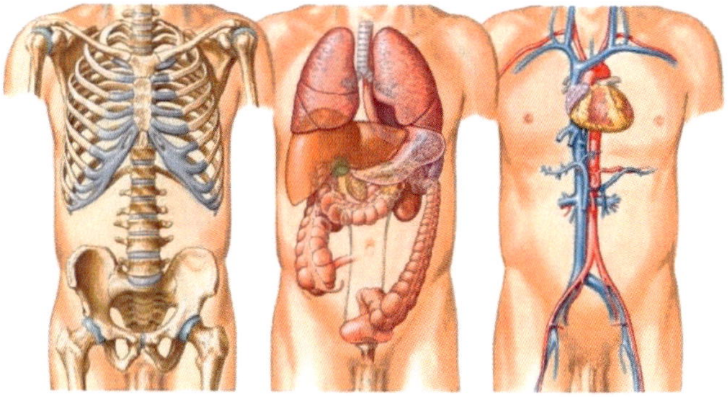

Normalization of Metabolic Processes

Increased solute levels in blood

By stimulating consumption of oxygen and nutrients, SCENAR therapy increases the metabolic rate, increases venous flow and improves the removal of the products of metabolism. Lymphatic flow will increase as well. Normalization of cell, tissue and system function - SCENAR treatment triggers the release of neuropeptides. These are further metabolized to produce a cascade of new bio-active compounds. Neuropeptides and the breakdown products help correct and balance the relationship between biochemical and functional systems in cells and tissues distant from the site being treated.

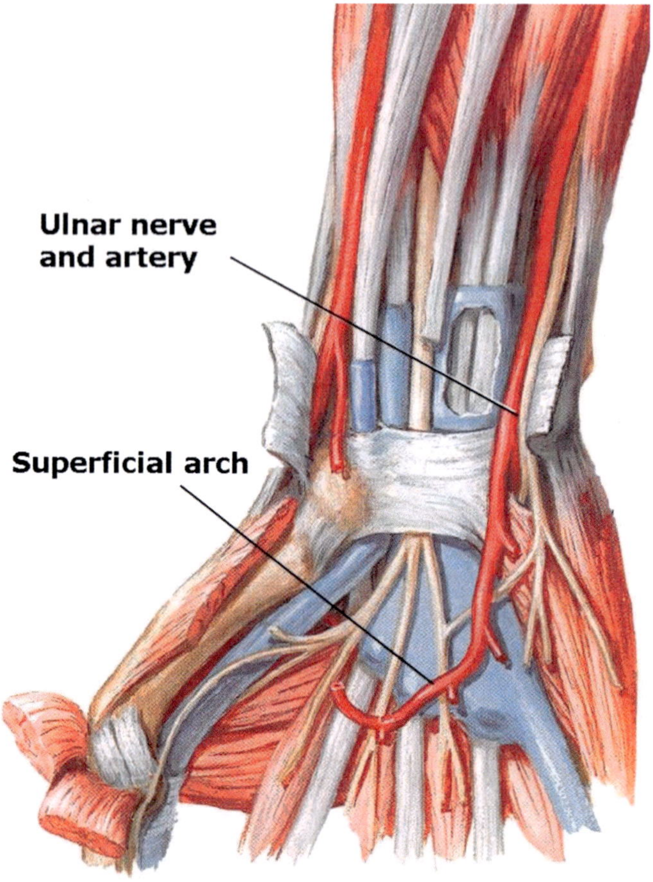
Ulnar nerve
and artery
Superficial arch

Normalization of Hormone Balance

Faster wound healing due to faster regeneration of tissues.

General Effect

Good sleep, good appetite and good sense of well-being due to higher levels of energy and immunity.

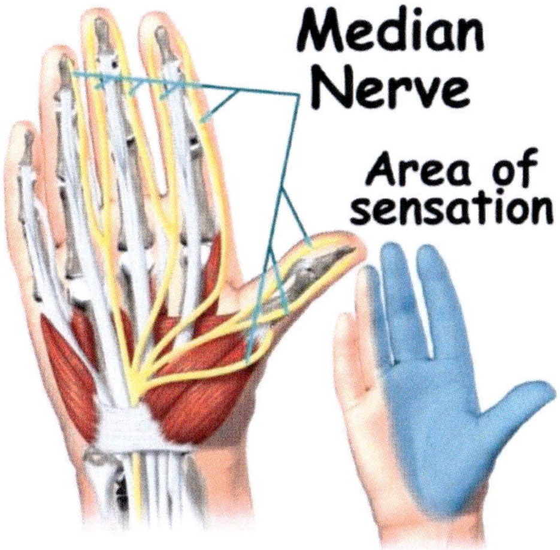
Median
Nerve
Area of
sensation

Chapter 4.
Diagnosis with the SCENAR

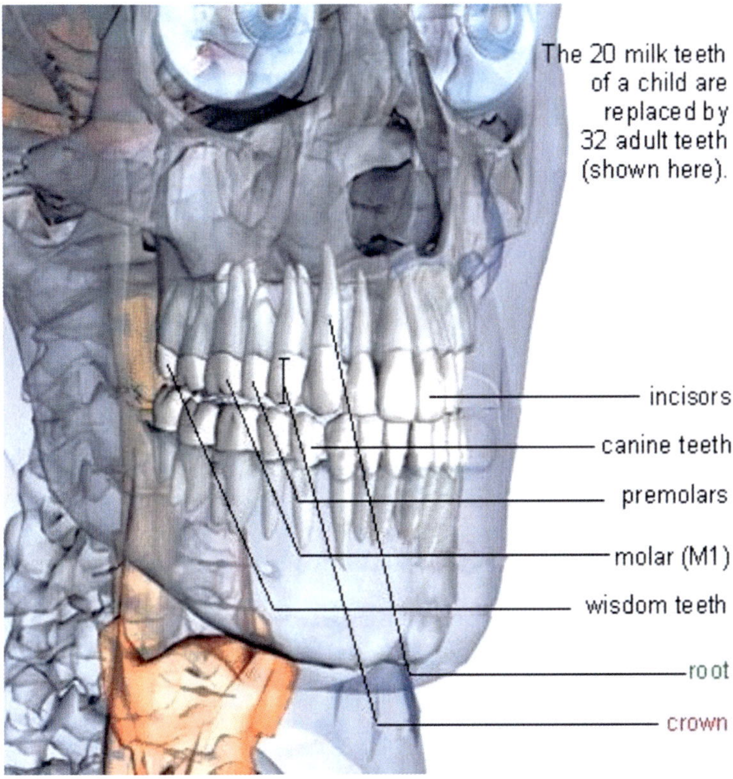
The 20 milk teeth
of a child are
replaced by
32 adult teeth
(shown here).
incisors
canine teeth
premolars
molar (M1)
wisdom teeth
root
crown

Diagnostic / Treatment

Ask the patient to point with one finger (if possible) to what is the most pressing problem RIGHT NOW (usually pain).

Ask the patient to recall anything about the pain, e.g., character, severity, timing, radiation, etc.

Is there a movement which triggers or regenerates the pain?

If possible, make the patient elicit/demonstrate the pain. Where appropriate compare with the opposite side. Test any weaknesses.

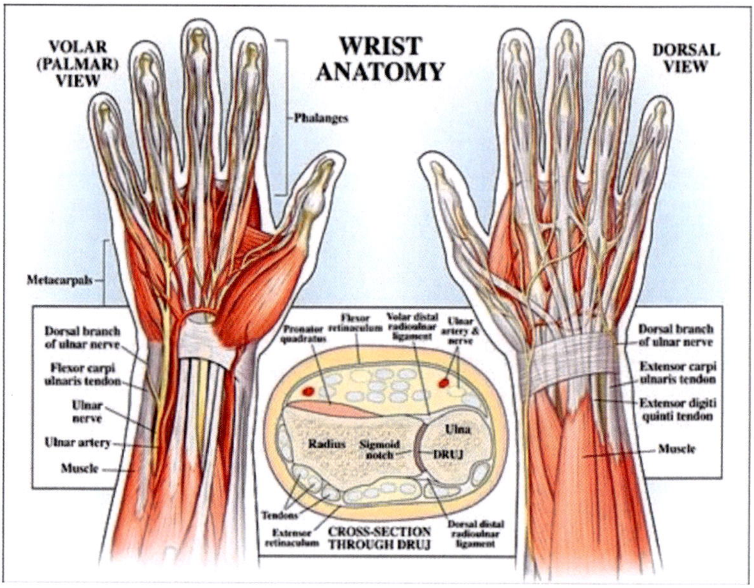
VOLAR (PALMAR) VIEW
WRIST ANATOMY
DORSAL VIEW
Phalanges
Metacarpals
Dorsal branch of ulnar nerve
Flexor carpi ulnaris tendon
Ulnar nerve
Ulnar artery
Muscle
Pronator quadratus
Flexor retinaculum
Volar distal radioulnar ligament
Ulnar artery & nerve
Radius
Sigmoid notch
Ulna
DRUJ
Tendons
Extensor retinaculum
CROSS-SECTION THROUGH DRUJ
Dorsal distal radioulnar ligament
Dorsal branch of ulnar nerve
Extensor carpi ulnaris tendon
Extensor digiti quinti tendon
Muscle

Primary Signs

Differences in the skin that are apparent before treatment.

Color, Itching, Rash, Scales, Pigmentation, Erosions, Spots, Sores, Scars

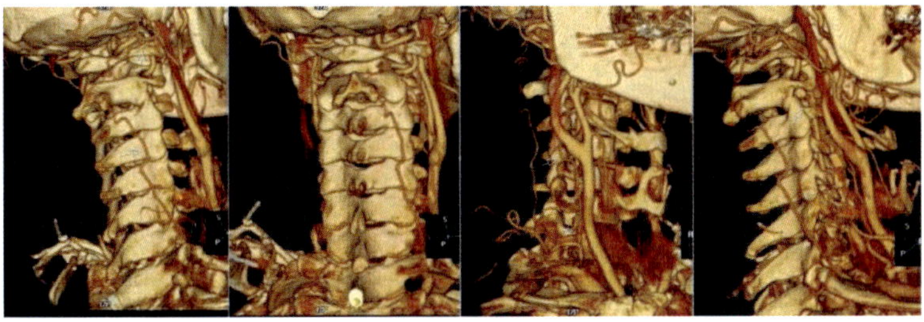

Secondary Factors

Differences which appear during and after the treatment outside treatment area:

Hyperemia / pallor Focal pain, Itching / Rash, Local pain after treatment, another topical complaint.

Microvibromassaging modes (1:1, 2:1) are very effective in cosmetology for working on mimic muscles and tissues of the neck area. Regular 'electronic massage' procedures improve tone of muscles and blood circulation in the area, which in turn positively influences the general state of health.

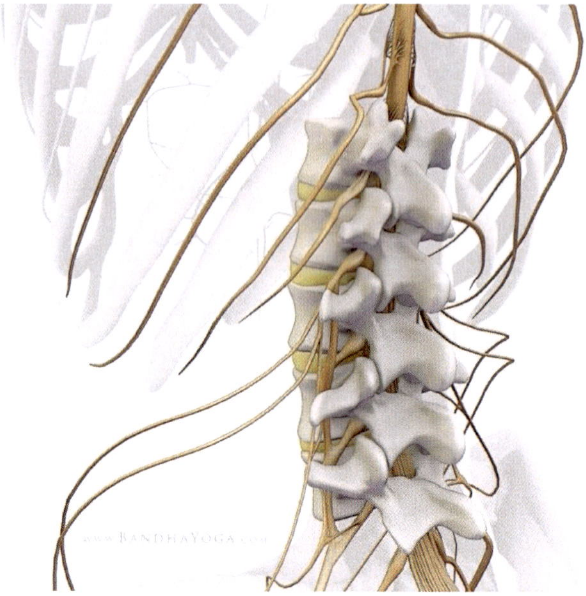

High energy levels are used in emergency situations, to deal with a problem with maximum efficiency (pain killing effect/CPR); during assessment of low sensitivity areas; and also when the state of low body reactivity is present (to 'wake up' the body response). It makes sense to utilize various energy levels during therapy, in order to enhance the body's response through diversity.

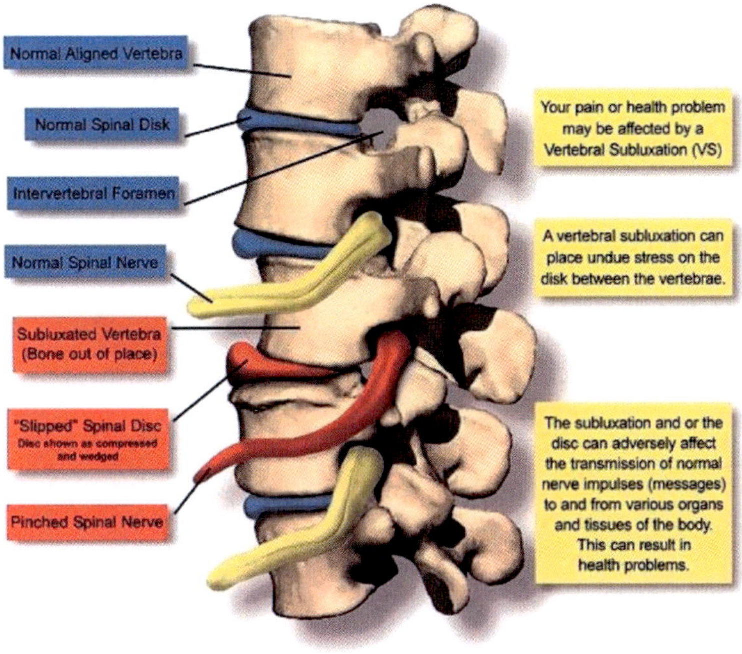
Normal Aligned Vertebra
Normal Spinal Disk
Intervertebral Foramen
Normal Spinal Nerve
Subluxated Vertebra
(Bone out of place)
"Slipped" Spinal Disc
Disc shown as compressed and wedged
Pinched Spinal Nerve
Your pain or health problem may be affected by a Vertebral Subluxation (VS)
A vertebral subluxation can place undue stress on the disk between the vertebrae.
The subluxation and or the disc can adversely affect the transmission of normal nerve impulses (messages) to and from various organs and tissues of the body. This can result in health problems.

Symmetrical Treatment

In order to increase the benefits of treatment, work on the symmetrical zones. It is not possible to work on pain spots because of open wounds, plaster, or bandages; you should work on zones symmetrical to the painful areas.

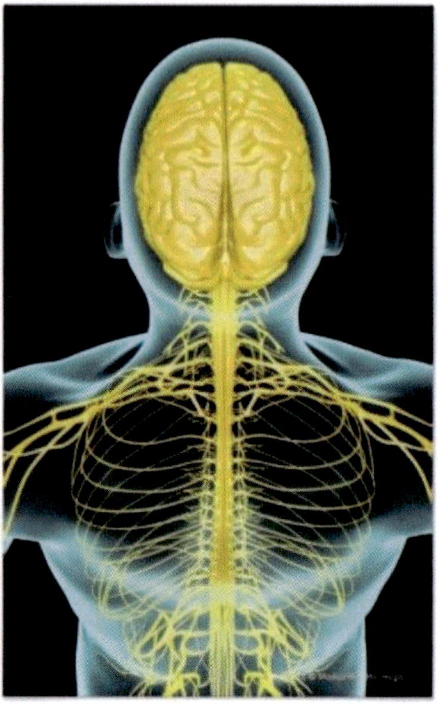

Main Diagnostic Symptoms:

A Large Diagnostic Symptom

This is the skin area, which appears during SCENAR application and differs from the surrounding skin surface by its color, moisture, pain or tactile sensibility, and so on. It also includes the areas where there is a change in the device's slide and sound tone.

There are five large diagnostic symptoms in SCENAR: sticking, sensitivity alteration, skin alteration, sound alteration, and change in numerical output display.

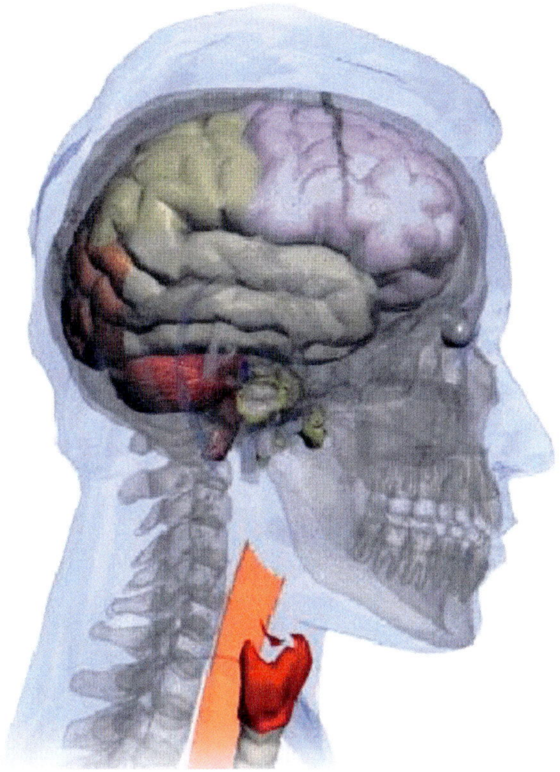

Stickiness

When you draw the device over the skin, it can "**stick**" so that you cannot get it moving forward without applying force. It means there is a pathological nidus over there, "Sticking" area needs to be treated additionally for 2 - 3 minutes.

Sensitivity Alteration

During treatment, the device electrodes contact parts of the skin with different sensitivity. Highly sensitive skin area coincides with the projection of the pathological nidus and is optimal for SCENAR application.

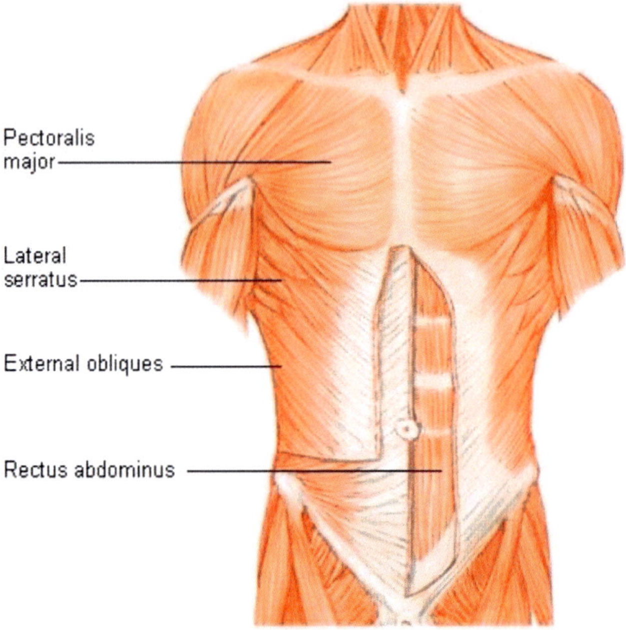
Pectoralis
major
Lateral
serratus
External obliques
Rectus abdominus

Skin Alteration

Skin reddening during SCENAR application indicates the increased functions in this area and is up for additional treatment. If a pale skin area stands out against the red background, it indicates the decreased functions in this area and is also up for additional treatment.

Upon revealing any uncharacteristic changes in the skin (blister, spot, scar, and so on), apply the device directly to the altered skin area.

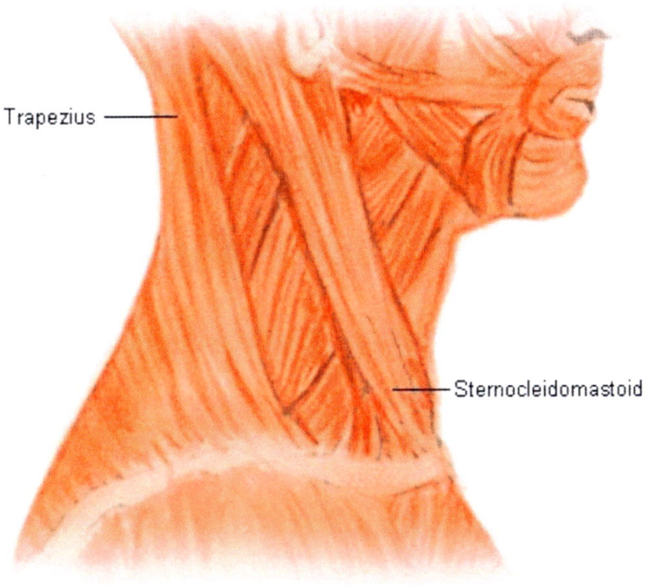
Trapezius
Sternocleidomastoid

Sound Alteration

Any change in **tonal sound** during SCENAR application indicates a pathological nidus. Skin area of the altered sound is up for additional treatment for 2-3 minutes.

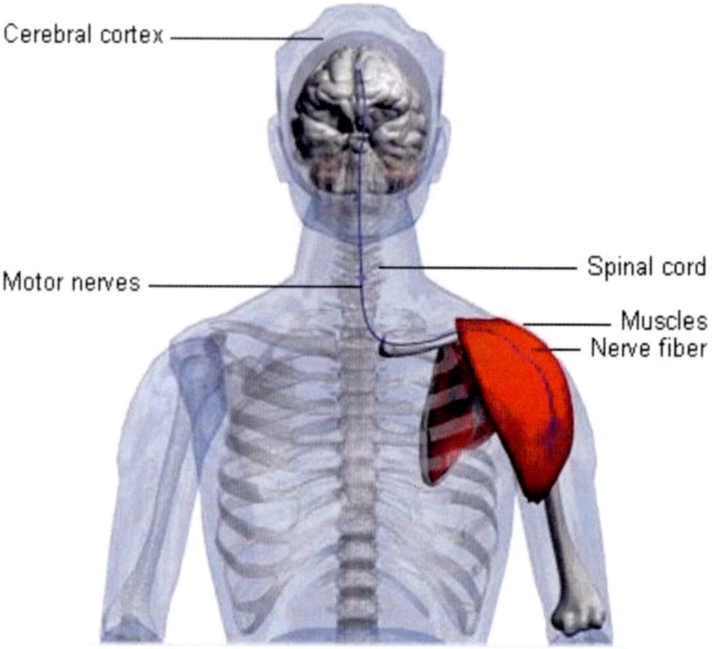
Cerebral cortex
Spinal cord
Motor nerves
Muscles
Nerve fiber

Change in Numerical Output Display.

Small Diagnostic Symptom

This is the most distinct and **well-marked small skin area**, which appears on the skin surface within the large diagnostic symptom area during SCENAR application.

This is the easy-to-identify and vivid diagnostic symptom and optimal skin area for Scenar application. Small diagnostic symptom must be up for additional treatment until it disappears.

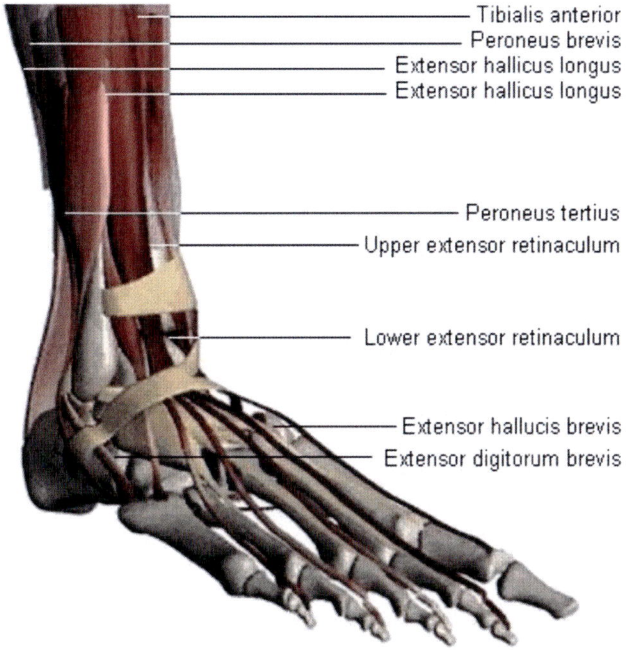
Tibialis anterior
Peroneus brevis
Extensor hallicus longus
Extensor hallicus longus
Peroneus tertius
Upper extensor retinaculum
Lower extensor retinaculum
Extensor hallucis brevis
Extensor digitorum brevis

Extra Diagnostic Symptoms:

Extra primary diagnostic symptom- this is the small skin area which initially, prior to SCENAR application, differs by some of its features from the other skin surface irrespectively of device treatment, i.e., the visually observed symptoms, such as skin coloration, sensation (itch, and others), **scar, wound, erosion, pigmentation**, and so on.

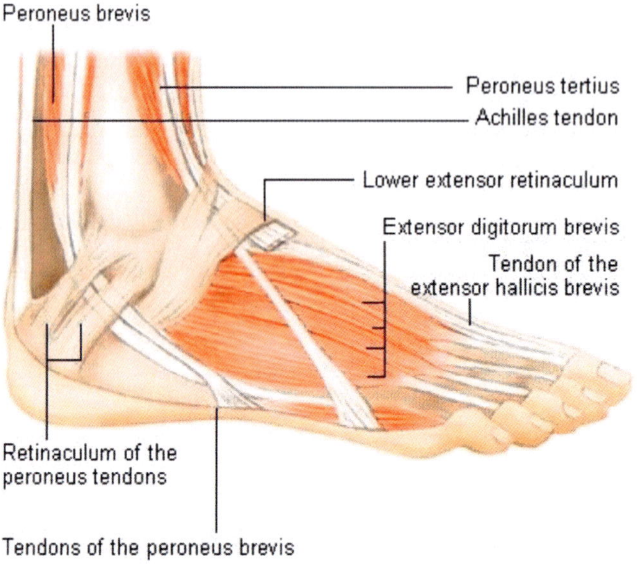
Peroneus brevis
Peroneus tertius
Achilles tendon
Lower extensor retinaculum
Extensor digitorum brevis
Tendon of the
extensor hallicis brevis
Retinaculum of the
peroneus tendons
Tendons of the peroneus brevis

Extra primary diagnostic symptom is also up for additional Scenar application according to the symmetric treatment method: right - left, top - bottom, etc.

Extra secondary diagnostic symptom- this is the skin area, which appears in the process of SCENAR application and differs from the other skin surface. It is located outside the areas applied by the SCENAR devices. The secondary symptom is also up for additional treatment. It should disappear with patient's recovery. If the "main small" and "extra secondary" symptoms are located over the endocrine glands, the therapy will be more effective.

Asymmetries

These are local changes that occur in, and only inside, the area that is being treated or as a result of a treatment.

- In the color of the skin: flushing / pallor
- In the client's sensations: numbness / hypersensitivity
- In the sound of the SCENAR when working: louder/ quieter
- In the stickiness or "drag" of the electrode when moved over the skin.
- In pain sensation: pain / no pain
- In Diagnosis 1: Highest IR / Highest Dose /Highest "0"

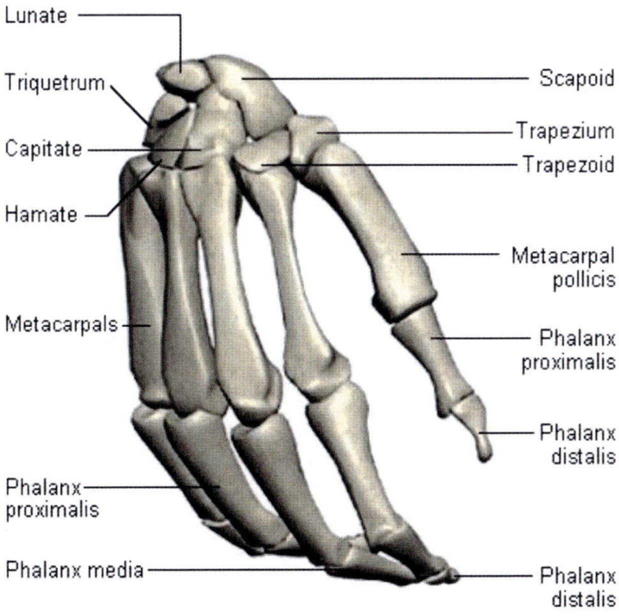

Lunate
Triquetrum
Capitate
Hamate
Metacarpals
Phalanx proximalis
Phalanx media
Scapoid
Trapezium
Trapezoid
Metacarpal pollicis
Phalanx proximalis
Phalanx distalis
Phalanx distalis

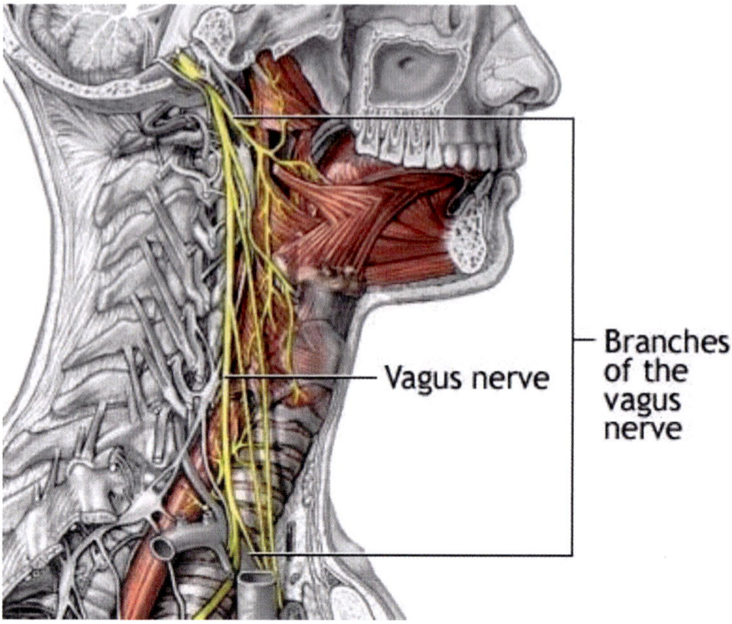
Vagus nerve
Branches of the vagus nerve

Small Asymmetry

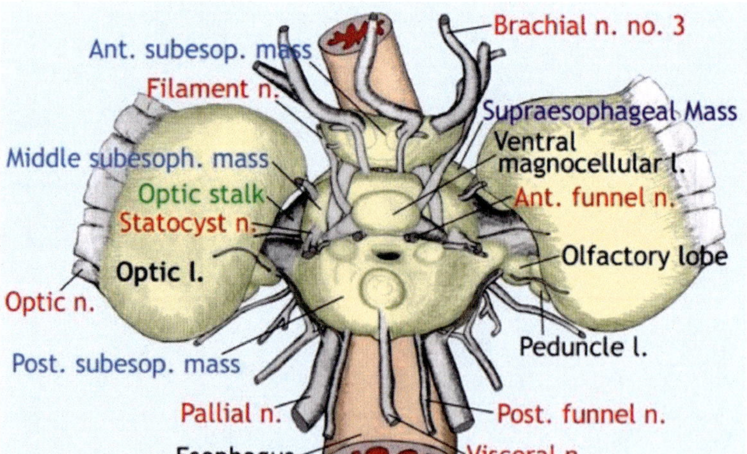
Brachial n. no. 3
Ant. subesop. mass
Filament n.
Supraesophageal Mass
Ventral magnocellular l.
Middle subesoph. mass
Optic stalk
Ant. funnel n.
Statocyst n.
Olfactory lobe
Optic l.
Optic n.
Peduncle l.
Post. subesop. mass
Pallial n.
Post. funnel n.
Esophagus
Visceral n.

When working in **Diagnosis 0,** skin coloration changes in two directions: redness and pallor. A small white patch within a red area or vice versa, is called a small asymmetry and it is important to treat this. This is perhaps the most significant treatment indicator and is very much a part of the SCENAR language. It describes a small area of difference within the area already showing secondary signs or asymmetries. For example: when working in Diag. 0 treatment mode, **the color of the skin changes in two directions: redness and pallor**. Thus a small white patch appears within a red circumscribed area or vice versa. The smaller difference in the middle of the first treatment indicator is called a Small Asymmetry and it is extremely important to treat this sign. **In Diag 1, a higher IR is a Small Asymmetry**. This type of reaction will also dictate your best frequency for treatment.

Vagus Nerve (X)
Schema - Enlargement of Distal Portions

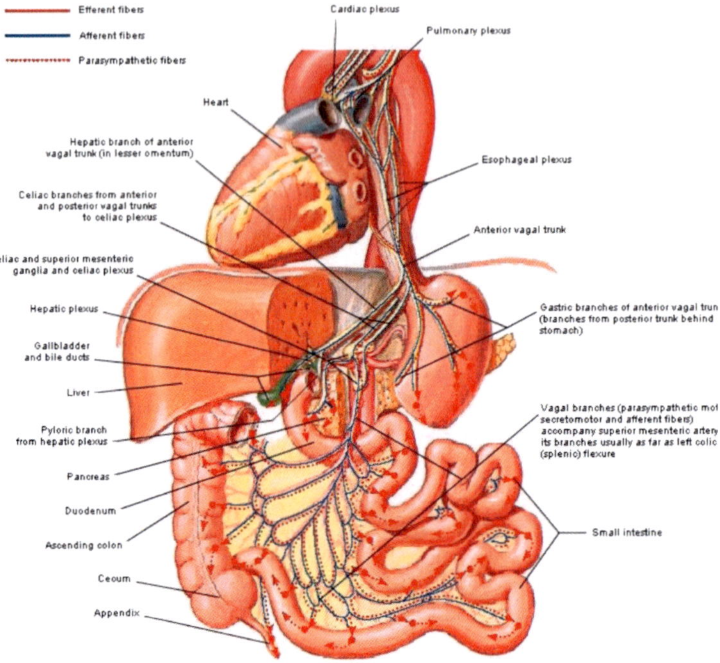
Efferent fibers
Afferent fibers
Parasympathetic fibers
Cardiac plexus
Pulmonary plexus
Heart
Hepatic branch of anterior vagal trunk (in lesser omentum)
Esophageal plexus
Celiac branches from anterior and posterior vagal trunks to celiac plexus
Anterior vagal trunk
Celiac and superior mesenteric ganglia and celiac plexus
Hepatic plexus
Gastric branches of anterior vagal trun (branches from posterior trunk behind stomach)
Gallbladder and bile ducts
Liver
Vagal branches (parasympathetic mot secretomotor and afferent fibers) accompany superior mesenteric artery its branches usually as far as left colic (splenic) flexure
Pyloric branch from hepatic plexus
Pancreas
Duodenum
Small intestine
Ascending colon
Cecum
Appendix

Asymmetry Techniques:

Asymmetry techniques are based on the subjective detection of the localizations of dissimilar expression, i.e., something different is detected. It could be as simple as you can turn your head one way but not the other- the concept is deceivingly simple yet profoundly influential. A sliding, stroking subjective **Diag. 0** technique in which signs such as spots of stickiness, redness, loud electrode sound and pronounced patient sensation. It is very important to also recognize the opposites as well, meaning spots of **non-stickiness in an area of general stickiness, blanched/whiteness in an area of general redness, a drop in sound of the electrode in an area of**

generally louder electrode sound and a lack of sensation in area of generally normal sensation. There is also the consideration of any localized, non-symmetrical sign such as a pimple, rash, roughness of skin, strange hair growth, etc. The numerical based system of measurements found in the Diag. 1 setting – many **algorithmic** procedures have been developed that coax out in increments the locations and patterns of dissimilar expressions - phasic stimulations are combined with a progressive hierarchy of relationships - a truly impressive consideration of system wide responses to localized activations - patterns also lead us to specific horizontal processes and procedures for the next session - furthermore, the relative values of the measurements lend important information as to the state of general self-regulation - the so called "corridors" of values are profound both in their indications

Follow these guidelines:

Work from higher numbers to lower numbers on the readings.

Work from the point of most pain to the point of less pain. Always look for dynamic changes in complaints, in sensations, in skin conditions both during and between treatments. Any change, even an apparent worsening is dynamic and positive. Work from simple techniques and protocols to the more complicated ones. Always look for **dynamic changes** in complaints, in sensations, in skin conditions both during and between treatments. Any change, even an apparent worsening is dynamic and positive. Work from simple techniques and protocols to the more complicated ones.

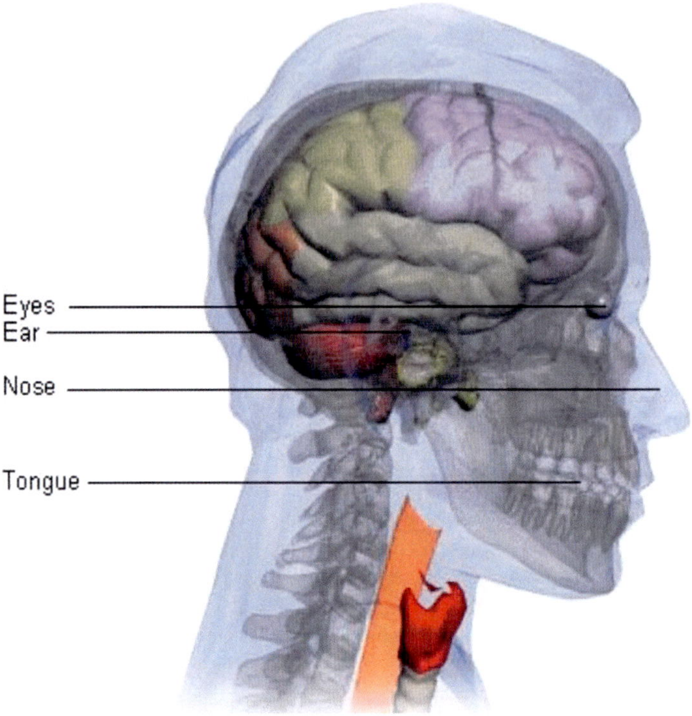
Eyes
Ear
Nose
Tongue

How to Use DIAG 1

Primary diagnostic symptoms would include localized pain, discoloration of a localized area of the skin, an itch, cicatrices, small wounds, necrosis, nevus pigmentosa or other spots, trophic disturbances (cellulitis, deformation of joints, etc.), which might be present before the beginning of the treatment procedure.

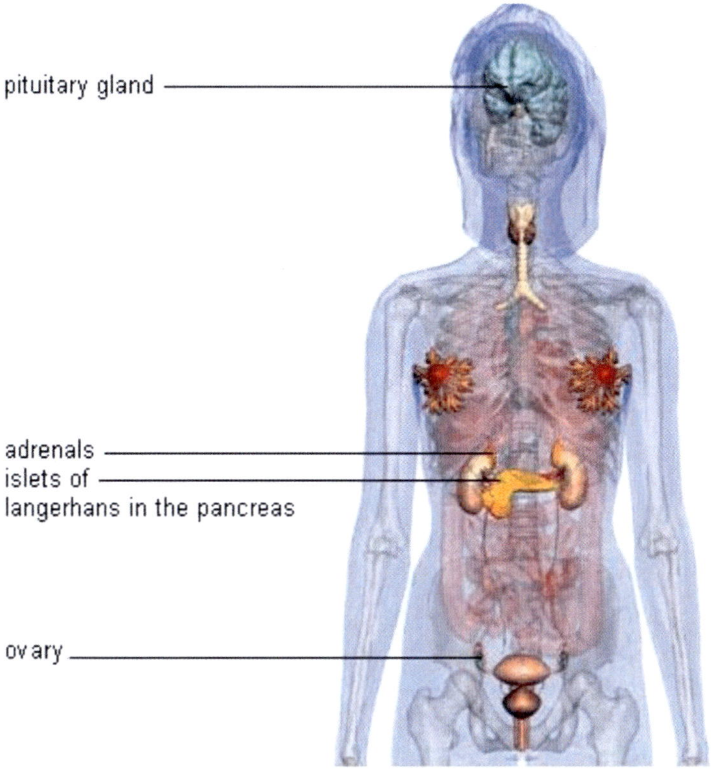
pituitary gland
adrenals
islets of
langerhans in the pancreas
ovary

Major diagnostic symptoms would include the appearance within the treatment area of differing qualities of the skin. These different qualities would include:

- Skin color change
- Sticking

Sticking is defined as hindered or restricted movement of the electrode over the skin. Any area(s) of stickiness need additional treatment.

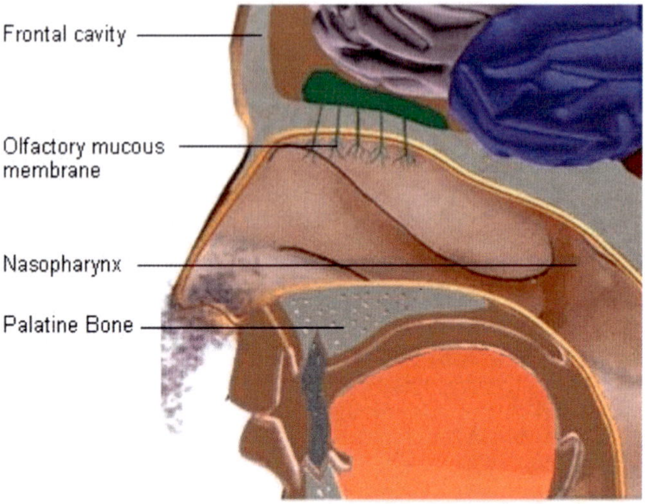
Frontal cavity
Olfactory mucous membrane
Nasopharynx
Palatine Bone

Skin sensitivity changes either increased or decreased

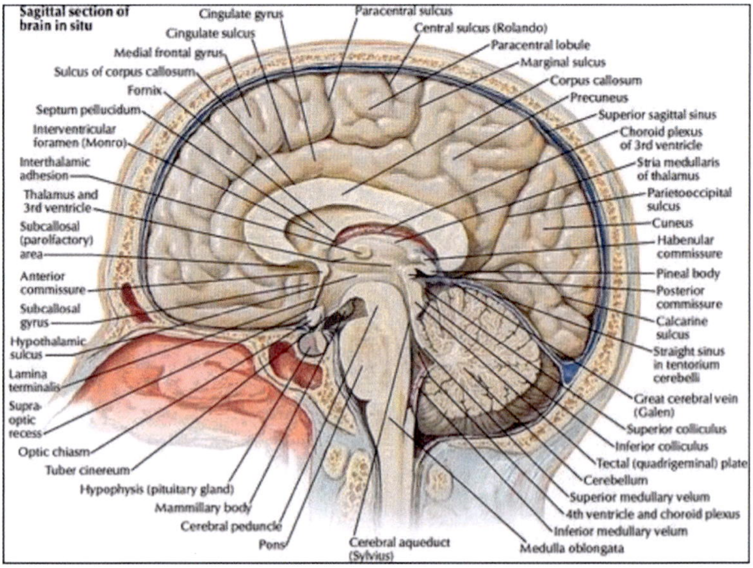
Sagittal section of brain in situ
Cingulate gyrus
Cingulate sulcus
Medial frontal gyrus
Sulcus of corpus callosum
Fornix
Septum pellucidum
Interventricular foramen (Monro)
Interthalamic adhesion
Thalamus and 3rd ventricle
Subcallosal (parolfactory) area
Anterior commissure
Subcallosal gyrus
Hypothalamic sulcus
Lamina terminalis
Supra-optic recess
Optic chiasm
Tuber cinereum
Hypophysis (pituitary gland)
Mammillary body
Cerebral peduncle
Pons
Cerebral aqueduct (Sylvius)
Paracentral sulcus
Central sulcus (Rolando)
Paracentral lobule
Marginal sulcus
Corpus callosum
Precuneus
Superior sagittal sinus
Choroid plexus of 3rd ventricle
Stria medullaris of thalamus
Parietooccipital sulcus
Cuneus
Habenular commissure
Pineal body
Posterior commissure
Calcarine sulcus
Straight sinus in tentorium cerebelli
Great cerebral vein (Galen)
Superior colliculus
Inferior colliculus
Tectal (quadrigeminal) plate
Cerebellum
Superior medullary velum
4th ventricle and choroid plexus
Inferior medullary velum
Medulla oblongata

Sound changes of the SCENAR device as it is moved over the patients' skin

During the session you may notice that the sound being emitted from the SCENAR device differs from that which you hear in the rest of the treatment areas.

These sound changes indicate that an area requires additional treatment.

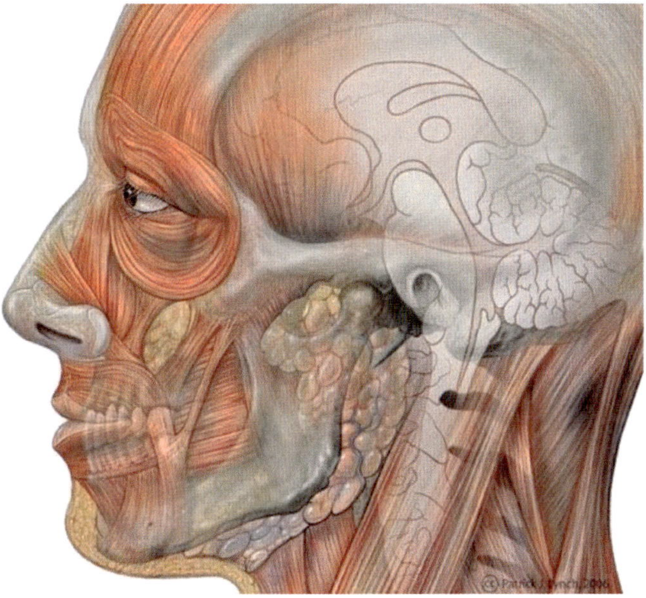

DIAG 1 Initial Response IR

When comparing **IRs**, we need a difference of +4 or higher.

When comparing Doses and '0's, we work on a difference of +1 or higher.

For the first Dose, the IR should be ±4 or greater than the following (preceding) IR.

After you give the first Dose on higher reading, any subsequent IR which is greater than the IR you have just dosed by +4 should be also dosed when working on the vertical line and greater by +1 when working on the horizontal line.

Choose the highest Dose within the route and bring the speed of reaction down to '0' (give 0 / Dose 2).

Get several different '0' s completing treatment on the back and then on the highest 0 reading set FmVar / Altemat for 2 minutes .

- Complete the procedure on the face using the principles above.
- Treat any one zone applying the same principles.
- If you did not get any "0"s, move on to the next zone.

Skin Signs in Scenar Therapy

Examine the skin properly before, during and after the treatment. The signs or treatment indicators will show where to work and dynamics of the treatment process.

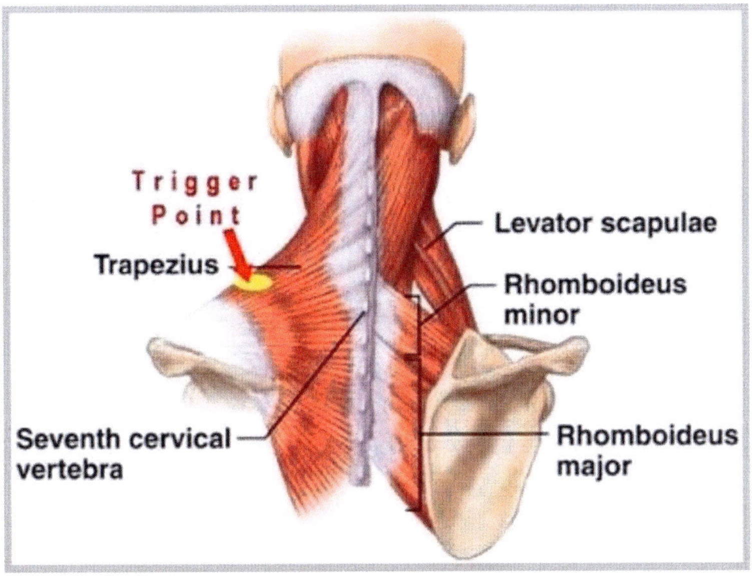
Trigger Point
Trapezius
Levator scapulae
Rhomboideus minor
Seventh cervical vertebra
Rhomboideus major

Primary Signs

Differences in the skin that is apparent before treatment.

- Color, Itching, Erosions, Sores
- Rash, Pigmentation, Spots, Scars
- Scales

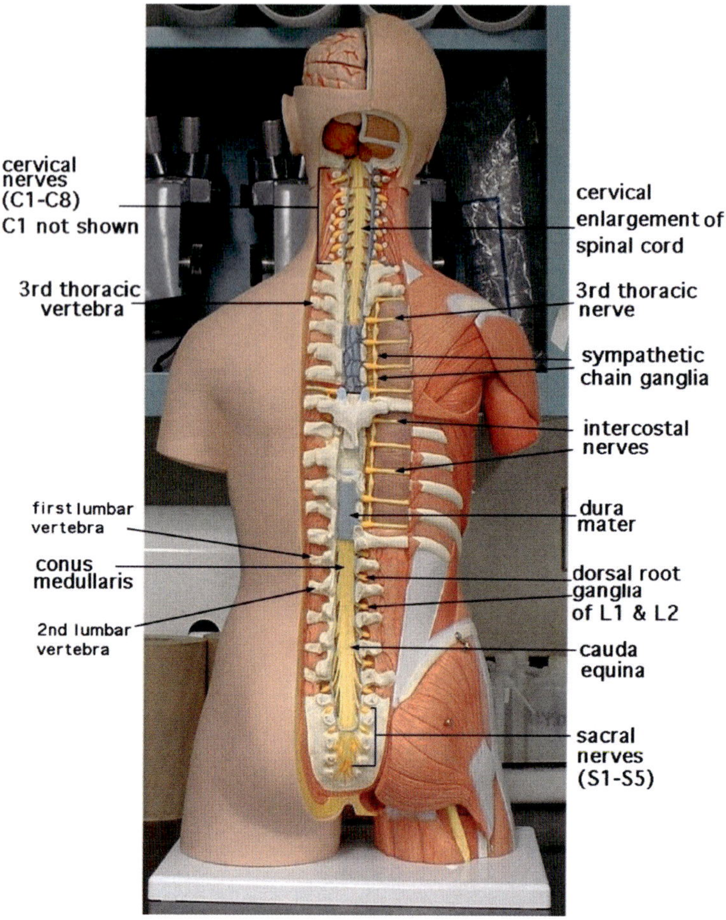
cervical nerves (C1-C8)
C1 not shown
3rd thoracic vertebra
first lumbar vertebra
conus medullaris
2nd lumbar vertebra
cervical enlargement of spinal cord
3rd thoracic nerve
sympathetic chain ganglia
intercostal nerves
dura mater
dorsal root ganglia of L1 & L2
cauda equina
sacral nerves (S1-S5)

Secondary Factors

Differences which appear during and after the treatment outside treatment area:

- Hyperemia / pallor
- Focal pain
- Itching / Rash
- Local pain after treatment
- Another topical complaint

Thorax

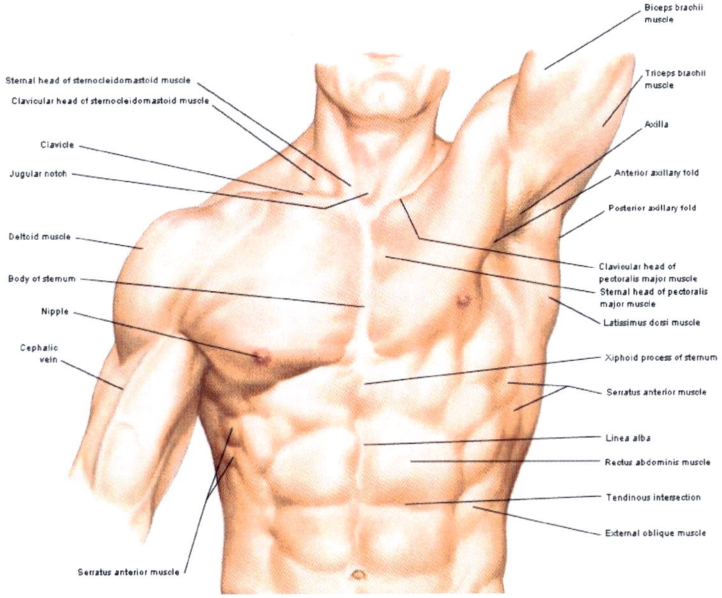
Sternal head of sternocleidomastoid muscle
Clavicular head of sternocleidomastoid muscle
Clavicle
Jugular notch
Deltoid muscle
Body of sternum
Nipple
Cephalic vein
Serratus anterior muscle
Biceps brachii muscle
Triceps brachii muscle
Axilla
Anterior axillary fold
Posterior axillary fold
Clavicular head of pectoralis major muscle
Sternal head of pectoralis major muscle
Latissimus dorsi muscle
Xiphoid process of sternum
Serratus anterior muscle
Linea alba
Rectus abdominis muscle
Tendinous intersection
External oblique muscle

Diagnostic 0

Set the SCENAR to the lowest possible power.

Place the SCENAR on the skin outside the area selected for treatment.

Increase the power to an appropriate level whilst on the skin.

Move to the area selected for treatment.

In Diagnosis = 0, move the SCENAR over the skin with firm pressure looking for signs of asymmetry -- redness, stickiness etc.

Continue rubbing with the SCENAR until the redness, stickiness etc. goes away.

NERVOUS SYSTEM OF THORAX AND UPPER LIMB (ANTERIOR VIEW)

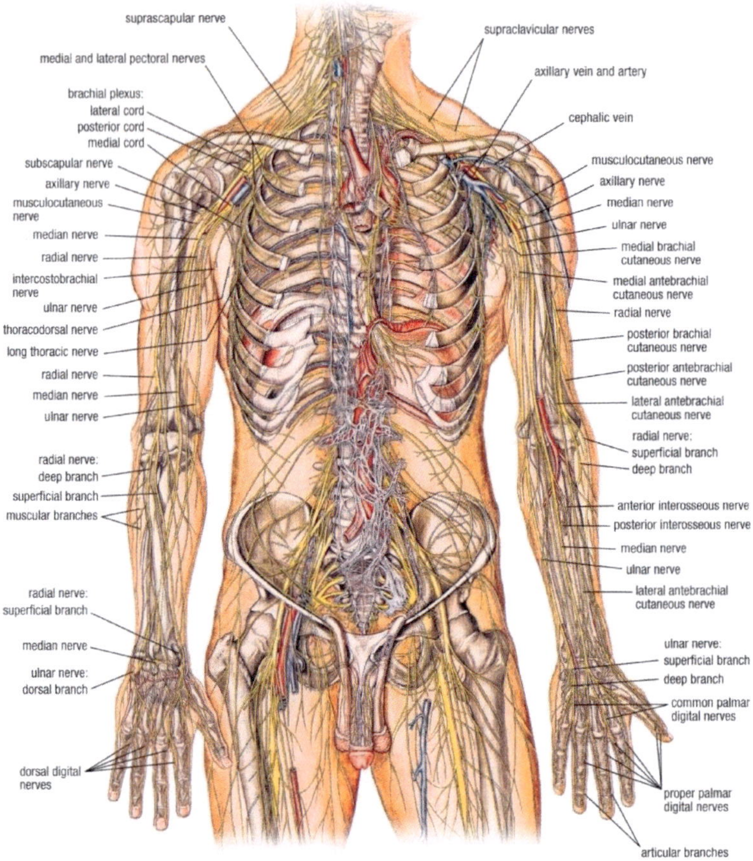

suprascapular nerve
medial and lateral pectoral nerves
brachial plexus:
lateral cord
posterior cord
medial cord
subscapular nerve
axillary nerve
musculocutaneous nerve
median nerve
radial nerve
intercostobrachial nerve
ulnar nerve
thoracodorsal nerve
long thoracic nerve
radial nerve
median nerve
ulnar nerve
radial nerve:
deep branch
superficial branch
muscular branches
radial nerve:
superficial branch
median nerve
ulnar nerve:
dorsal branch
dorsal digital nerves
supraclavicular nerves
axillary vein and artery
cephalic vein
musculocutaneous nerve
axillary nerve
median nerve
ulnar nerve
medial brachial cutaneous nerve
medial antebrachial cutaneous nerve
radial nerve
posterior brachial cutaneous nerve
posterior antebrachial cutaneous nerve
lateral antebrachial cutaneous nerve
radial nerve:
superficial branch
deep branch
anterior interosseous nerve
posterior interosseous nerve
median nerve
ulnar nerve
lateral antebrachial cutaneous nerve
ulnar nerve:
superficial branch
deep branch
common palmar digital nerves
proper palmar digital nerves
articular branches

Diagnostic 1

Measure the initial reactions

Look for the highest of the initial reactions.

Replace the SCENAR on the area with the highest number and treat until the multitone bell rings. (Hold still for 3 seconds before removing from skin). This is called a 'dose'.

Then compare areas that have had a 'dose'. The one with the highest dose (threshold of the reaction) (see page 23) is treated again until the relative speed of the reaction (second number from left on the top line) becomes 0 (often a few minutes).

Then by comparing areas that have been taken to zero, we choose the one on which to set FM Var (often for 2 minutes).

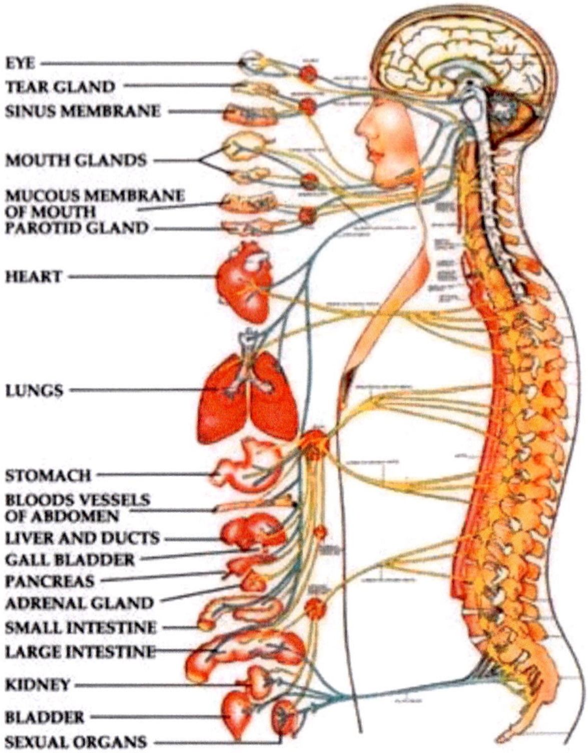
EYE
TEAR GLAND
SINUS MEMBRANE
MOUTH GLANDS
MUCOUS MEMBRANE OF MOUTH
PAROTID GLAND
HEART
LUNGS
STOMACH
BLOODS VESSELS OF ABDOMEN
LIVER AND DUCTS
GALL BLADDER
PANCREAS
ADRENAL GLAND
SMALL INTESTINE
LARGE INTESTINE
KIDNEY
BLADDER
SEXUAL ORGANS

Using DIAG 1:

When you place the device on the skin and by applying equal pressure the "Initial Reaction reading" will appear. Keep the electrode lengthwise.

Take two IP readings at the area you have chosen for this exercise.

At the position where the higher IR, place the RITM Scenar and keep it on the skin until the multi-tone bell rings. This mean you treated to Dose*.

Example: IR1 = 19 IR2 = 30

19 <30 30 / 49*

Now, choose exactly same area on other arm and follow the same principle: take readings of two IRs. Higher readings of IR treat to Dose*

Example: IR1 =27

27<31

IR2 = 31

31/49*

Now compare on each arm value of the Dose*. The higher readings of the Dose* treat to Zero by placing thes Scenar at the position of highest Dose* and waiting for the second bell to ring while response rate (the last number in the bottom row) reaches 0 or/and @ appears in the second box.

In principle the SCENAR (Self-Controlled Energy Neuron Adaptive Regulation) device works as a catalyst on the body's immune system. The SCENAR reads the resistance level of the skin and relays this information to the brain via the skin itself. This accelerates the body's healing mechanism through stimulation of the neuropeptides in each damaged cell. In addition the SCENAR could be used to treat individuals whose bodies do not repair them properly as a result of chronic illness. A classic example of this is suffers of fibromyalgia where SCENAR may act as a regeneration and pain management tool.

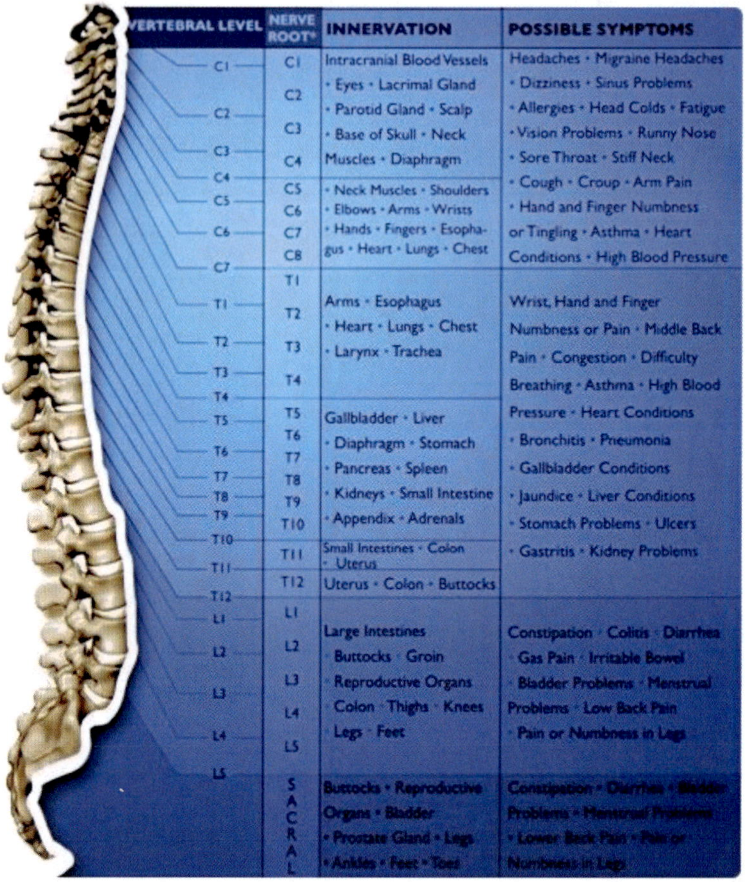

VERTEBRAL LEVEL	NERVE ROOT*	INNERVATION	POSSIBLE SYMPTOMS
C1, C2, C3	C1, C2, C3, C4	Intracranial Blood Vessels • Eyes • Lacrimal Gland • Parotid Gland • Scalp • Base of Skull • Neck Muscles • Diaphragm	Headaches • Migraine Headaches • Dizziness • Sinus Problems • Allergies • Head Colds • Fatigue • Vision Problems • Runny Nose • Sore Throat • Stiff Neck
C4, C5, C6, C7	C5, C6, C7, C8	• Neck Muscles • Shoulders • Elbows • Arms • Wrists • Hands • Fingers • Esophagus • Heart • Lungs • Chest	• Cough • Croup • Arm Pain • Hand and Finger Numbness or Tingling • Asthma • Heart Conditions • High Blood Pressure
T1, T2, T3, T4	T1, T2, T3, T4	Arms • Esophagus • Heart • Lungs • Chest • Larynx • Trachea	Wrist, Hand and Finger Numbness or Pain • Middle Back Pain • Congestion • Difficulty Breathing • Asthma • High Blood Pressure • Heart Conditions
T5, T6, T7, T8, T9, T10	T5, T6, T7, T8, T9, T10	Gallbladder • Liver • Diaphragm • Stomach • Pancreas • Spleen • Kidneys • Small Intestine • Appendix • Adrenals	• Bronchitis • Pneumonia • Gallbladder Conditions • Jaundice • Liver Conditions • Stomach Problems • Ulcers • Gastritis • Kidney Problems
T11	T11	Small Intestines • Colon • Uterus	
T12	T12	Uterus • Colon • Buttocks	
L1, L2, L3, L4	L1, L2, L3, L4, L5	Large Intestines • Buttocks • Groin • Reproductive Organs • Colon • Thighs • Knees • Legs • Feet	Constipation • Colitis • Diarrhea • Gas Pain • Irritable Bowel • Bladder Problems • Menstrual Problems • Low Back Pain • Pain or Numbness in Legs
L5	SACRAL	Buttocks • Reproductive Organs • Bladder • Prostate Gland • Legs • Ankles • Feet • Toes	Constipation • Diarrhea • Bladder Problems • Menstrual Problems • Lower Back Pain • Pain or Numbness in Legs

Start with twice a day and as things improve, go to once a day, then every other day.

Start from the healthy side.

Treat the area where the nerve leaves the skull- always moving towards the ear.

Treat star nodule on the neck

Work on temporal arteries

At first two-three sessions do not touch the most painful area.

Treat closed eyelids until visible contractions noted, Treat similarly for lips.

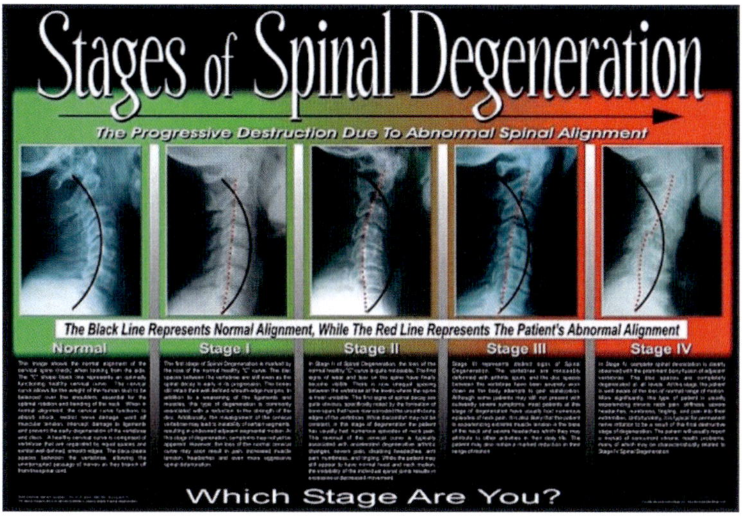
Stages of Spinal Degeneration
The Progressive Destruction Due To Abnormal Spinal Alignment
The Black Line Represents Normal Alignment, While The Red Line Represents The Patient's Abnormal Alignment
Normal
Stage I
Stage II
Stage III
Stage IV
Which Stage Are You?

When to use:

To localize symptoms

To save time when looking for asymmetry

To avoid healing crisis

To optimize the action time

In the presence of clearly defined local symptoms.

In an emergency for achieving functional changes in organs/systems.

When large surfaces are being treated.

Shoulder Anatomy

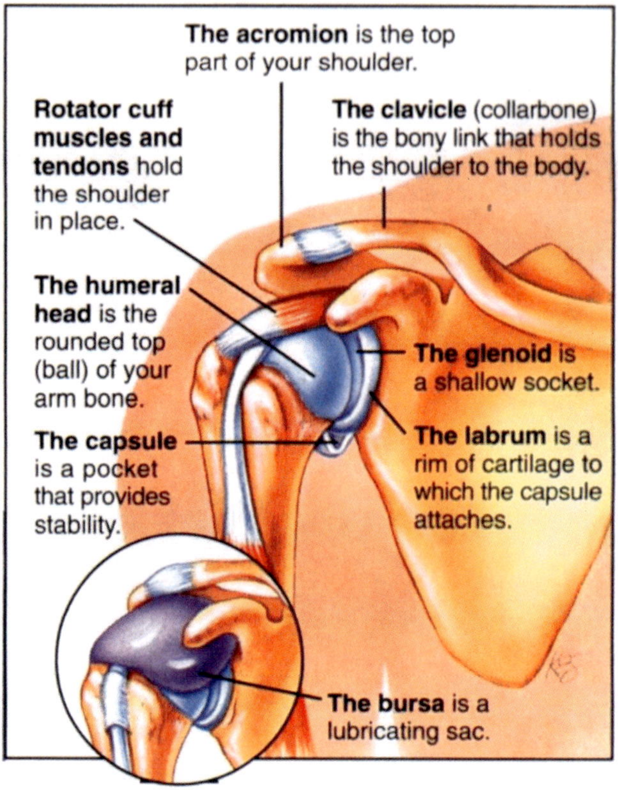
The acromion is the top part of your shoulder.
The clavicle (collarbone) is the bony link that holds the shoulder to the body.
Rotator cuff muscles and tendons hold the shoulder in place.
The humeral head is the rounded top (ball) of your arm bone.
The glenoid is a shallow socket.
The capsule is a pocket that provides stability.
The labrum is a rim of cartilage to which the capsule attaches.
The bursa is a lubricating sac.

If areas of small asymmetry have been revealed during the treatment in Diagnosis 0, you may work on them again in Diagnosis 1. Place the device electrode on the area under investigation. Remain in skin contact without moving. Relative speed of the reaction t 8 c c[1] Initial 32 34* Reaction t = Timer C = coefficient of form of C1=ongoing coefficient Dose = Threshold of the reaction. The higher the **Initial Reaction**, the better that electrode position is to treat. By comparing readings from various areas, it is possible to choose the best places to dose for optimum effect. When an area is chosen to dose, the electrode is placed on the skin and a 'dose' is given. When the 'dose' is completed, the machine emits an audio signal and a '*' appears in the bottom right corner. The number in the bottom right is also recorded and can be compared to others for further treatment. If the SCENAR is placed on the skin and the sound of the multi-tone rings immediately, remove the SCENAR from the skin and place it back. Continue to do this until contact is established and treat this area. When the IR (left bottom corner) and Dose (bottom right corner) are the same in two areas, i.e. there is no difference between areas, choose the area for treatment with the lowest dynamic based on the form coefficient. **SCENAR therapy is a medical technology, which is directed towards activation of the body's own reserves**. The SCENAR influences the body in a non-invasive way via skin. The skin plays a very important role in regulating body systems, as it is the interface between the body and the environment. **The SCENAR influences, and is influenced by, the reaction of the skin**. The skin resistance varies with changes in the internal environment, which is a very finely balanced combination of chemicals of assorted nature. The SCENAR reacts to these skin changes and inputs an electrical signal similar to a natural neuron impulse. By continuously using biofeedback, the SCENAR modifies each successive input to either amplify or dampen the form of the pathological signals that exist in the body. Schema of how the SCENAR interface with the **Pathological signals**. So every impulse is actually different from the preceding input. The organism is unable to accommodate to the stimuli and the reaction to the impulses does not diminish, i.e., there is no process of habituation.

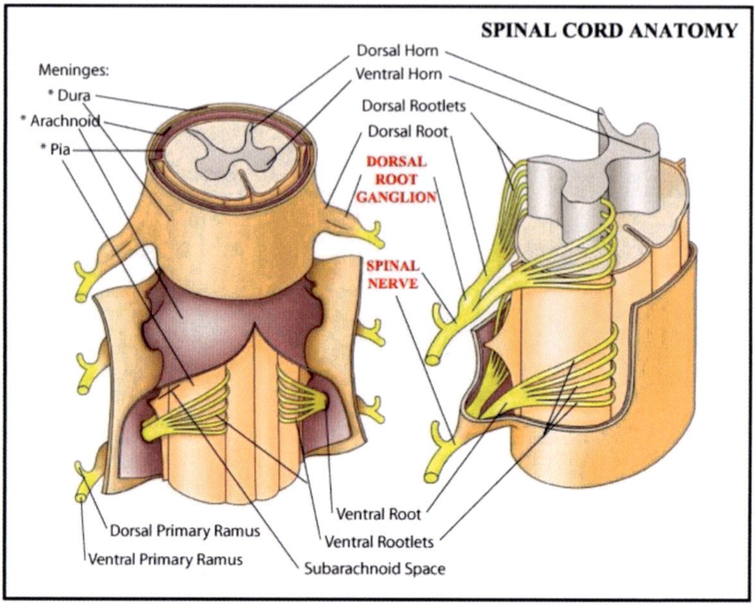
SPINAL CORD ANATOMY
Meninges:
* Dura
* Arachnoid
* Pia
Dorsal Horn
Ventral Horn
Dorsal Rootlets
Dorsal Root
DORSAL ROOT GANGLION
SPINAL NERVE
Dorsal Primary Ramus
Ventral Primary Ramus
Ventral Root
Ventral Rootlets
Subarachnoid Space

Current Complaints

Ask the patient to point with one finger (if possible) to what is the most pressing problem right now. (usually pain). Ask the patient to recall anything about the pain, e.g., character, severity, timing, radiation etc. Is there a movement which triggers or regenerates the pain?

If possible, make the patient elicit/demonstrate the pain. Where appropriate compare with the opposite side. Test any weaknesses.

SPINAL AND CRANIAL NERVES

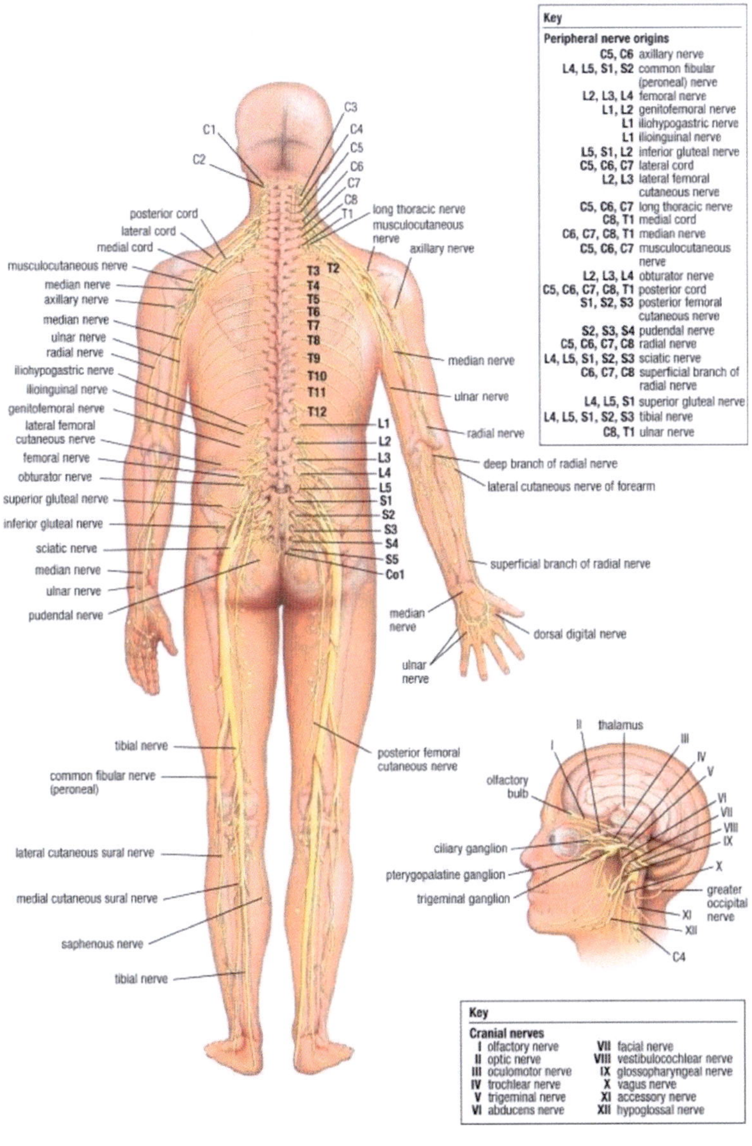
Key
Peripheral nerve origins
C5, C6 axillary nerve
L4, L5, S1, S2 common fibular (peroneal) nerve
L2, L3, L4 femoral nerve
L1, L2 genitofemoral nerve
L1 iliohypogastric nerve
L1 ilioinguinal nerve
L5, S1, L2 inferior gluteal nerve
C5, C6, C7 lateral cord
L2, L3 lateral femoral cutaneous nerve
C5, C6, C7 long thoracic nerve
C8, T1 medial cord
C6, C7, C8, T1 median nerve
C5, C6, C7 musculocutaneous nerve
L2, L3, L4 obturator nerve
C5, C6, C7, C8, T1 posterior cord
S1, S2, S3 posterior femoral cutaneous nerve
S2, S3, S4 pudendal nerve
C5, C6, C7, C8 radial nerve
L4, L5, S1, S2, S3 sciatic nerve
C6, C7, C8 superficial branch of radial nerve
L4, L5, S1 superior gluteal nerve
L4, L5, S1, S2, S3 tibial nerve
C8, T1 ulnar nerve
C1
C2
C3
C4
C5
C6
C7
C8
T1
T2
T3
T4
T5
T6
T7
T8
T9
T10
T11
T12
L1
L2
L3
L4
L5
S1
S2
S3
S4
S5
Co1
posterior cord
lateral cord
medial cord
musculocutaneous nerve
median nerve
axillary nerve
median nerve
ulnar nerve
radial nerve
iliohypogastric nerve
ilioinguinal nerve
genitofemoral nerve
lateral femoral cutaneous nerve
femoral nerve
obturator nerve
superior gluteal nerve
inferior gluteal nerve
sciatic nerve
median nerve
ulnar nerve
pudendal nerve
long thoracic nerve
musculocutaneous nerve
axillary nerve
median nerve
ulnar nerve
radial nerve
deep branch of radial nerve
lateral cutaneous nerve of forearm
superficial branch of radial nerve
median nerve
dorsal digital nerve
ulnar nerve
tibial nerve
common fibular nerve (peroneal)
posterior femoral cutaneous nerve
lateral cutaneous sural nerve
medial cutaneous sural nerve
saphenous nerve
tibial nerve
I
II
thalamus
III
IV
V
VI
VII
VIII
IX
X
XI
XII
C4
olfactory bulb
ciliary ganglion
pterygopalatine ganglion
trigeminal ganglion
greater occipital nerve
Key
Cranial nerves
I olfactory nerve
II optic nerve
III oculomotor nerve
IV trochlear nerve
V trigeminal nerve
VI abducens nerve
VII facial nerve
VIII vestibulocochlear nerve
IX glossopharyngeal nerve
X vagus nerve
XI accessory nerve
XII hypoglossal nerve

Move the device steadily (speed) and firmly (pressure) in one direction. Start treatment at any presenting primary signs. In the presence of active complaints (especially in combination with primary signs) start treating here.

Treat one site at a time, until any small asymmetry (or secondary sign) appears. When you have achieved an asymmetry, change the action regime (Freq, Mod, z, Dmpf, Intensity or any combination of these). Work, looking for a **small asymmetry**.

Then work on the area of small asymmetry, varying the direction of the electrode (4 directions), attempting to achieve a dynamic change (in the pain, in the color, in stickiness of the electrode, in the local sensation, in the sound from the device). Ideally work until the sign disappears or until an opposite sign appears. Finish the procedure when you have achieved a subjective improvement of the patient's condition.

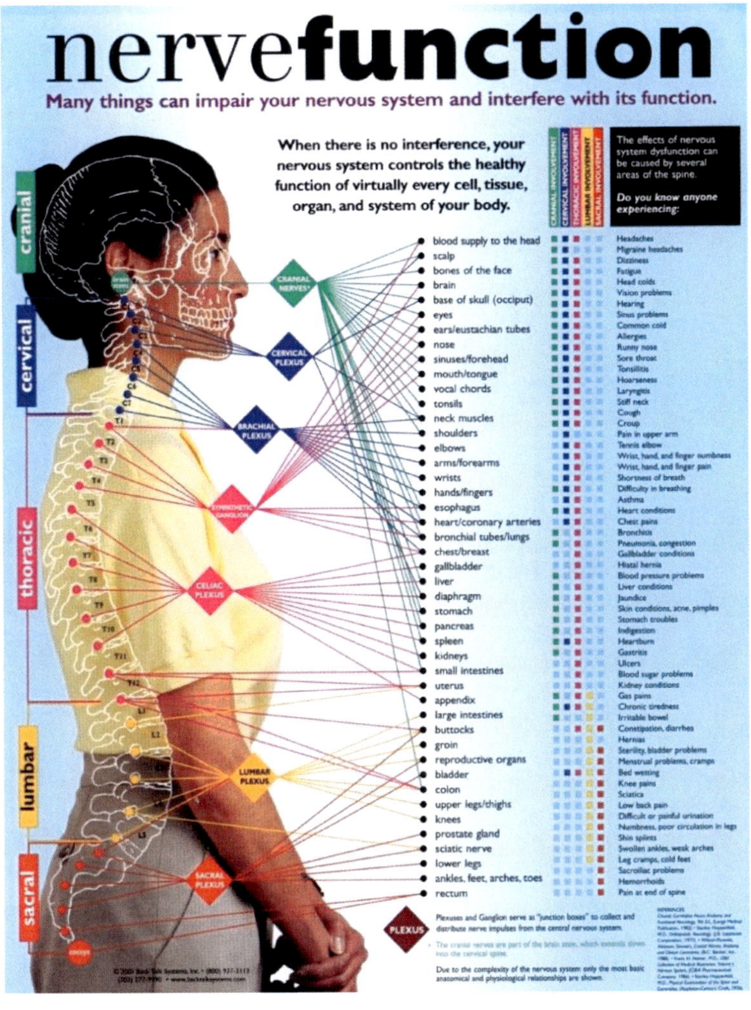

nervefunction
Many things can impair your nervous system and interfere with its function.
When there is no interference, your nervous system controls the healthy function of virtually every cell, tissue, organ, and system of your body.
CRANIAL INVOLVEMENT
CERVICAL INVOLVEMENT
THORACIC INVOLVEMENT
LUMBAR INVOLVEMENT
SACRAL INVOLVEMENT
The effects of nervous system dysfunction can be caused by several areas of the spine.
Do you know anyone experiencing:
cranial
cervical
thoracic
lumbar
sacral
CRANIAL NERVES*
CERVICAL PLEXUS
BRACHIAL PLEXUS
SYMPATHETIC GANGLION
CELIAC PLEXUS
LUMBAR PLEXUS
SACRAL PLEXUS
blood supply to the head
scalp
bones of the face
brain
base of skull (occiput)
eyes
ears/eustachian tubes
nose
sinuses/forehead
mouth/tongue
vocal chords
tonsils
neck muscles
shoulders
elbows
arms/forearms
wrists
hands/fingers
esophagus
heart/coronary arteries
bronchial tubes/lungs
chest/breast
gallbladder
liver
diaphragm
stomach
pancreas
spleen
kidneys
small intestines
uterus
appendix
large intestines
buttocks
groin
reproductive organs
bladder
colon
upper legs/thighs
knees
prostate gland
sciatic nerve
lower legs
ankles, feet, arches, toes
rectum
Headaches
Migraine headaches
Dizziness
Fatigue
Head colds
Vision problems
Hearing
Sinus problems
Common cold
Allergies
Runny nose
Sore throat
Tonsillitis
Hoarseness
Laryngitis
Stiff neck
Cough
Croup
Pain in upper arm
Tennis elbow
Wrist, hand, and finger numbness
Wrist, hand, and finger pain
Shortness of breath
Difficulty in breathing
Asthma
Heart conditions
Chest pains
Bronchitis
Pneumonia, congestion
Gallbladder conditions
Hiatal hernia
Blood pressure problems
Liver conditions
Jaundice
Skin conditions, acne, pimples
Stomach troubles
Indigestion
Heartburn
Gastritis
Ulcers
Blood sugar problems
Kidney conditions
Gas pains
Chronic tiredness
Irritable bowel
Constipation, diarrhea
Hernias
Sterility, bladder problems
Menstrual problems, cramps
Bed wetting
Knee pains
Sciatica
Low back pain
Difficult or painful urination
Numbness, poor circulation in legs
Shin splints
Swollen ankles, weak arches
Leg cramps, cold feet
Sacroiliac problems
Hemorrhoids
Pain at end of spine
PLEXUS
Plexuses and Ganglion serve as "junction boxes" to collect and distribute nerve impulses from the central nervous system.
Due to the complexity of the nervous system only the most basic anatomical and physiological relationships are shown.

When there are no more reactions or there is an insignificant subjective effect:

Change the action regime and extend the area of action along a horizontal line or along a segment.

Include the general action area (3 paths).

Continue to reveal areas of small asymmetry and secondary signs.

Chapter 5. Priority Areas for Treatment

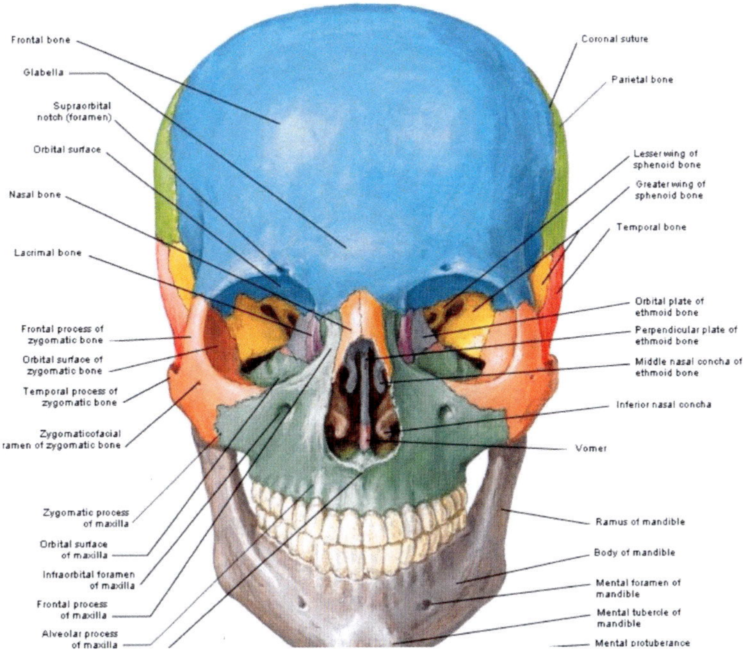

Frontal bone
Glabella
Supraorbital notch (foramen)
Orbital surface
Nasal bone
Lacrimal bone
Frontal process of zygomatic bone
Orbital surface of zygomatic bone
Temporal process of zygomatic bone
Zygomaticofacial ramen of zygomatic bone
Zygomatic process of maxilla
Orbital surface of maxilla
Infraorbital foramen of maxilla
Frontal process of maxilla
Alveolar process of maxilla
Coronal suture
Parietal bone
Lesser wing of sphenoid bone
Greater wing of sphenoid bone
Temporal bone
Orbital plate of ethmoid bone
Perpendicular plate of ethmoid bone
Middle nasal concha of ethmoid bone
Inferior nasal concha
Vomer
Ramus of mandible
Body of mandible
Mental foramen of mandible
Mental tubercle of mandible
Mental protuberance

Direct Projection of the Pain.

Primary signs as described in the "Treatment Reaction Indicators" above:

- **Asymmetry**
- **Small Asymmetry**
- **Horizontals**
- **General Zones**
- **Symmetrical Areas**

- **Reciprocal areas**
- **Gloves and Socks** – back and front of hands and wrists and top and bottom of feet and ankles as well as Auricular points. (see charts below)

The channel or meridian relevant to the current symptoms

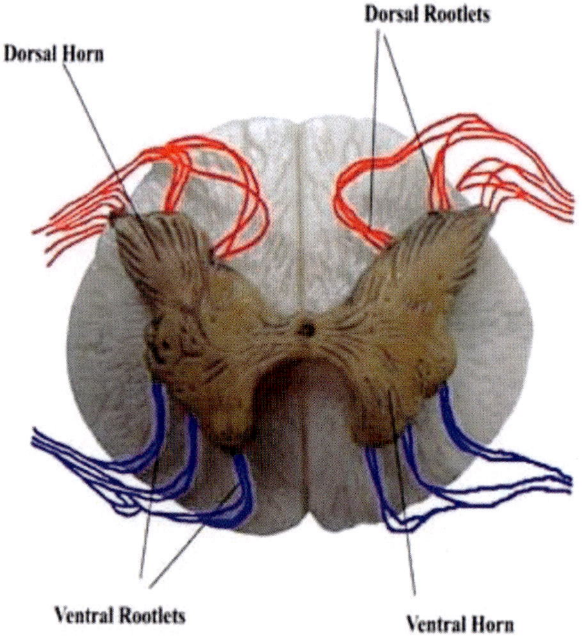

Dorsal Rootlets
Dorsal Horn
Ventral Rootlets
Ventral Horn

Set the electrode on a patient's skin for several seconds, well away from the intended treatment area, to make sure that there are no unpleasant sensations. When contact with the patient's skin is detected by the device the short sound signal will beep (only in DIAGN modes), the NOBODY sign changes to ++++++, in the up-left screen corner the stopwatch resets and begins to count the stimulating duration. The stopwatch operates either automatically (starts at the beginning of every new skin contact detection and stops on the skin contact loss) or manually.

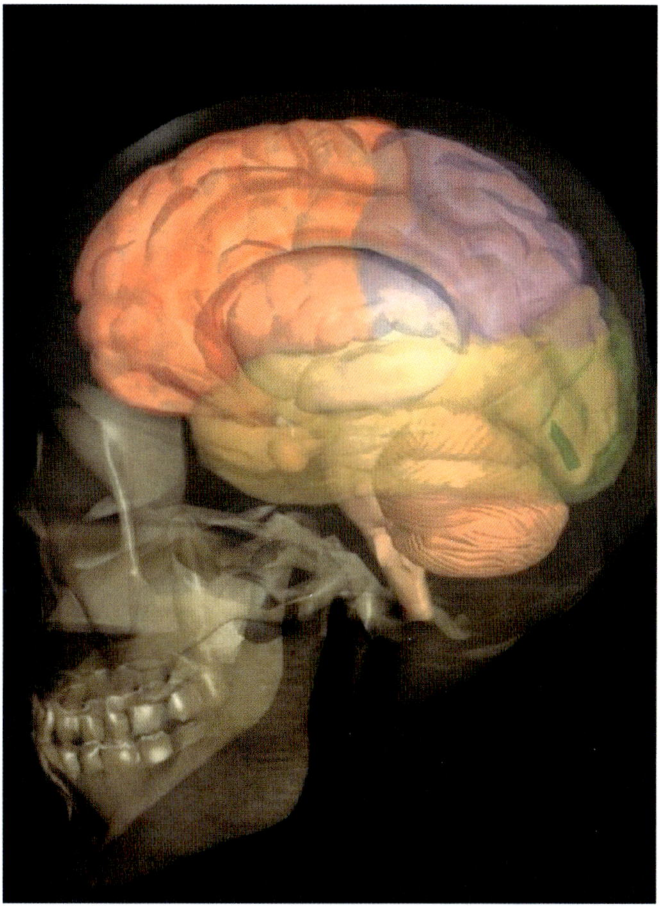

Press and keep pressing button (+) up to the client's first sensations such as gentle prickling or vibration. Do not allow uncomfortable or painful sensations to occur by hurrying.

Scenar Effects

Anti-inflammatory effect

A leucocyte cuff surrounds an inflammatory focus in order to prevent the inflammation from spreading to the surrounding tissues. Eventually this cuff will be in the way of reorganization and recovery, as new leucocytes cannot reach the focus of inflammation. The action of the SCENAR reduces the cuff and speeds recovery. In acute situations, maximum benefit is obtained if treatment is given every two hours.

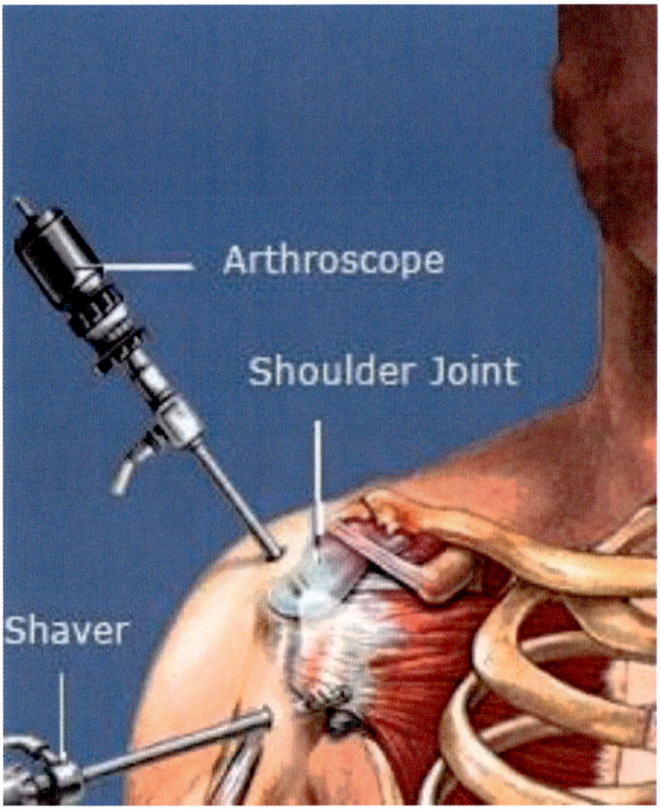
Arthroscope
Shoulder Joint
Shaver

The anti-inflammatory effect is realized through improved microcirculation.

Anti-edema effect

Helps reduce swelling by redistributing the fluid between the lymphatic and vascular systems. Again, in acute situations, treat twice hourly for maximum effect.

Hemostatic effect

Blood is routed through a collateral blood supply leading to a reduction of pressure in the main vessel which allows bleeding to stop. Bleeding may increase before it stops as treatment will initiate an increased circulation to the area to facilitate healing.

Anti-shock/Anti-allergic effect

Localized or general reactions can be observed with food allergy, drug reactions and insect bites, and may manifest as urticarial rashes, edema (including that of the larynx), rhinitis, bronchospasm and so on. These symptoms are treated as they occur according to the first rule of SCENAR.

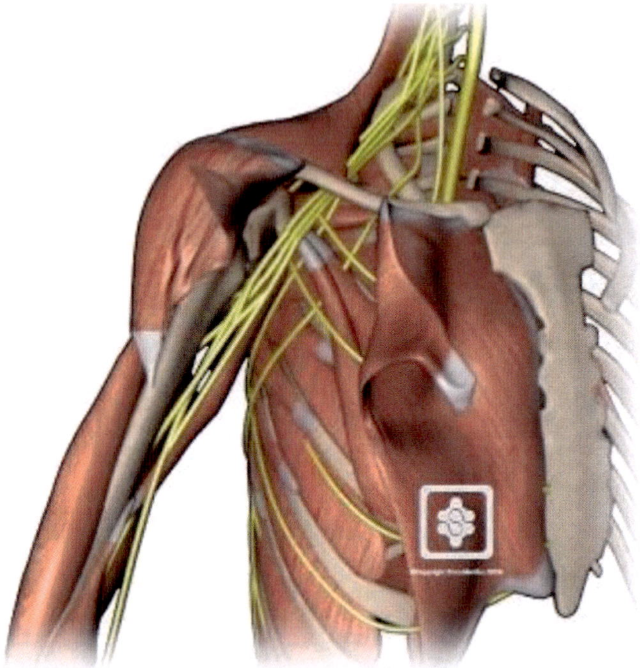

Antipyretic effect

Lowering of high temperatures can be obtained by treating the main blood vessels of the neck. It's best to treat only very high temperatures, as slight pyrexia is usually a normal adaptive reaction.

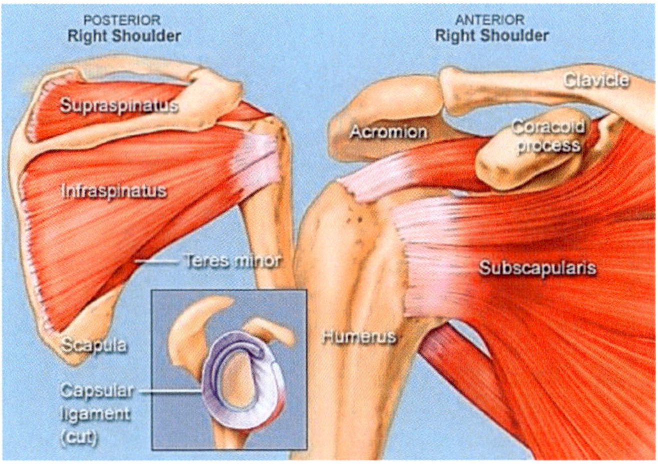
POSTERIOR
Right Shoulder
ANTERIOR
Right Shoulder
Clavicle
Supraspinatus
Acromion
Coracoid process
Infraspinatus
Teres minor
Subscapularis
Humerus
Scapula
Capsular ligament (cut)

Normalization of metabolic processes:

SCENAR therapy increases the metabolic rate, increases venous flow and improves the removal of the by-products of metabolism. Lymphatic flow will increase as well. Stimulating consumption of oxygen and nutrients increases solute levels in the blood.

SCENAR treatment triggers the release of neuropeptides. These are further metabolized to produce a cascade of new bioactive compounds. Some of the Neuropeptides and by-products have a regulative role in cellular function; i.e. they help correct and balance the relationship between the biochemical and functional systems in cells and tissues. These **regulative peptides** often function within more than one tissue, which explains distant effects from the site being treated. This results in normalization of cell, tissue and system functions.

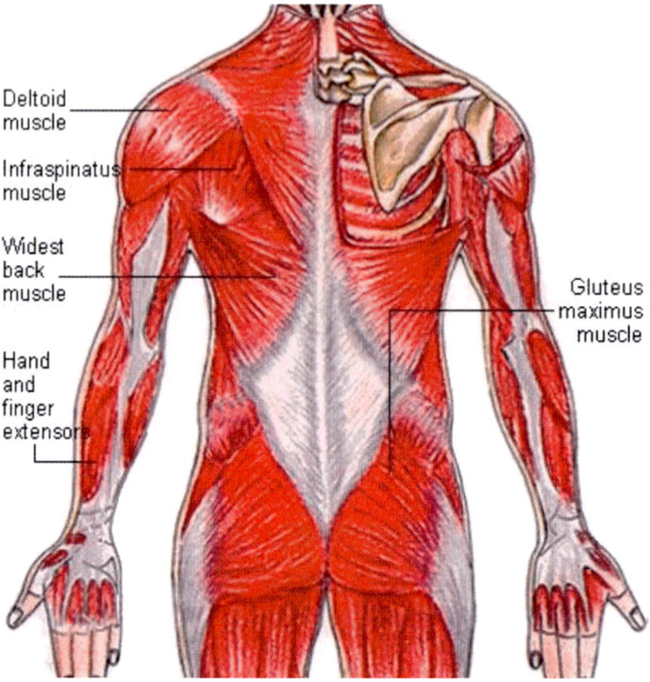
Deltoid muscle
Infraspinatus muscle
Widest back muscle
Hand and finger extensors
Gluteus maximus muscle

Faster wound healing

This is due to faster regeneration of tissues as a result of the above processes.

General effects

- Normal sleep patterns
- Better appetite
- Improved sense of well-being due to higher levels of energy

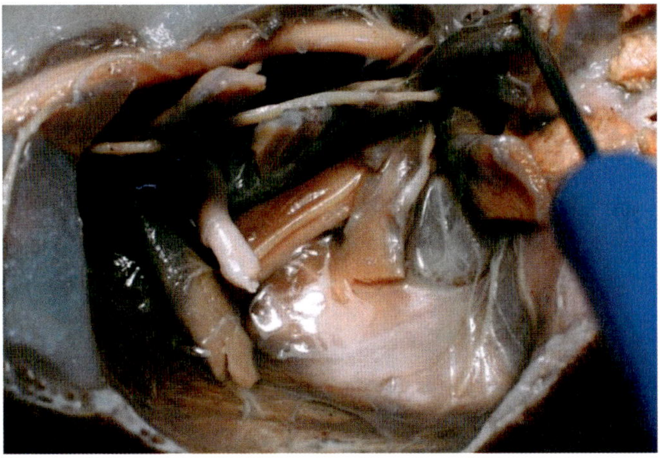

Pain Killing Effects

- Blocks transmission of the pain impulses due to refraction in the nerve endings of the peripheral nerve fibers.
- Establishes a new dominant center in the cortex of the brain, which suppresses the pain focus.
- Considerably reduces edema around the nerve fibers hence reducing pressure effects and helping to alleviate pain

The Brachial Plexus

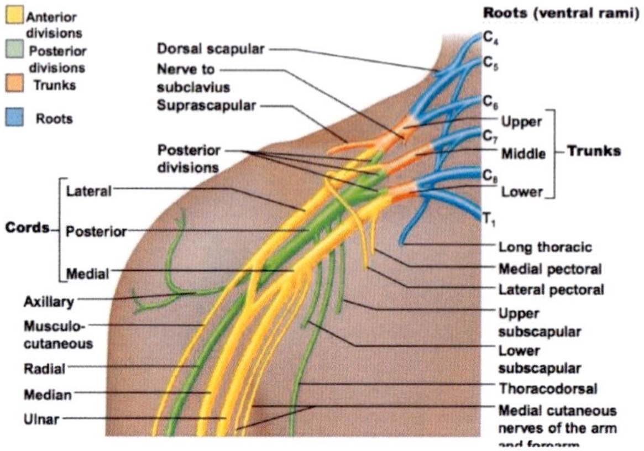

Anterior divisions
Posterior divisions
Trunks
Roots
Roots (ventral rami)
C_4
C_5
C_6
C_7
C_8
T_1
Dorsal scapular
Nerve to subclavius
Suprascapular
Posterior divisions
Upper
Middle
Lower
Trunks
Cords
Lateral
Posterior
Medial
Axillary
Musculo-cutaneous
Radial
Median
Ulnar
Long thoracic
Medial pectoral
Lateral pectoral
Upper subscapular
Lower subscapular
Thoracodorsal
Medial cutaneous nerves of the arm

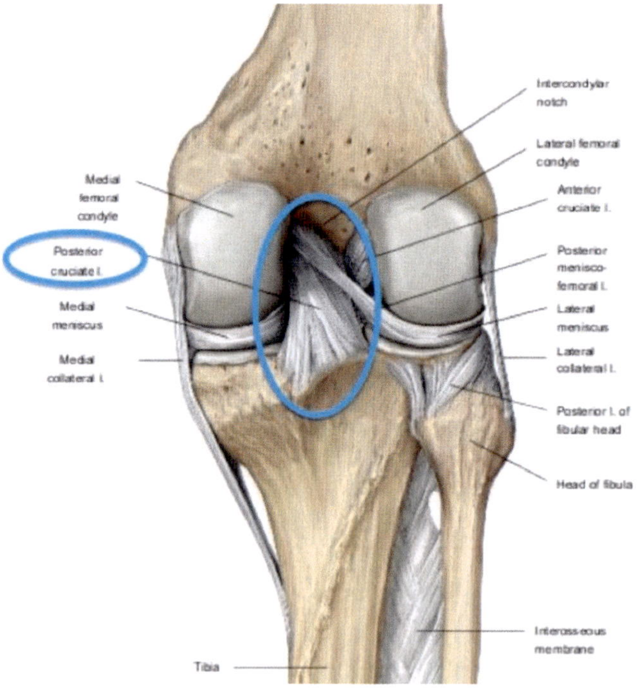

Intercondylar notch
Lateral femoral condyle
Medial femoral condyle
Anterior cruciate l.
Posterior cruciate l.
Posterior menisco-femoral l.
Medial meniscus
Lateral meniscus
Medial collateral l.
Lateral collateral l.
Posterior l. of fibular head
Head of fibula
Interosseous membrane
Tibia

Anti-allergic effect

The anti-allergic effect is achieved by intensified production of corticosteroid hormones and biologically active substances.

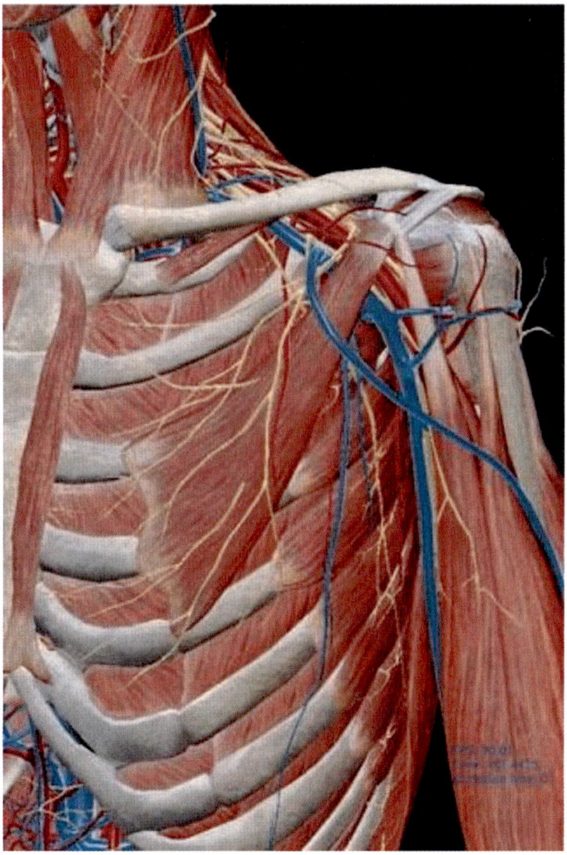

Dehydration effect

This effect helps fluids come out of the organism.

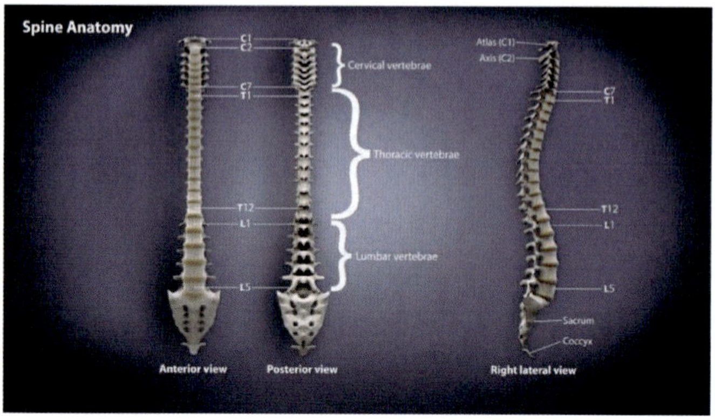
Spine Anatomy
C1
C2
C7
T1
Cervical vertebrae
Thoracic vertebrae
T12
L1
Lumbar vertebrae
L5
Atlas (C1)
Axis (C2)
C7
T1
T12
L1
L5
Sacrum
Coccyx
Anterior view
Posterior view
Right lateral view

Immunoregulating effect

This occurs due to stimulation of the immune system. If patient has a low immunity, SCENAR application helps increase it. But if there is an autoimmune process in the organism, then the SCENAR application helps reduce the immune response.

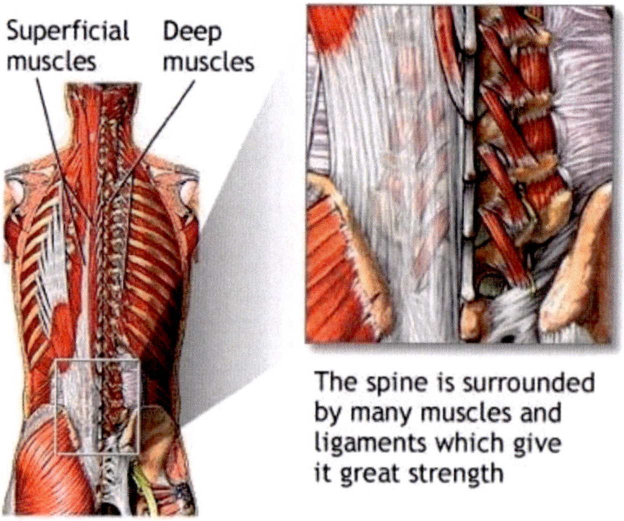
Superficial muscles
Deep muscles

The spine is surrounded by many muscles and ligaments which give it great strength

Vascular effect

Normalizes vascular tone, improves hemodynamics, and activates microcirculation due to elimination of spasm in vessels.

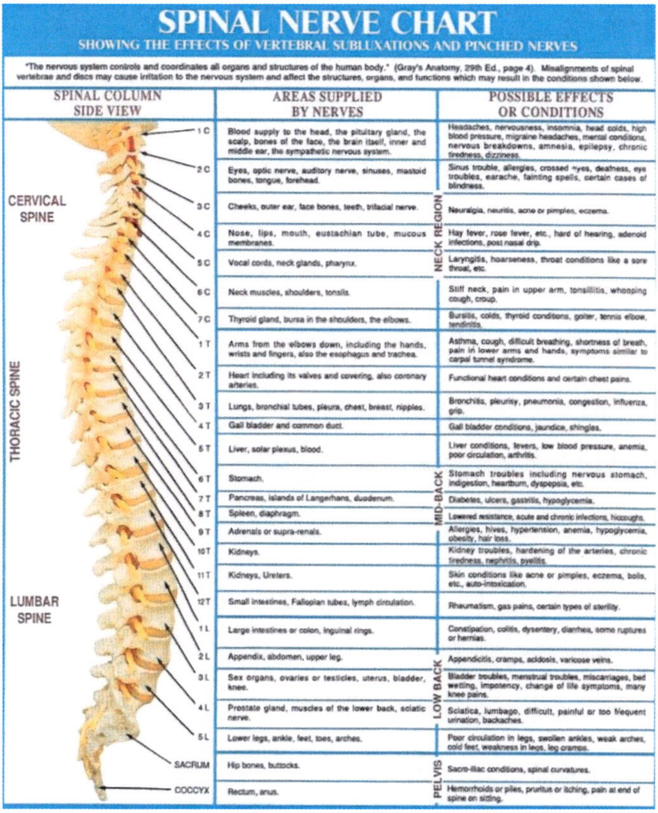
CERVICAL SPINE
THORACIC SPINE
LUMBAR SPINE
NECK REGION
MID-BACK
LOW BACK
PELVIS

SPINAL NERVE CHART

SHOWING THE EFFECTS OF VERTEBRAL SUBLUXATIONS AND PINCHED NERVES

"The nervous system controls and coordinates all organs and structures of the human body." (Gray's Anatomy, 29th Ed., page 4). Misalignments of spinal vertebrae and discs may cause irritation to the nervous system and affect the structures, organs, and functions which may result in the conditions shown below.

SPINAL COLUMN SIDE VIEW	AREAS SUPPLIED BY NERVES	POSSIBLE EFFECTS OR CONDITIONS
1 C	Blood supply to the head, the pituitary gland, the scalp, bones of the face, the brain itself, inner and middle ear, the sympathetic nervous system.	Headaches, nervousness, insomnia, head colds, high blood pressure, migraine headaches, mental conditions, nervous breakdowns, amnesia, epilepsy, chronic tiredness, dizziness.
2 C	Eyes, optic nerve, auditory nerve, sinuses, mastoid bones, tongue, forehead.	Sinus trouble, allergies, crossed eyes, deafness, eye troubles, earache, fainting spells, certain cases of blindness.
3 C	Cheeks, outer ear, face bones, teeth, trifacial nerve.	Neuralgia, neuritis, acne or pimples, eczema.
4 C	Nose, lips, mouth, eustachian tube, mucous membranes.	Hay fever, rose fever, etc., hard of hearing, adenoid infections, post nasal drip.
5 C	Vocal cords, neck glands, pharynx.	Laryngitis, hoarseness, throat conditions like a sore throat, etc.
6 C	Neck muscles, shoulders, tonsils.	Stiff neck, pain in upper arm, tonsillitis, whooping cough, croup.
7 C	Thyroid gland, bursa in the shoulders, the elbows.	Bursitis, colds, thyroid conditions, goiter, tennis elbow, tendinitis.
1 T	Arms from the elbows down, including the hands, wrists and fingers, also the esophagus and trachea.	Asthma, cough, difficult breathing, shortness of breath, pain in lower arms and hands, symptoms similar to carpal tunnel syndrome.
2 T	Heart including its valves and covering, also coronary arteries.	Functional heart conditions and certain chest pains.
3 T	Lungs, bronchial tubes, pleura, chest, breast, nipples.	Bronchitis, pleurisy, pneumonia, congestion, influenza, grip.
4 T	Gall bladder and common duct.	Gall bladder conditions, jaundice, shingles.
5 T	Liver, solar plexus, blood.	Liver conditions, fevers, low blood pressure, anemia, poor circulation, arthritis.
6 T	Stomach.	Stomach troubles including nervous stomach, indigestion, heartburn, dyspepsia, etc.
7 T	Pancreas, islands of Langerhans, duodenum.	Diabetes, ulcers, gastritis, hypoglycemia.
8 T	Spleen, diaphragm.	Lowered resistance, acute and chronic infections, hiccoughs.
9 T	Adrenals or supra-renals.	Allergies, hives, hypertension, anemia, hypoglycemia, obesity, hair loss.
10 T	Kidneys.	Kidney troubles, hardening of the arteries, chronic tiredness, nephritis, pyelitis.
11 T	Kidneys, Ureters.	Skin conditions like acne or pimples, eczema, boils, etc., auto-intoxication.
12 T	Small intestines, Fallopian tubes, lymph circulation.	Rheumatism, gas pains, certain types of sterility.
1 L	Large intestines or colon, inguinal rings.	Constipation, colitis, dysentery, diarrhea, some ruptures or hernias.
2 L	Appendix, abdomen, upper leg.	Appendicitis, cramps, acidosis, varicose veins.
3 L	Sex organs, ovaries or testicles, uterus, bladder, knee.	Bladder troubles, menstrual troubles, miscarriages, bed wetting, impotency, change of life symptoms, many knee pains.
4 L	Prostate gland, muscles of the lower back, sciatic nerve.	Sciatica, lumbago, difficult, painful or too frequent urination, backaches.
5 L	Lower legs, ankle, feet, toes, arches.	Poor circulation in legs, swollen ankles, weak arches, cold feet, weakness in legs, leg cramps.
SACRUM	Hip bones, buttocks.	Sacro-iliac conditions, spinal curvatures.
COCCYX	Rectum, anus.	Hemorrhoids or piles, pruritus or itching, pain at end of spine on sitting.

Hemostatic effect

This occurs due to activated collateral blood supply and relieved stress in the arterial vessel.

Spinal Cord in Situ

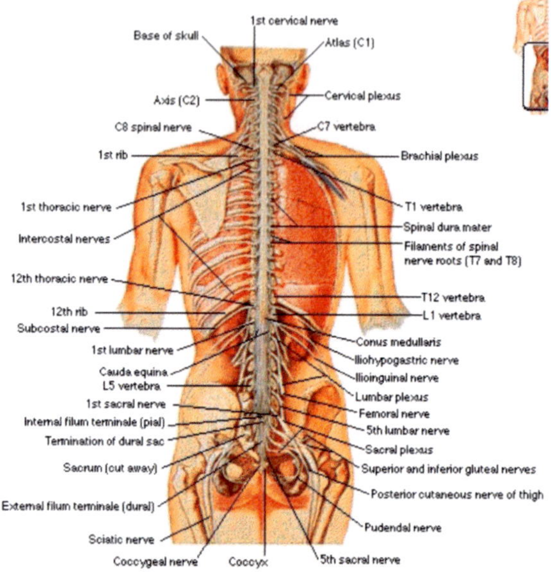
1st cervical nerve
Base of skull
Atlas (C1)
Axis (C2)
Cervical plexus
C8 spinal nerve
C7 vertebra
1st rib
Brachial plexus
1st thoracic nerve
T1 vertebra
Intercostal nerves
Spinal dura mater
Filaments of spinal nerve roots (T7 and T8)
12th thoracic nerve
T12 vertebra
12th rib
L1 vertebra
Subcostal nerve
Conus medullaris
1st lumbar nerve
Iliohypogastric nerve
Cauda equina
Ilioinguinal nerve
L5 vertebra
Lumbar plexus
1st sacral nerve
Femoral nerve
Internal filum terminale (pial)
5th lumbar nerve
Termination of dural sac
Sacral plexus
Sacrum (cut away)
Superior and inferior gluteal nerves
Posterior cutaneous nerve of thigh
External filum terminale (dural)
Pudendal nerve
Sciatic nerve
Coccygeal nerve
Coccyx
5th sacral nerve

Improved collateral blood circulation effect

This occurs involuntarily due to direct electrical current application to the sensitive and vegetative nerve fibers.

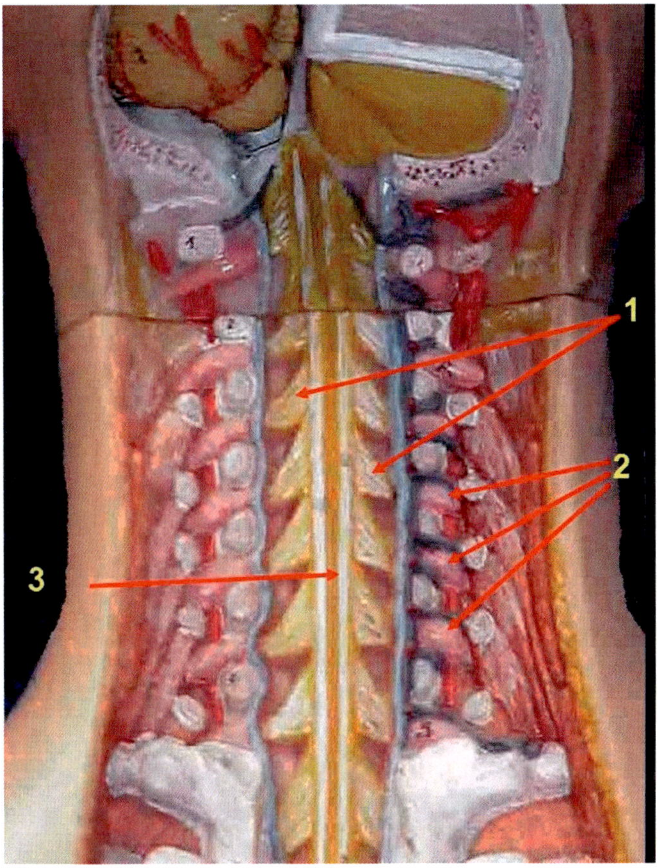
1
2
3

Normalized metabolic (albuminous, fatty, carbohydrate, mineral) effect to be due to improved functions of the kidneys, skin, sweat glands, lungs, liver, internal secretion glands and central nervous system.

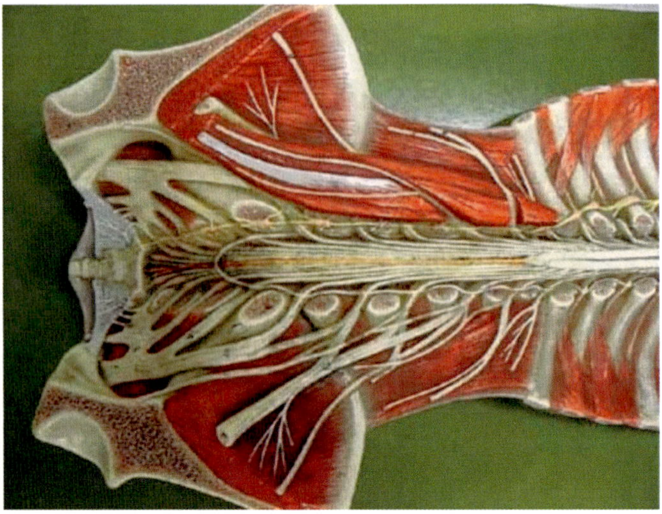

Anti-shock effect

This effect becomes apparent under any form of shock: traumatic, pain, anaphylactic, etc.

Chapter 6.
Aims in Scenar Therapy

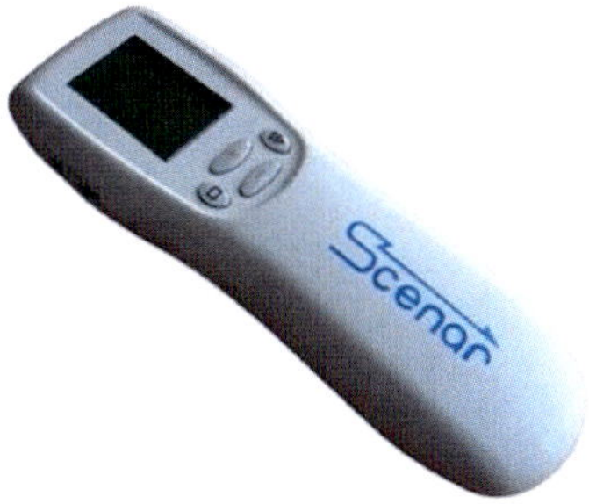
Scenar

Relieve pain

Stimulate the system's energy and boost the immune system.

Balance homeostasis.

Eradicate repetitive Central Nervous System patterns.

Assessment of the patient's complaints.

Analysis of the patient history.

Assessment of previous treatments.

Assessment of compatibility of other therapies with SCENAR therapy.

Development of the plan of action, combination of zones and regime for action.

Assessment of the prognosis of the case.

Search for Primary signs.

Analysis of the presenting complaints of the patient and treatment based on teaching their neurology how to function differently.

Search for any asymmetry work on it search for on the small asymmetry with consequent treatment. This gives the most efficient action, i.e., maximum effect in minimum time.

Observation and search and treatment any for Secondary Factor.

Initial Reaction analysis to enable decisions to be made about the regime for action.

Individual dosing during the procedure, progressing to "0" and treating on FmVar.

Stabilization of the patient's condition when necessary.

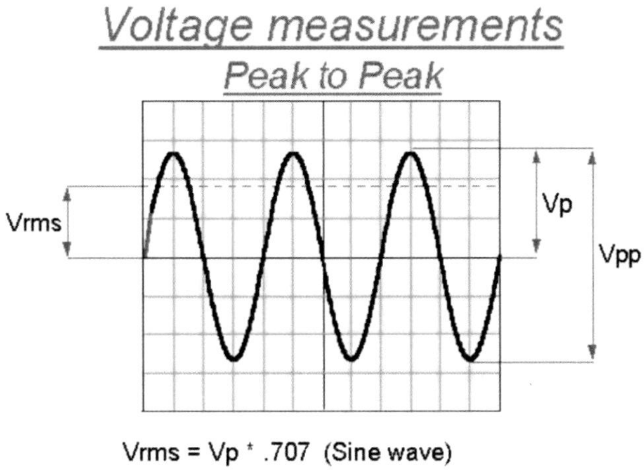
Voltage measurements
Peak to Peak
Vrms
Vp
Vpp
Vrms = Vp * .707 (Sine wave)

Always look for dynamic changes: at examination, in complaints, in sensations, skin condition and between treatments. Any change, even a worsening, is regarded as dynamic and useful.

Measuring DC Voltage

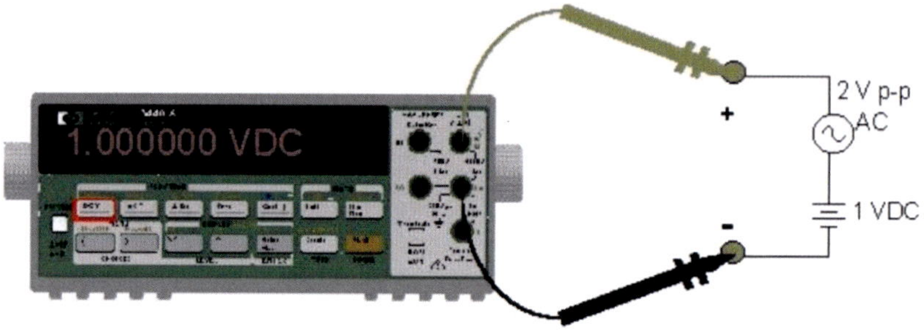
1.000000 VDC
+
-
2 V p-p
AC
1 VDC

* Note measurement indicates only DC portion of signal

Reflexogenic zones, i.e. the body regions with a certain reflex caused by adequate receptors stimulation. Reflexogenic zones take an active part in the regulation of the body's vital functions and allow to use various effects on them for treatment purposes. **Projection zones, i.e. the zones projected by internal organs, blood and lymphatic vessels, nerves and nerve plexuses**. Anatomic regions receive their names depending on their disposition on the human body, and there are a lot of them. Special attention should be paid to the distal parts of extremities taking into account their abundant neurotropic innervation as well as the fact that the majority of meridians (energy channels) are originating and ending over there. **Reflexogenic zones** are located along the major nerve trunks, at the nerve-muscle joints, along the cranial satures, over the sensitive tendon areas (there are acupuncture points over there), over the projection of major lymphatic and blood vessels.

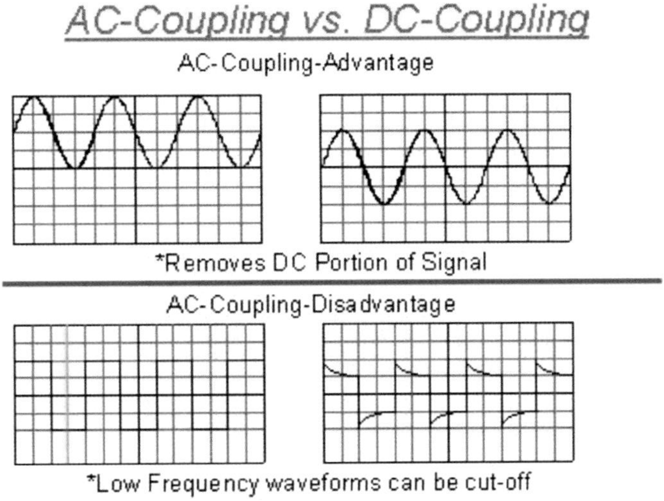
AC-Coupling vs. DC-Coupling
AC-Coupling-Advantage
*Removes DC Portion of Signal
AC-Coupling-Disadvantage
*Low Frequency waveforms can be cut-off

Reciprocal treatment, i.e. treatment of the symmetric area.

Analysis of cyclic changes in the pathological system.

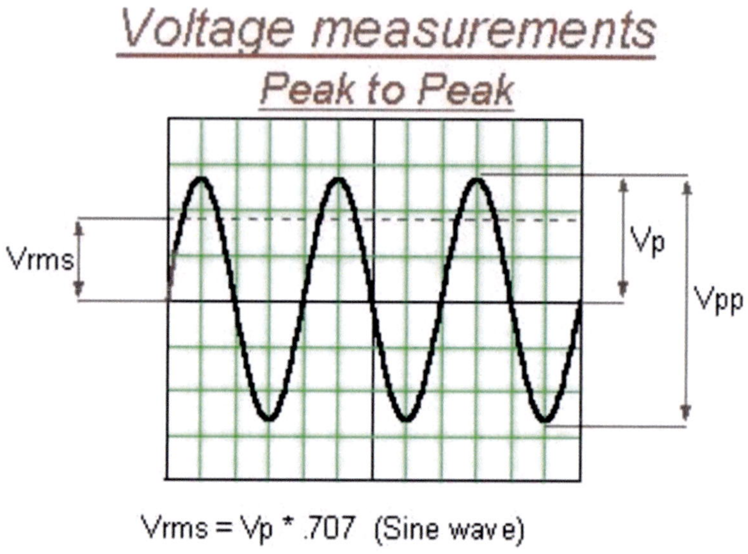
Voltage measurements
Peak to Peak
Vrms
Vp
Vpp
Vrms = Vp * .707 (Sine wave)

You can analyze them on patient's complaints and device treatment modes. Certain dynamic changes indicate the recovery process is under way. Let's, for instance, take coughing because of bronchi disorders. Initially, there was no cough, then it became dry, and moist the next day, then the phlegm began discharging, and then cough and phlegm considerably decreased and completely disappeared, i.e. the whole cycle is observed: from 0 to 0. It is this cyclic change that must always be analyzed by the SCENAR user.

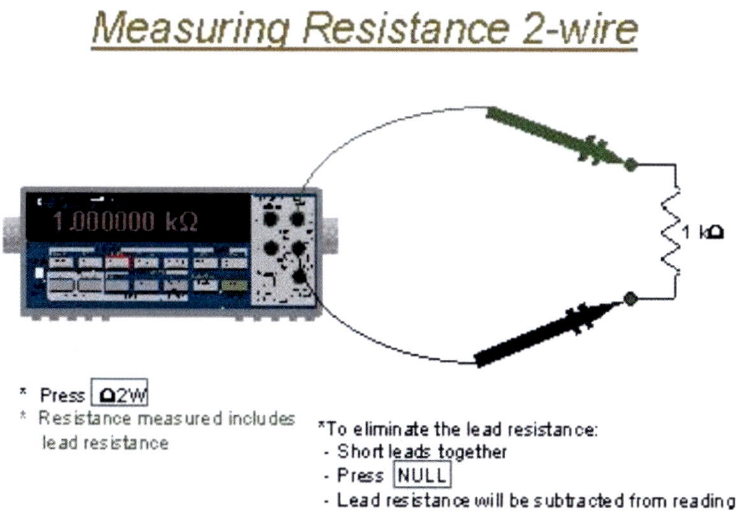
Measuring Resistance 2-wire
1 kΩ
* Press Ω2W
* Resistance measured includes lead resistance
*To eliminate the lead resistance:
- Short leads together
- Press NULL
- Lead resistance will be subtracted from reading

Analysis of dynamic changes in patient's complaints, sensations and skin. SCENAR-user should notice, analyze and use these changes to stabilize patient's condition.

Optimal and efficient treatment.

Optimal and efficient treatment means a search for the optimal treatment zone to gain the best possible healing effect, i.e. revealing of the diagnostic symptoms.

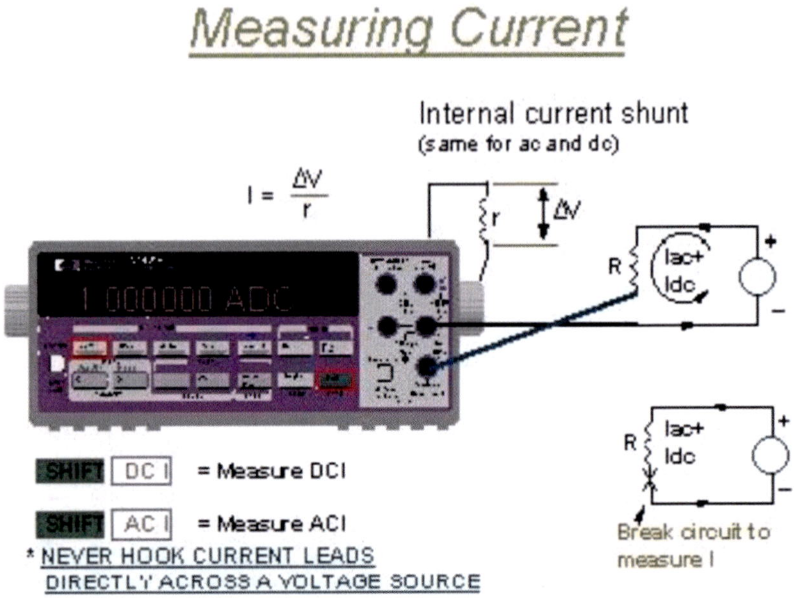
Measuring Current
Internal current shunt
(same for ac and dc)
I = ΔV / r
r
ΔV
1 000000 ADC
R
Iac+
Idc
+
–
R
Iac+
Idc
+
–
Break circuit to
measure I
SHIFT DC I = Measure DCI
SHIFT AC I = Measure ACI
* NEVER HOOK CURRENT LEADS
DIRECTLY ACROSS A VOLTAGE SOURCE

Repetition factor

Procedure repetition factor depends on patient's disease condition. Acute disease conditions and first aid patients are treated according to the following principle: **the more acute (dangerous) is the disease condition, the more significant should be the treatment dose, and more lengthy and frequent treatment sessions. Every-two-hour sessions are possible to help patient out of this condition.** If the disease condition has a positive dynamic change, the intervals between sessions may be increased up to 6-7 hours or completely stopped. Repeat diagnostics and sessions in about 8 to 10 hours.

INFRASPINATUS

YOUR TWO INFRASPINATUS muscles are found in your shoulders. They help to stabilize the shoulder joints, and turn the arms away from the body. Each infraspinatus muscle is attached at one end to the shoulder blade, and at the other to the upper arm bone.

Chronic and sluggish disorders are usually treated once a day or every other day, but even every two days or once a week treatment is possible. Try to treat patients at the same hour and situation for the entire course. Paroxysm-type disorders are treated by relieving each case of paroxysm and by conducting prophylactic therapy courses planned in between paroxysms. It is recommended to conduct 3-4 therapy courses a year, each one consisting of 7-15 sessions. If you are able to determine the paroxysm recurrence rate, it is advisable to conduct prophylactic therapy courses 10 – 14 days prior to paroxysm.

Interconnecting Neurons

INTERCONNECTING neurons, or interneurons, make up 99 percent of the nerve cells in your body. They are found in the central nervous system.

Interconnecting neurons form the link between motor neurons and sensory neurons; receiving, processing, and relaying messages around your body.

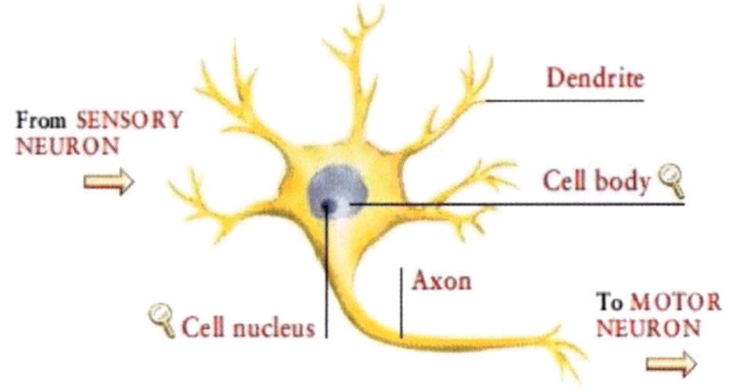

Dendrite
From SENSORY NEURON
Cell body
Axon
Cell nucleus
To MOTOR NEURON

SCENAR affects selectively, i.e. only on pathological systems (organs and tissues), and does not affect healthy ones. SCENAR features are as follows:

Try to initiate therapy when there is an active complaint from patient.

SCENAR quickly restores functional disorders in the body. Organic disorders take more time to treat.

Repeat **SCENAR** course if there are new complaints from patient. For instance, patient took treatment course for hypertension, and later on he caught cold and began coughing. In this case, treatment for his new complaints must be repeated. Due to no adaptation to treatment, there is no need to continuously increase power level during each SCENAR session.

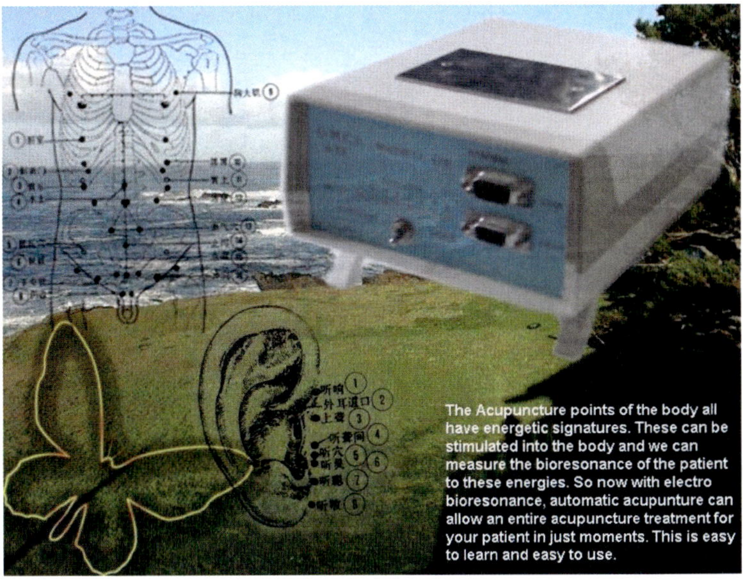
The Acupuncture points of the body all have energetic signatures. These can be stimulated into the body and we can measure the bioresonance of the patient to these energies. So now with electro bioresonance, automatic acupunture can allow an entire acupuncture treatment for your patient in just moments. This is easy to learn and easy to use.

Relieve pain

- Stimulate the system's energy and boost the immune system
- Balance homeostasis
- Eradicate repetitive Central Nervous System patterns
- Assessment of the patients complains
- Analysis of the patient history
- Assessment of previous treatments.
- Assessment of compatibility of other therapies with SCENAR therapy.
- Development of the plan of action, combination of zones and regime for action.

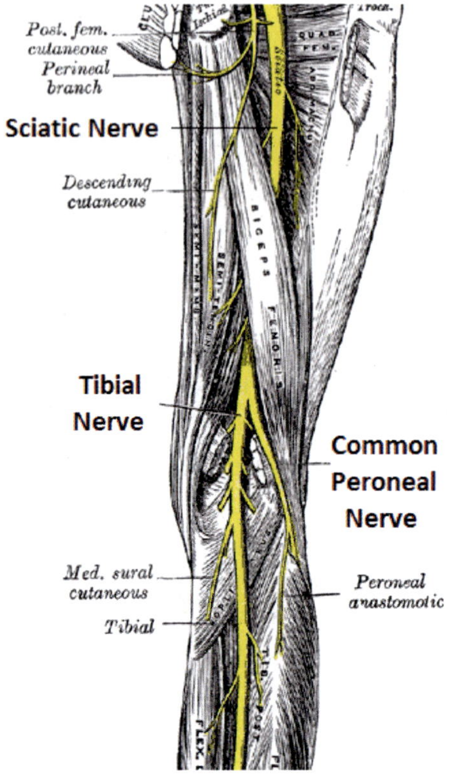
Post. fem. cutaneous
Perineal branch
Sciatic Nerve
Descending cutaneous
BICEPS
Tibial Nerve
Common Peroneal Nerve
Med. sural cutaneous
Peroneal anastomotic
Tibial

Search for Primary Signs

Analysis of the presenting complaints of the patient, and treatment based on teaching their neurology how to function differently.

Search for any asymmetry; work on it - search for the small asymmetry with consequent treatment.

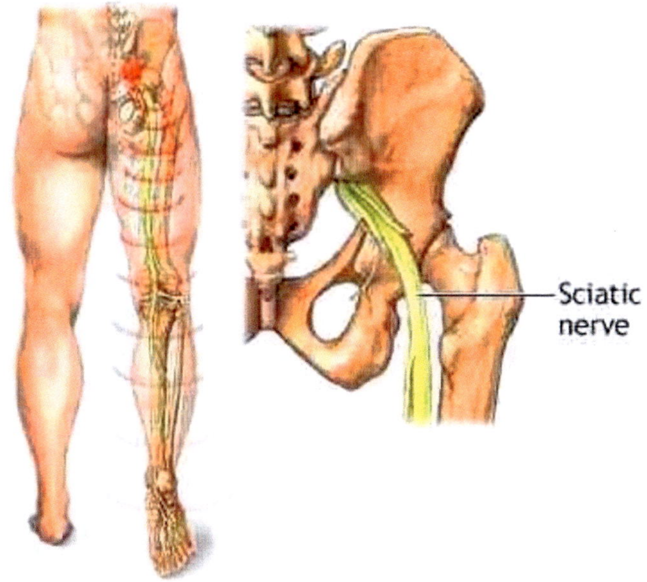
Sciatic
nerve

This gives the most efficient action, i.e., maximum effect in minimum time.

Observation and search and treatment any for Secondary Factors.

Initial Reaction analysis to enable decisions to be made about the regime for action.

Individual dosing during the procedure, progressing to “0” and treating on FmVar.

Stabilization of the patient’s condition when necessary.

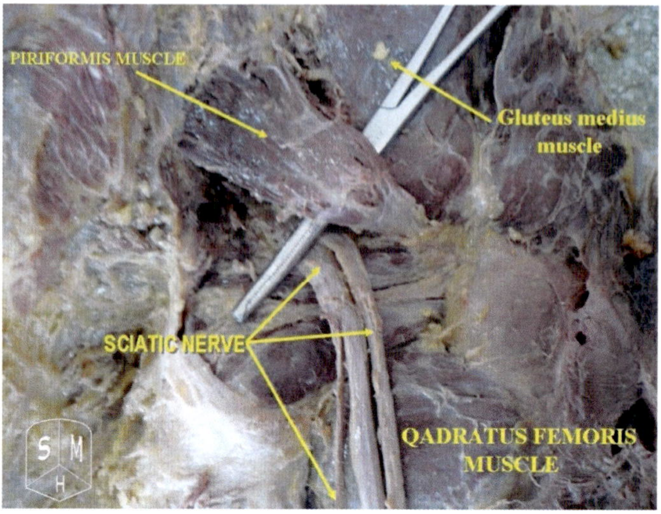
PIRIFORMIS MUSCLE
Gluteus medius muscle
SCIATIC NERVE
QADRATUS FEMORIS MUSCLE

The SCENAR devices can produce the following power levels:

Comfortable power level, i.e., the power level which does not cause any unpleasant irritative sensations (pain, sharp “tingling”, burning, etc.) in patient.

High (increased) power level, i.e., the power level which causes some unpleasant irritative sensations (slight pain, “pricking”, burning, etc.) in patient. The device application should not cause patient's unbearable sensations. If, nevertheless, the application of high power level is required, it is necessary to determine the patient's individual sensitivity (threshold) on the skin area to be treated, first, and start applying the device only after that step.

Stimulate the system's energy and boost the immune system

Salivary Glands
Dissection

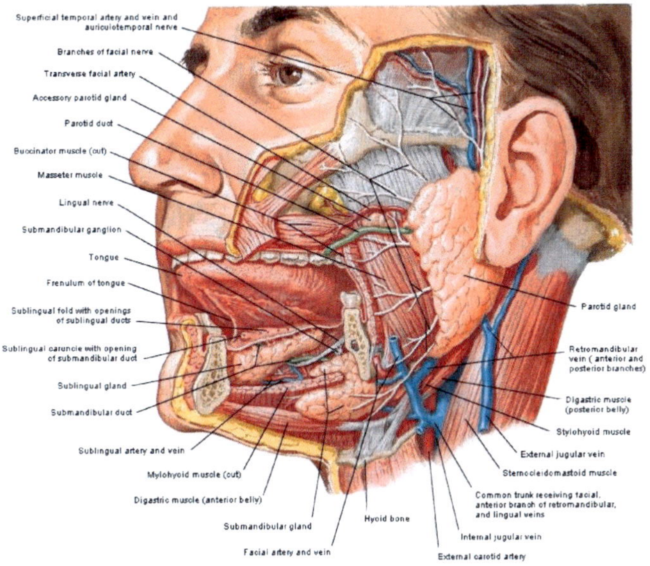
Superficial temporal artery and vein and auriculotemporal nerve
Branches of facial nerve
Transverse facial artery
Accessory parotid gland
Parotid duct
Buccinator muscle (cut)
Masseter muscle
Lingual nerve
Submandibular ganglion
Tongue
Frenulum of tongue
Sublingual fold with openings of sublingual ducts
Sublingual caruncle with opening of submandibular duct
Sublingual gland
Submandibular duct
Sublingual artery and vein
Mylohyoid muscle (cut)
Digastric muscle (anterior belly)
Submandibular gland
Facial artery and vein
Hyoid bone
Parotid gland
Retromandibular vein (anterior and posterior branches)
Digastric muscle (posterior belly)
Stylohyoid muscle
External jugular vein
Sternocleidomastoid muscle
Common trunk receiving facial, anterior branch of retromandibular, and lingual veins
Internal jugular vein
External carotid artery

Balance homeostasis

Eradicate repetitive Central Nervous System patterns

This principle of regularity at the development of the adaptive reactions allows the organism to react on any action of the irritant at a wide range of intensity. It provides fine-tuning of homeostasis at small changes in the strength of the irritants.

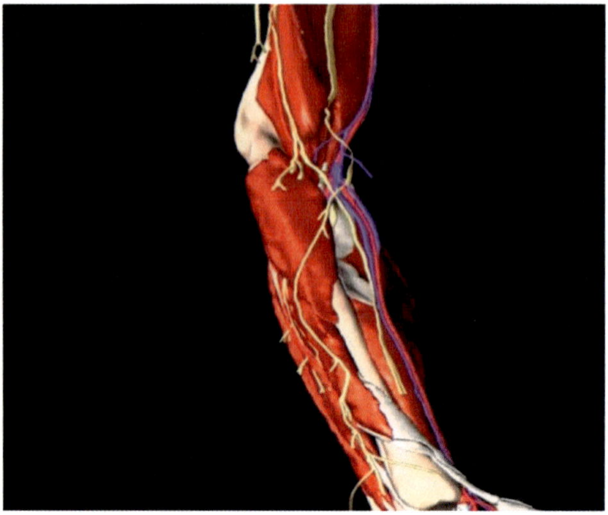

The main goal of RITM SCENAR therapy is to activate maximum number of C Fibers to induce the secretion of a sufficient amount of neuropeptides. This is achieved by active feedback, bipolar electric impulse and individually dosed influence.

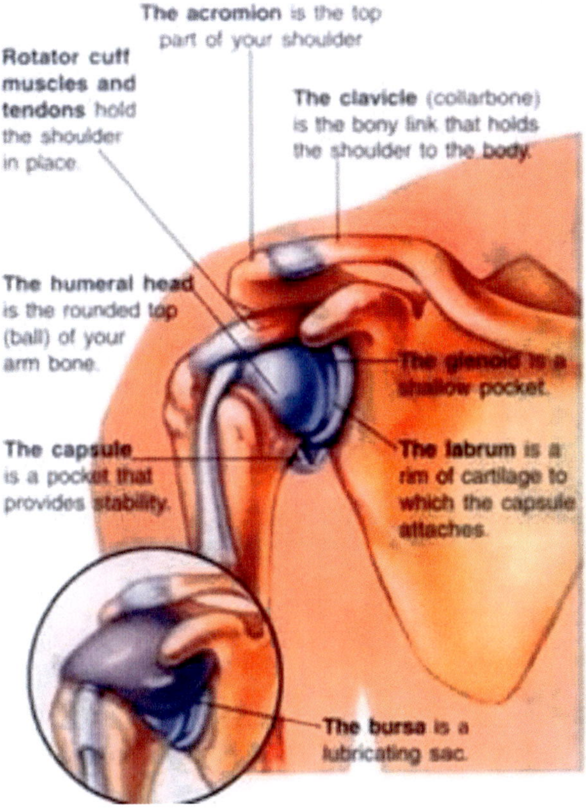
The acromion is the top part of your shoulder
Rotator cuff muscles and tendons hold the shoulder in place.
The clavicle (collarbone) is the bony link that holds the shoulder to the body.
The humeral head is the rounded top (ball) of your arm bone.
The glenoid is a shallow pocket.
The capsule is a pocket that provides stability.
The labrum is a rim of cartilage to which the capsule attaches.
The bursa is a lubricating sac.

Active feedback

The most unique characteristic of RITM SCENAR is that it can induce changes in the parameters of its impulse automatically and in accordance with the body's response to the device. Scenar does this by monitoring the skin's impedance and then changes the electric impulse it is sending out in accordance with the changes in the **skin's impedance.**

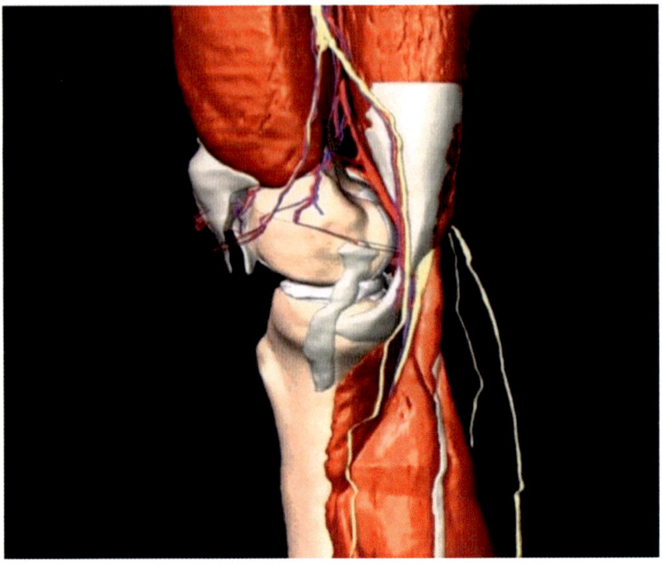

The body creates **electromagnetic and acoustic fields**. In a pathological state these fields are modified. It is these signals that are detected by Scenar and are used to form the therapeutic impulses from Scenar. Scenar therefore enables a unique interaction between it and the patient's body. The electrical signals generated by the Scenar are similar in form to the body's own endogenous neurological impulses. In this way the body does not recognize them as foreign.

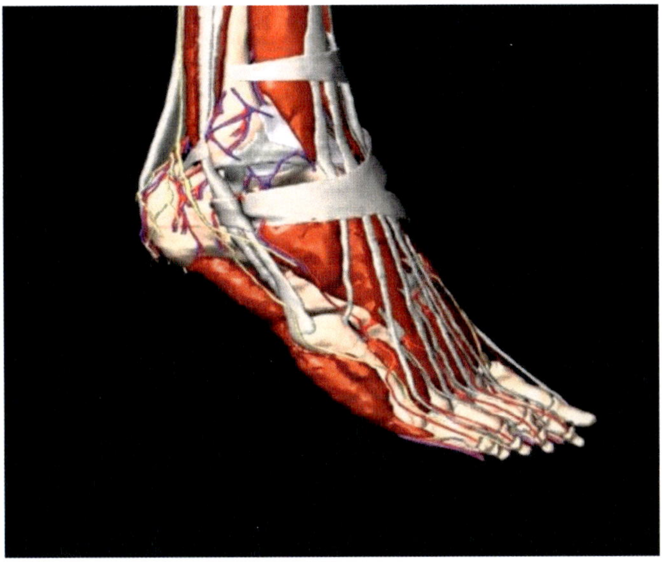

The Scenar Professional series devices measure the electrical activity of the body (skin impedance) and display the information on a LCD screen. This allows the practitioner to view current readings and choose the most appropriate mode of operation and zone of treatment.

Chapter 7. Physiological Effects on Pain Relief

Three mechanisms are involved in the pain relieving effect:

Neurophysiological

SCENAR impulse causes impulses in thick and thin nerve fibers and in the brain this prevents the passage of pain impulses. SCENAR impulses act on A Fibers which activate the substantial gelatinous in the spinal cord and in its excited state it depolarizes the pain impulses arriving at this time. This prevents transmission of the pain impulses from the periphery to the brain, that is, it closes the gate (gate theory).

Cutaneous Nerves of Head and Neck

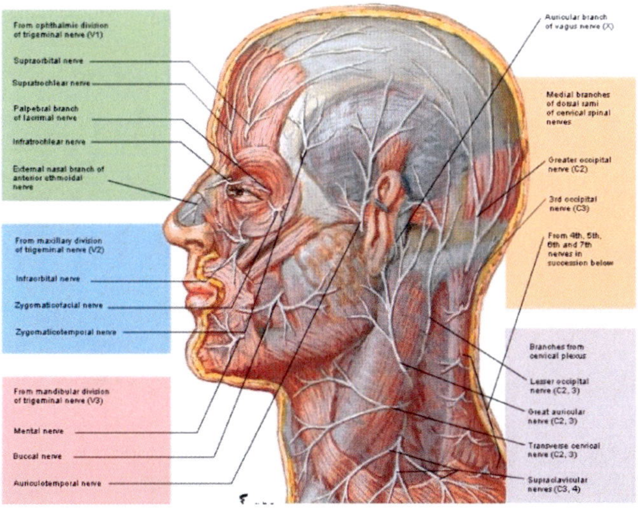

From ophthalmic division of trigeminal nerve (V1)
Supraorbital nerve
Supratrochlear nerve
Palpebral branch of lacrimal nerve
Infratrochlear nerve
External nasal branch of anterior ethmoidal nerve
From maxillary division of trigeminal nerve (V2)
Infraorbital nerve
Zygomaticofacial nerve
Zygomaticotemporal nerve
From mandibular division of trigeminal nerve (V3)
Mental nerve
Buccal nerve
Auriculotemporal nerve
Auricular branch of vagus nerve (X)
Medial branches of dorsal rami of cervical spinal nerves
Greater occipital nerve (C2)
3rd occipital nerve (C3)
From 4th, 5th, 6th and 7th nerves in succession below
Branches from cervical plexus
Lesser occipital nerve (C2, 3)
Great auricular nerve (C2, 3)
Transverse cervical nerve (C2, 3)
Supraclavicular nerves (C3, 4)

Neuro-chemical pain-killing effect

Usually lasts for at least four hours and gives a more profound effect than narcotics and will potentate the effects of administered narcotics.

Refraction in the nerve endings of the peripheral nerve fibers blocks the transmission of the pain impulse.

A new dominant focus is established in the cortex of the brain, which suppresses the pain focus.

SCENAR action considerably reduces edema around the nerve fibers and so reduces the pressure on nociceptors.

Three factors are involved.

- Neurophysiological
- Neuro-chemical
- Psycho-emotional

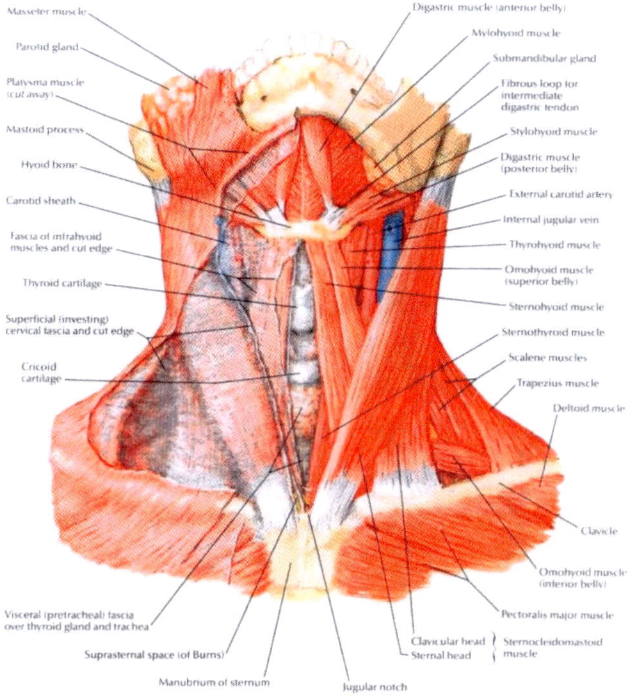
Masseter muscle
Parotid gland
Platysma muscle
(cut away)
Mastoid process
Hyoid bone
Carotid sheath
Fascia of infrahyoid
muscles and cut edge
Thyroid cartilage
Superficial (investing)
cervical fascia and cut edge
Cricoid
cartilage
Visceral (pretracheal) fascia
over thyroid gland and trachea
Suprasternal space (of Burns)
Manubrium of sternum
Jugular notch
Digastric muscle (anterior belly)
Mylohyoid muscle
Submandibular gland
Fibrous loop for
intermediate
digastric tendon
Stylohyoid muscle
Digastric muscle
(posterior belly)
External carotid artery
Internal jugular vein
Thyrohyoid muscle
Omohyoid muscle
(superior belly)
Sternohyoid muscle
Sternothyroid muscle
Scalene muscles
Trapezius muscle
Deltoid muscle
Clavicle
Omohyoid muscle
(inferior belly)
Pectoralis major muscle
Clavicular head
Sternal head
Sternocleidomastoid
muscle

Nociceptors are pain receptors and in the brain there is a nociceptive system, which is counteracted by an antagonistic system, the anti-nociceptive system.

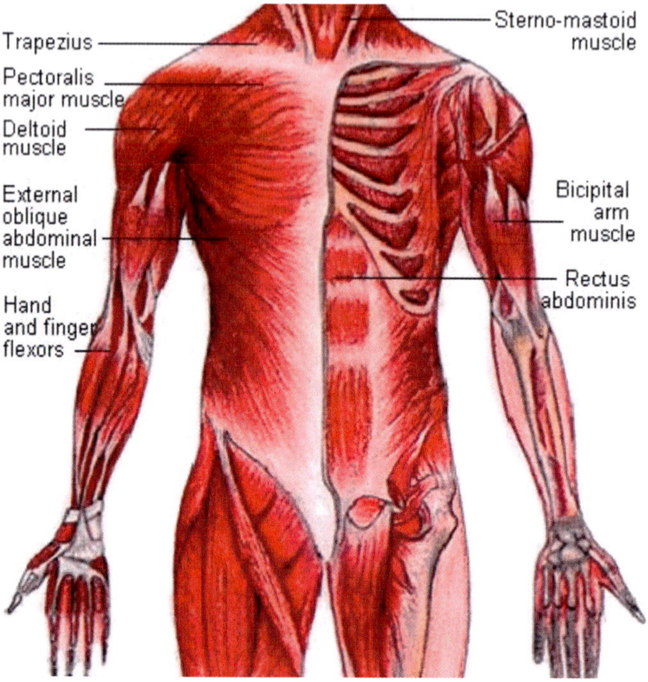
Trapezius
Pectoralis major muscle
Deltoid muscle
External oblique abdominal muscle
Hand and finger flexors
Sterno-mastoid muscle
Bicipital arm muscle
Rectus abdominis

Pain impulses begin in free nerve endings. These endings are called nociceptors. Sharp pain is conducted via delta fibers, which terminate in lamina 1 and V of the spinal cord. Prolong often burning pain is conducted via C fibers, which terminate in laminar II and V of the cord. The neurotransmitter of these pain **afferent endings**, is called **substance P**. The neurons of these laminar contribute to the formation of the lateral spine - thalamic tract. This pathway not only projects fibers directly to the thalamus but also provides collaterals at every level of the spinal cord and brain stem. **Synaptic interaction** of these collaterals at this (**mencephalic**) level, results in an enhanced state of readiness without conscious awareness of pain stimulus.

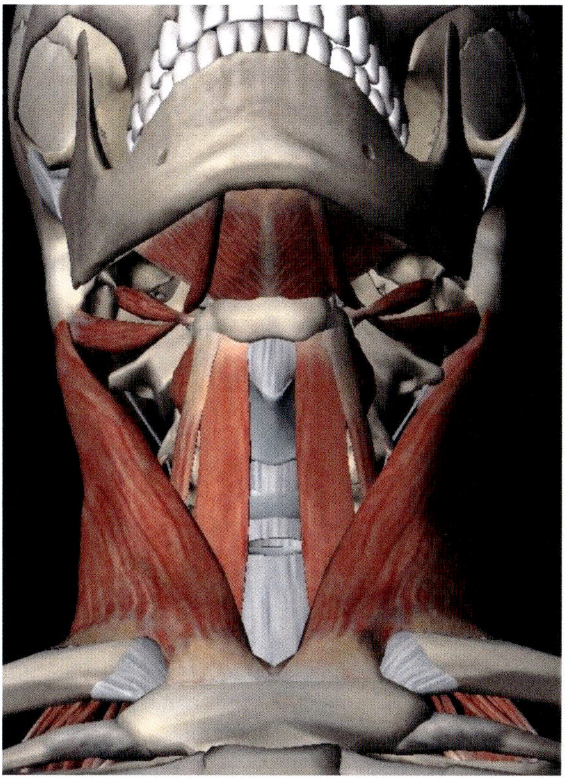

Then from **thalamic level** begins non-localized conscious pain level. From the cortex descending pain inhibitory pathways begin. Fibers follow towards thalamus, then to **midbrain region** and to the reticular formation which allows a mixing of other systems and changes **neurotransmitters** to enhance and refine the degree of inhibition. Descending pathways fibers synapse with inter-neurons with both incoming **primary pain afferents** and cells whose axons form the lateral spin thalamic tract, closing the inhibitory arch. All of these areas involved in descending pathways and other parts of the brain as well, are rich in opiate receptors, such as morphine, codeine meperidines as well as very impotent endogenous opiates encephalin and endorphins, where **encephalin**may alter the degree to which the calcium channel of synaptic zones permit to release substance P. SCENAR therapy is aiming to amplify these pain controlling mechanisms. There are three hormone systems in the **anti-nociceptive system**, **opiate, serotonin and adrenalin systems,** all of which influence each other.

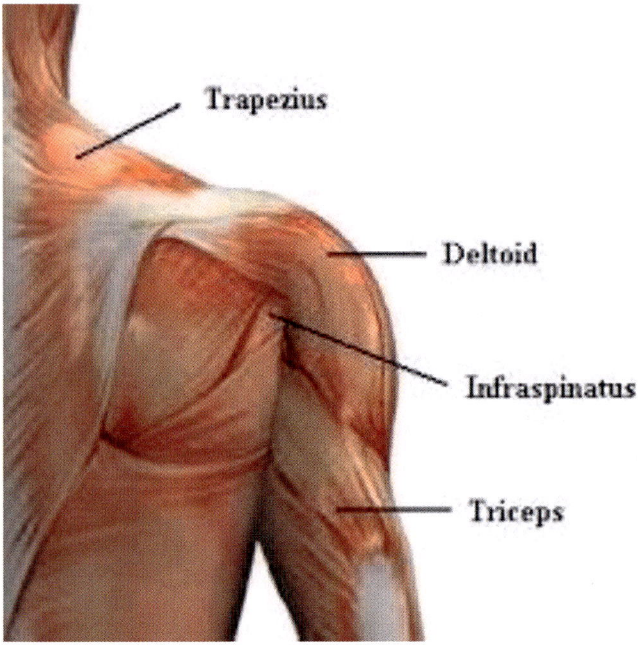
Trapezius
Deltoid
Infraspinatus
Triceps

Electrical stimulation from the device acting on peripheral nerve fibers influences both nociceptive and anti-nociceptive systems. This releases opioid-like compounds which block release of compound P at the level of the **substantia gelatinousa** and block transmission of the pain impulses chemically. The SCENAR acts mainly on the serotoninergic mechanism rather than directly on the opiate mechanism. Oxygenation of tissues is often disturbed in pathological processes (**ischemia**). SCENAR also releases vasodilators locally, which enhances oxygen supply and eases pain. There are also released dopamine, **encephalin** and **noradrenaline a**nd these account for long-term **analgesia.**

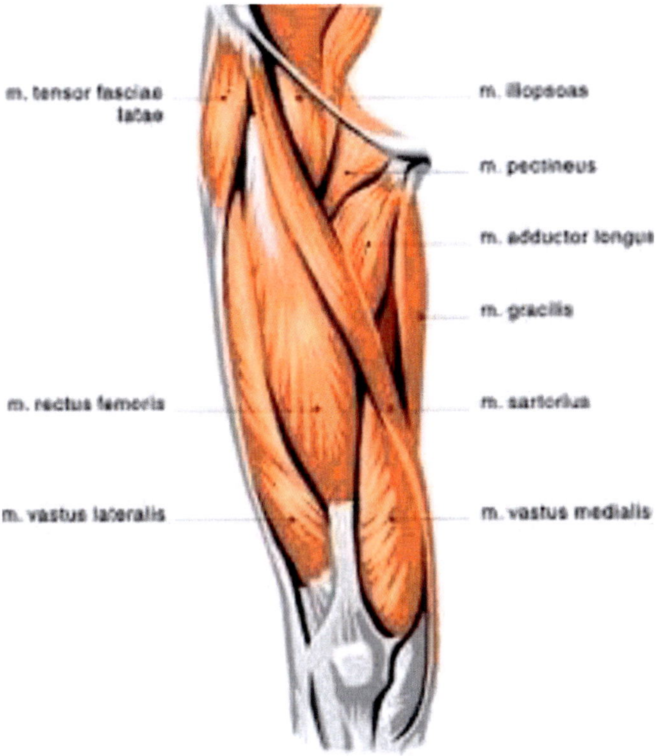
m. tensor fasciae latae
m. iliopsoas
m. pectineus
m. adductor longus
m. gracilis
m. rectus femoris
m. sartorius
m. vastus lateralis
m. vastus medialis

Psycho-emotional effects on the **reticular formation** of the stem of the brain may give sedative and analgesic effects. It is thought that there is an area here that, when stimulated, reduces pain sensitivity. There may be cells, which are self-stimulating and have a memory for chronic pain. SCENAR treatment may suppress their memory. Exacerbations caused by SCENAR appear gradually and appear at the place where the function is building up. Common exacerbations of the disease will progress slowly.

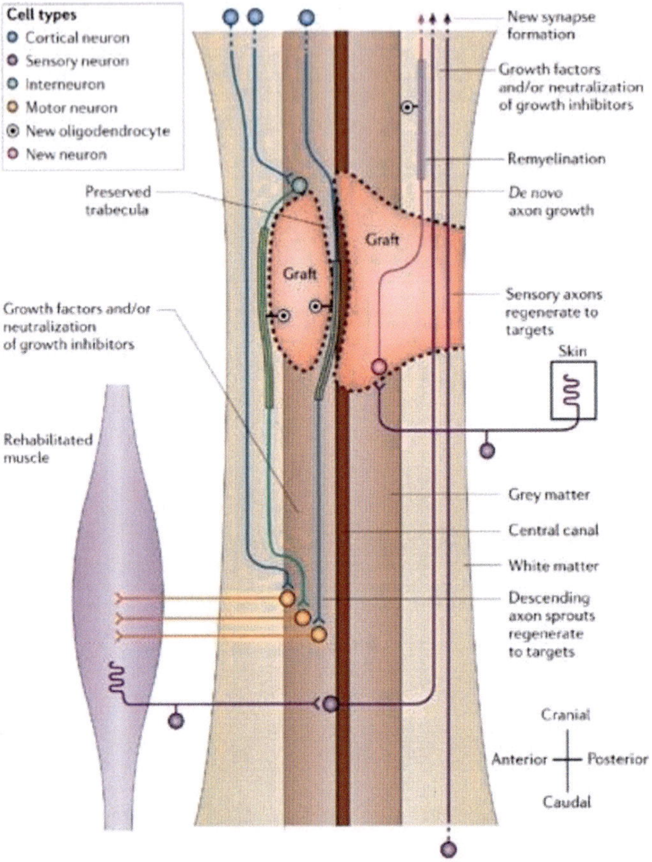
Cell types
Cortical neuron
Sensory neuron
Interneuron
Motor neuron
New oligodendrocyte
New neuron
New synapse formation
Growth factors and/or neutralization of growth inhibitors
Remyelination
De novo axon growth
Preserved trabecula
Graft
Graft
Sensory axons regenerate to targets
Skin
Growth factors and/or neutralization of growth inhibitors
Rehabilitated muscle
Grey matter
Central canal
White matter
Descending axon sprouts regenerate to targets
Cranial
Anterior
Posterior
Caudal

Exacerbations caused by SCENAR will have an expansion of:

- A zone of activity of the process
- A zone of pain
- An aggravation of any accompanying chronic conditions, but there will not -be aggravation in the patient's state.

SCENAR devices act at the cell level and rehabilitate respiratory enzyme chains of the mitochondria (i.e., respiratory ferments structure responsible for cell breathing), cytoplasmic membranes, etc. So they recover homeostasis of the cell media (its internal invariability). Generally, the cellular reactions help **restore respiratory capacity** in tissues and organs, lower concentration of hydrogen ions in tissues, restore or improve utilization of free oxygen by the cell (depending on how far gone is the pathological process), and restore and improve metabolic processes in the body. **This is the major SCENAR therapeutic effect**, which helps correct various disorders and pathological conditions. The next feature of SCENAR application is based on such neurophysiological concept as the new stimulus or the body response to the new stimulus (therapeutic effect due to the influence of some new physiotherapeutic factor).

As a rule, this response is shown only at the initial stages of impact, and accordingly same is the therapeutic effect. Major distinction of SCENAR devices in this area rests on the fact that the device impulse works according to the "**biological feedback**" principle.

Neurohumoral mechanisms initiate production of endorphins at the cerebrospinal level (dopamine, norepinephrine) to produce morphine-like effect. Their secretions under pulse treatment stand for a long analgesic effect; the processes that involve various neuropeptides hold an interim position between the mediator (neurotransmission) and modulator (hormonal) processes. These processes are of great importance for the body's brain functioning and adaptation reaction of an organism.

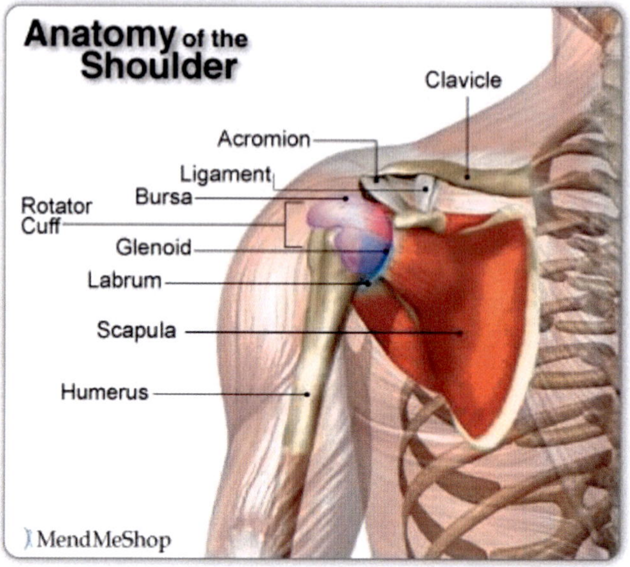
Anatomy of the Shoulder
Clavicle
Acromion
Ligament
Bursa
Rotator Cuff
Glenoid
Labrum
Scapula
Humerus
MendMeShop

Psychic factor

Cerebral structures receive afferents from the various points of the body. There is the conception which says that the pain information blocking is caused by inhibition effect of a certain truncus cerebri reticular formation on all the afferent system levels including the segmental mechanism of pain input control. The reticular formation is supposed to have the body's specific zones. The electric current stimulation of these zones activates the reticular formation which results in subsequent pain sensibility decrease. Chronic pain causes central neurons' activity change in presence of a cell self-excitation (cell self-excitation is a kind of memory). Transdermal electro stimulation can suppress this activity.

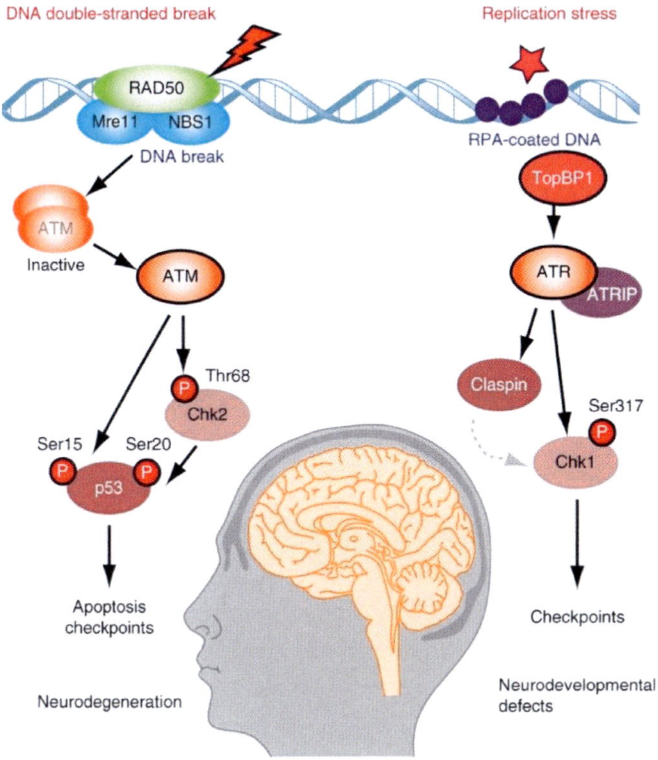
DNA double-stranded break
Replication stress
RAD50
Mre11
NBS1
DNA break
RPA-coated DNA
TopBP1
ATM
Inactive
ATM
ATR
ATRIP
Thr68
P
Chk2
Claspin
Ser317
Ser15
Ser20
P
p53
Chk1
Apoptosis
checkpoints
Checkpoints
Neurodegeneration
Neurodevelopmental
defects

As a rule, this response is shown only at the initial stages of impact, and accordingly same is the therapeutic effect. Major distinction of SCENAR devices in this area rests on the fact that the device impulse works according to the “**biological feedback**” principle.

Three Health State Levels

- Energy level, i.e., organism efficiency.
- Psycho-emotional level (mood, sleep, appetite).
- Mental level (thoughts, fantasies).

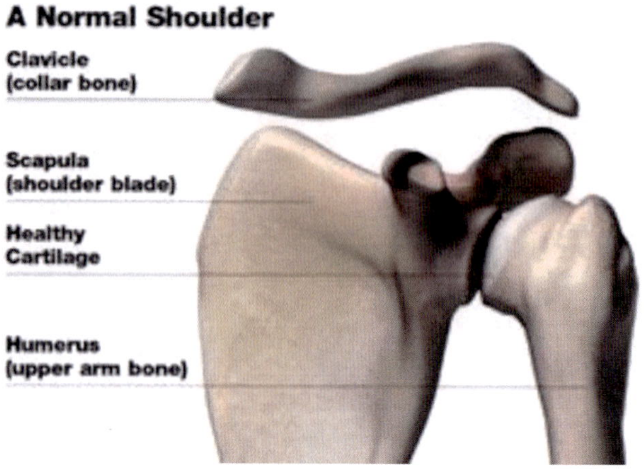
A Normal Shoulder
Clavicle
(collar bone)
Scapula
(shoulder blade)
Healthy
Cartilage
Humerus
(upper arm bone)

The general effect of the SCENAR influence on the organism may be interpreted as three G's: good sleep, good appetite and good mood. This is the effect of higher energy and reactivity levels and the state-of-health change on these levels would mean that the majority of the therapeutic work for patient's recovery was done successfully. Energy application level is the impact intensity measured by patient's subjective sensations.

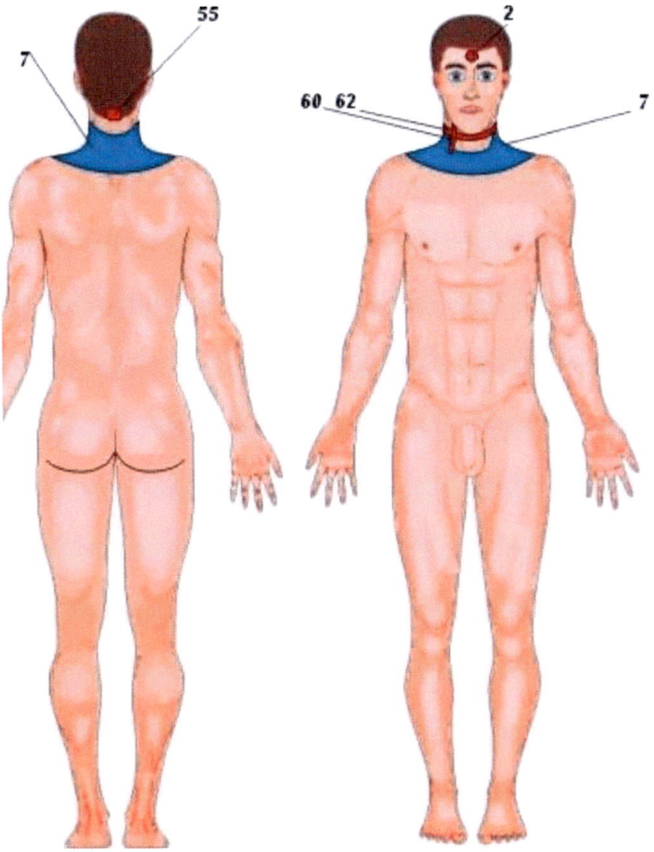
55
7
2
60 62
7

Patterns of Scenar Impulses

The skin develops from the same embryological layer as the nervous system. **Reflexology and acupuncture treat areas on the skin that represent internal organs and energy pathways**. Using the SCENAR, it is possible to influence every system of the body and to balance energy flow in the meridians SCENAR adds energy to the system, a system that may be depleted in its reserves as it attempts to heal itself. Normally the body undergoes adaptive reactions to changes in the environment and often these are suppressed by such things as cough mixtures, anti-inflammatory medicines etc. The signal received from the SCENAR, acting on the skin, causes a regulating adaptive reaction within a short period of time. This may restore lost functions and goes some way to explain how unresolved problems from the past resurface to be dealt with.

Chapter 8. Choosing an Area for Treatment

Work according to the first rule, i.e., work on any complaint (usually pain). Determine the **pathological focus** and the **projection of the pain**. Work locally and towards any **referred pain**.

Look for any **asymmetry** and work on all **asymmetries,** trying to achieve dynamics, i.e. aiming for the disappearance of the asymmetry or trying to achieve the opposite sign.

If there are many complaints, or none - use the second rule i.e. Three Pathways and Six Points. Find and note areas to set Doses (Dose 1), Zeros (Dose 2) and FM (Alternate). These will be the areas that need treatment.

Treat horizontals and segments

At any stage when a Secondary Factor appears, treat that area.

Remember the following options; Work on the symmetrical area. Use Reciprocal principles

Treat Meridians

How to Use Frequency

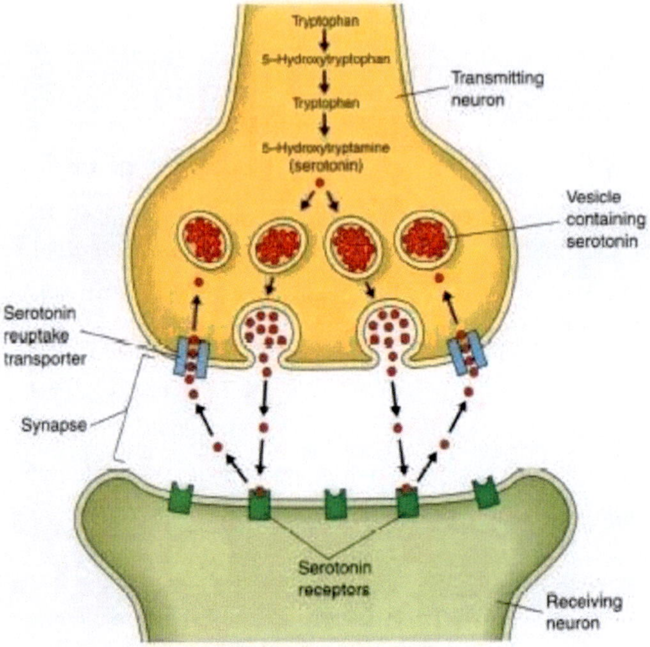
Tryptophan
5-Hydroxytryptophan
Tryptophan
5-Hydroxytryptamine
(serotonin)
Transmitting
neuron
Vesicle
containing
serotonin
Serotonin
reuptake
transporter
Synapse
Serotonin
receptors
Receiving
neuron

The condition is degenerative:

Acute pain, the ailment is chronic - use frequency modulation (FM) or frequency deviation (Freq dev) settings, in CONSTANT or FmVar (ALTERNAT) mode.

There is no pain, the ailment is not chronic - start on 15Hz - 50Hz, end on above 90Hz, in CONSTANT or Fm mode.

The condition is not degenerative:

Inflammation - treat on or above 120Hz

Acute pain in small muscles, joints, internal organs, viral infections - use 40Hz - 90Hz and 120Hz - 180Hz.

Acute pain in large muscles, joints, face muscles - use 200Hz - 350Hz, alternate with 15Hz - 90Hz.

Acute heart pain - use 190Hz - 230Hz.

Headache - 160Hz, 20Hz plus Intens.

Acute trauma and swelling -(use 350Hz)

Wounds - use 230Hz - 190Hz, 20Hz.

Constipation - use 20Hz plus Intens.

Scars - use 18Hz

Muscles, vessels, nerves stimulation - use 20Hz - 28Hz - 35Hz - 45Hz.

Children and Elderly - use 60Hz - 90Hz.

Chapter 9. How to Work With the SCENAR

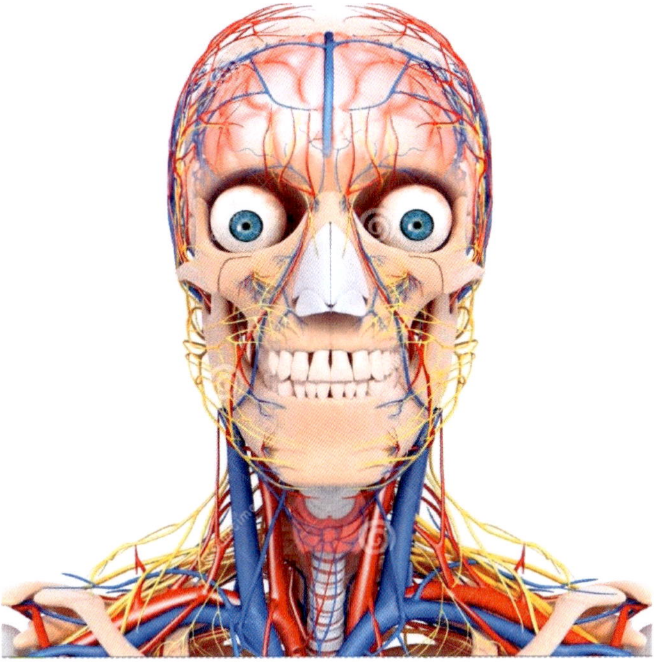

Move the device steadily (speed) and firmly (pressure) in one direction. Start treatment at any presenting primary signs. In the presence of active complaints (especially in combination with **primary signs**) start treating here.

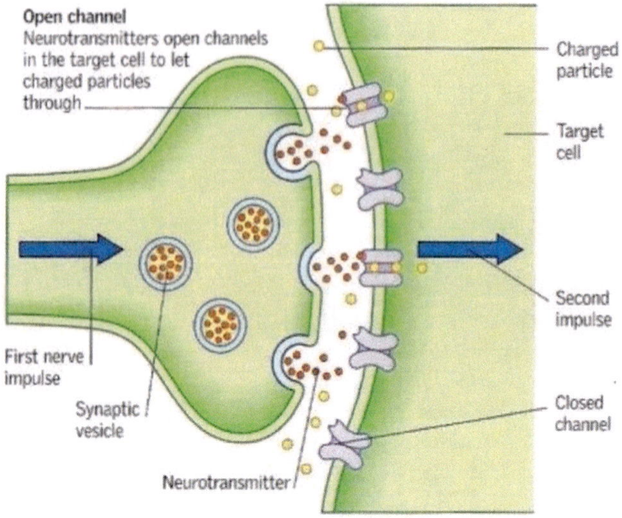
Open channel
Neurotransmitters open channels in the target cell to let charged particles through
Charged particle
Target cell
First nerve impulse
Synaptic vesicle
Neurotransmitter
Second impulse
Closed channel

Treat one site at a time, until any small asymmetry (or secondary sign) appears. When you have achieved an asymmetry, change the action regime (Freq, Mod, z, Dmpf, Intensity or any combination of these). Work, looking for a **small asymmetry.**

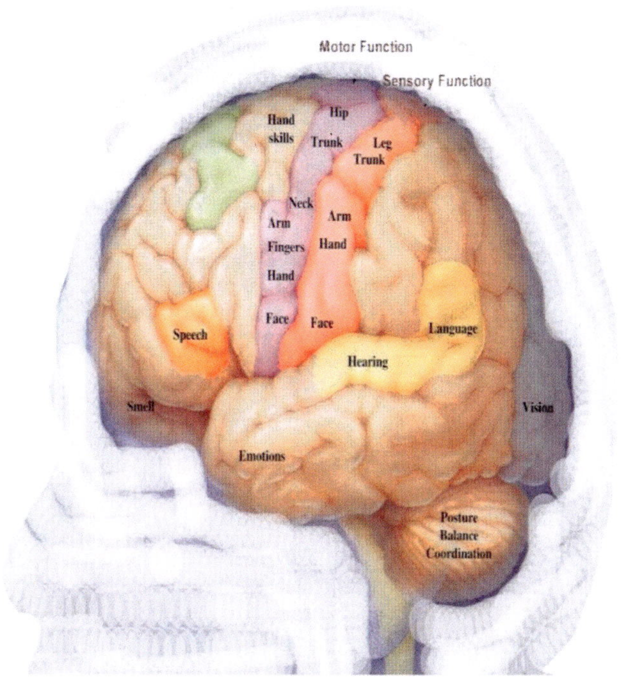
Motor Function
Sensory Function
Hand skills
Hip
Trunk
Leg
Trunk
Neck
Arm
Arm
Fingers
Hand
Hand
Face
Face
Speech
Language
Hearing
Smell
Vision
Emotions
Posture
Balance
Coordination

Then work on the area of small asymmetry, varying the direction of the electrode (4 directions), attempting to **achieve a dynamic change** (in the pain, in the color, in stickiness of the electrode, in the local sensation, in the sound from the device). Ideally work until the sign disappears or until an opposite sign appears. Finish the procedure when you have achieved a subjective improvement of the patient's condition.

When there are no more reactions or there is an insignificant subjective effect:

Change the action regime and extend the area of action along a horizontal line or along a segment. Include the general action area (3 paths).Continue to reveal areas of small asymmetry and secondary sign

Stickiness

When you draw the device over the skin, it can "stick" so that you cannot get it moving forward without applying force. It means there is a pathological nidus over there. "Sticking" area needs to be treated additionally for 2 – 3 minutes.

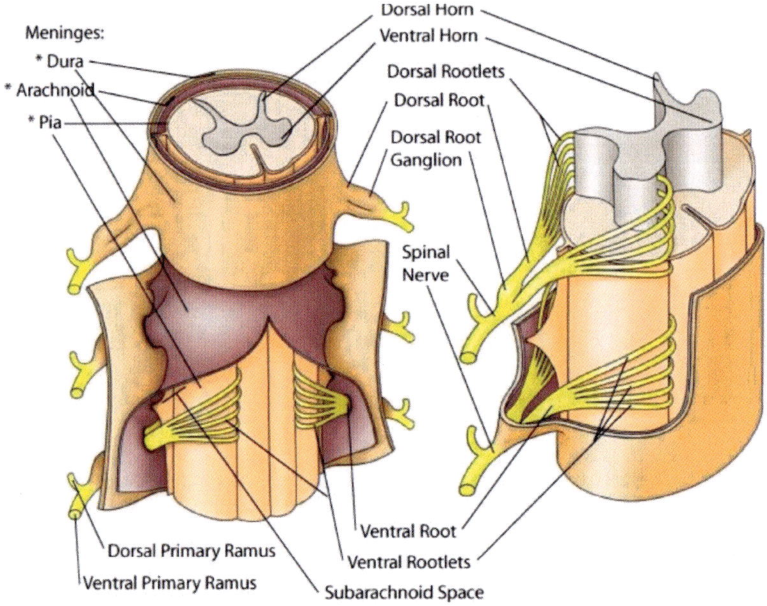

Meninges:
* Dura
* Arachnoid
* Pia
Dorsal Horn
Ventral Horn
Dorsal Rootlets
Dorsal Root
Dorsal Root Ganglion
Spinal Nerve
Dorsal Primary Ramus
Ventral Primary Ramus
Ventral Root
Ventral Rootlets
Subarachnoid Space

Sensitivity alteration.

During treatment, the device electrodes contact parts of the skin with different sensitivity. Highly sensitive skin area coincides with the projection of the pathological nidus and is optimal for SCENAR application.

Skin alteration.

Skin reddening during SCENAR application indicates the **increased functions** in this area and is up for additional treatment. If a pale skin area stands out against the red background, it indicates the decreased functions in this area and is also up for additional treatment. Upon revealing any uncharacteristic changes in the skin (blister, spot, scar, and so on), apply the device directly to the altered skin area.

Sound alteration.

Any change in tonal sound during SCENAR application indicates a pathological nidus. Skin area of the altered sound is up for additional treatment for 2 – 3 minutes.

Change in numerical output display.

Small diagnostic symptom

This is the most distinct and well-marked small skin area, which appears on the skin surface within the large diagnostic symptom area during SCENAR-application. This is the easy-to-identify and vivid diagnostic symptom and optimal skin area for SCENAR application. Small diagnostic symptom must be up for additional treatment until it disappears.

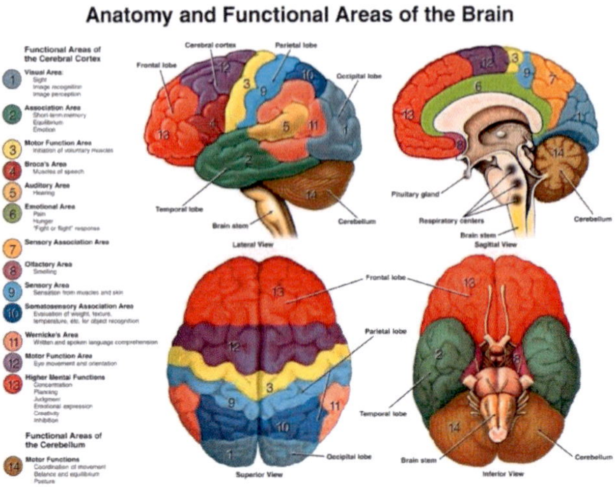
Anatomy and Functional Areas of the Brain
Functional Areas of the Cerebral Cortex
1 Visual Area
2 Association Area
3 Motor Function Area
4 Broca's Area
5 Auditory Area
6 Emotional Area
7 Sensory Association Area
8 Olfactory Area
9 Sensory Area
10 Somatosensory Association Area
11 Wernicke's Area
12 Motor Function Area
13 Higher Mental Functions
Functional Areas of the Cerebellum
14 Motor Functions
Frontal lobe
Temporal lobe

Extra primary diagnostic symptom

This is the small skin area which initially, prior to SCENAR application, differs by some of its features from the other skin surface irrespectively of device treatment, i.e., the visually observed symptoms, such as skin coloration, sensation (itch, and others), scar, wound, erosion, pigmentation, and so on. **Extra primary diagnostic symptom** is also up for additional SCENAR application according to the symmetric treatment method: right - left, top - bottom.

Extra secondary diagnostic symptom

This is the skin area, which appears in the process of SCENAR application and differs from the other skin surface. It is located outside the areas applied by the

SCENAR devices. The secondary symptom is also up for additional treatment. It should disappear with patient's recovery. If the main small and extra secondary symptoms are located over the endocrine glands, the therapy will be more effective. If the main diagnostic symptoms are revealed and diagnosed, maximum time should be spent on treating them. If you fail to reveal the main diagnostic symptoms, further treatment should be accented on the extra diagnostic symptoms (be satisfied with few), giving preference to the secondary symptoms because their treatment is more effective than that of the "primary" ones. If neither main nor extra symptoms are diagnosed, then go on with active complaint treatment method, and also apply the device to the general reflex zones. During a detailed examination of any person, one or pathology can be revealed next to always. Revealed disorders can be functional or organic. Functional disorders are reversible and temporal, with structure of tissues and organs being unbroken. Usually functional disorders are easy and quick to correct. If changes in tissues and organs are structural, then these are the organic disorders. **SCENAR devices can be used for both functional and organic disorders**.

SCENAR Users Should Be Guided by the Following Principles:

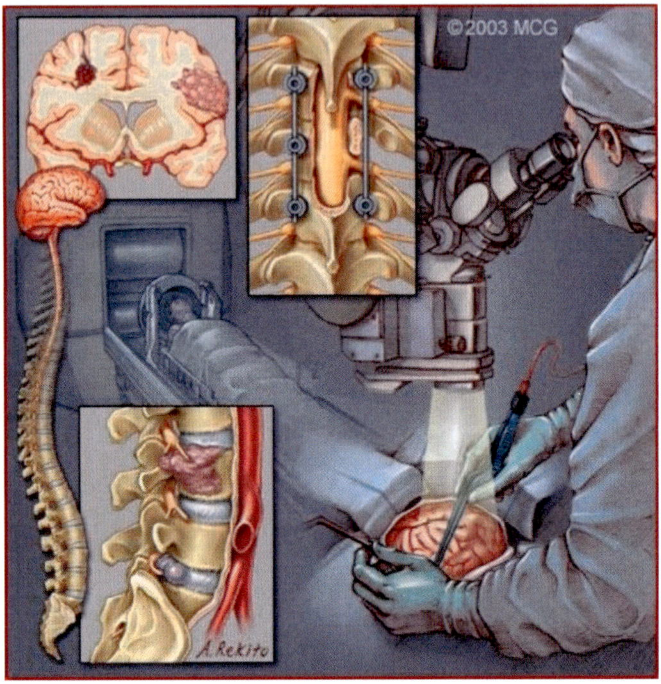
©2003 MCG
A.Rekito

Treatment upon active complaint.

Initiate treatment **"upon active complaint"** if patient shows the exact location of pain and only then decide on the next area. If there are multiple complaints from patient, initiate treatment from the general reflex zones.

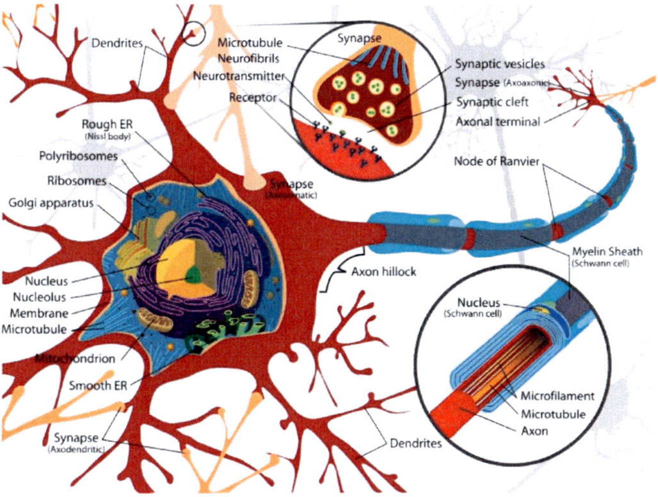
Dendrites
Microtubule
Neurofibrils
Neurotransmitter
Receptor
Synapse
Synaptic vesicles
Synapse (Axoaxonic)
Synaptic cleft
Axonal terminal
Node of Ranvier
Rough ER
(Nissl body)
Polyribosomes
Ribosomes
Golgi apparatus
Myelin Sheath
(Schwann cell)
Axon hillock
Nucleus
Nucleolus
Membrane
Microtubule
Nucleus
(Schwann cell)
Smooth ER
Microfilament
Microtubule
Axon
Synapse
(Axodendritic)
Dendrites

Elementary-to-complex treatment.

Initiate treatment with elementary methods: i.e. **apply the device to the location of pain and toward its irradiation** (eccentric pain), large diagnostic symptom, small diagnostic symptom, general reflex zones, and extra diagnostic symptoms. Use detachable electrode if there is no direct access to the treatment area.

Search for the large and localization of the small diagnostic symptoms (low adequacy principle), i.e. the more exact and accurate is the treatment area chosen by the SCENAR user, the higher will be the SCENAR effect; the less is the treatment area, the higher will be the healing effect.

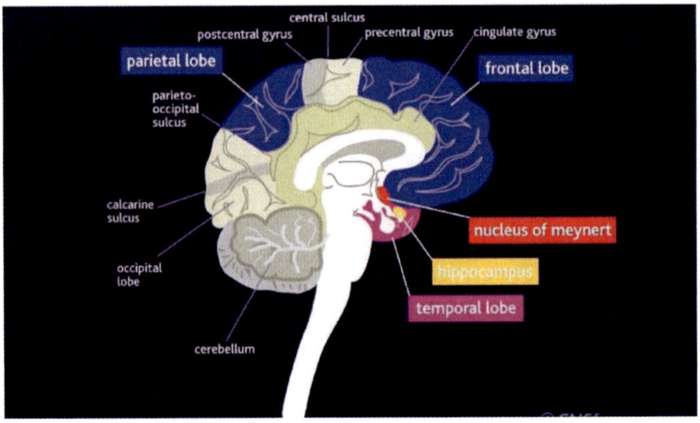
central sulcus
postcentral gyrus
precentral gyrus
cingulate gyrus
parietal lobe
frontal lobe
parieto-
occipital
sulcus
calcarine
sulcus
occipital
lobe
cerebellum
nucleus of meynert
hippocampus
temporal lobe

Treatment of the reflexogenic zones.

Reflexogenic zones are located along the major nerve trunks, at the nerve-muscle joints, along the cranial satures, over the sensitive tendon areas (there are acupuncture points over there), over the projection of major lymphatic and blood vessels.

Reciprocal treatment, i.e. treatment of the symmetric area.

Analysis of cyclic changes in the pathological system.

You can analyze them on patient's complaints and device treatment modes. Certain dynamic changes indicate the recovery process is under way. Let's, for instance, take coughing because of bronchi disorders. Initially, there was no cough, then it became dry, and moist the next day, then the phlegm began discharging, and then cough and phlegm considerably decreased and completely disappeared, i.e. the whole cycle is observed: from 0 to 0. It is this cyclic change that must always be analyzed by the SCENAR user.

Analysis of dynamic changes in patient's complaints

Sensations and skin. SCENAR-user should notice, analyze and use these changes to stabilize patient's condition.

Optimal and efficient treatment.

Optimal and efficient treatment means a search for the optimal treatment zone to gain the best possible healing effect, i.e. revealing of the diagnostic symptoms.

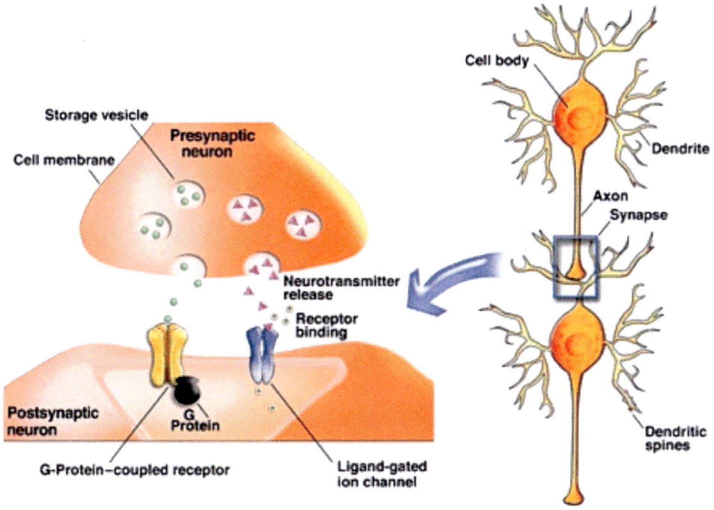

Storage vesicle
Presynaptic neuron
Cell membrane
Neurotransmitter release
Receptor binding
Postsynaptic neuron
G Protein
G-Protein-coupled receptor
Ligand-gated ion channel
Cell body
Dendrite
Axon
Synapse
Dendritic spines

Repetition factor

Procedure repetition factor depends on patient's disease condition. Acute disease conditions and first aid patients are treated according to the following principle: the more acute (dangerous) is the disease condition, the more significant should be the treatment dose, and more lengthy and frequent treatment sessions. Every-two-hour sessions are possible to help patient out of this condition. If the disease condition has a positive dynamic change, the intervals between sessions may be increased up to 6-7 hours or completely stopped. Repeat diagnostics and sessions in about 8 to 10 hours.

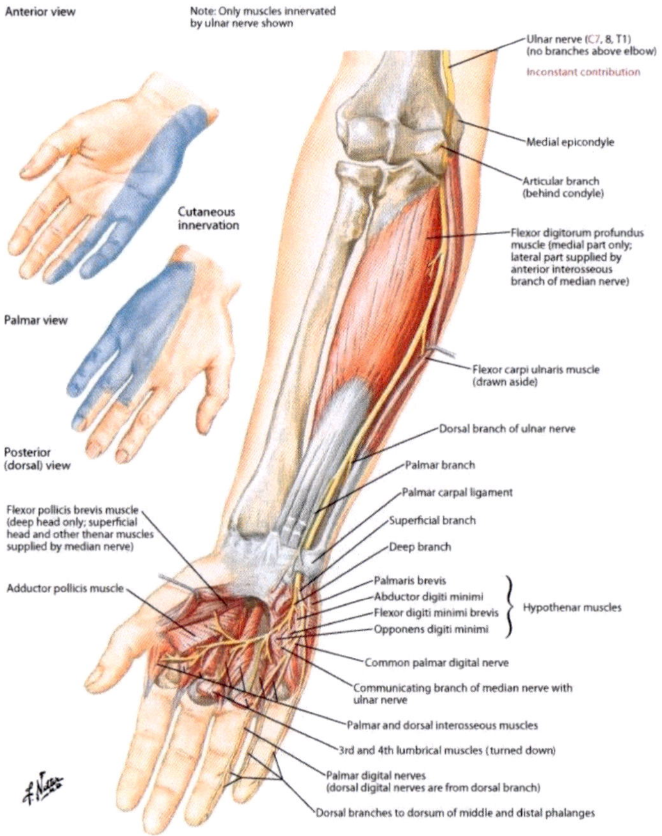

Anterior view
Note: Only muscles innervated by ulnar nerve shown
Ulnar nerve (C7, 8, T1) (no branches above elbow)
Inconstant contribution
Medial epicondyle
Articular branch (behind condyle)
Cutaneous innervation
Flexor digitorum profundus muscle (medial part only; lateral part supplied by anterior interosseous branch of median nerve)
Palmar view
Flexor carpi ulnaris muscle (drawn aside)
Dorsal branch of ulnar nerve
Posterior (dorsal) view
Palmar branch
Palmar carpal ligament
Flexor pollicis brevis muscle (deep head only; superficial head and other thenar muscles supplied by median nerve)
Superficial branch
Deep branch
Adductor pollicis muscle
Palmaris brevis
Abductor digiti minimi
Flexor digiti minimi brevis
Opponens digiti minimi
Hypothenar muscles
Common palmar digital nerve
Communicating branch of median nerve with ulnar nerve
Palmar and dorsal interosseous muscles
3rd and 4th lumbrical muscles (turned down)
Palmar digital nerves (dorsal digital nerves are from dorsal branch)
Dorsal branches to dorsum of middle and distal phalanges

Chronic and sluggish disorders are usually treated once a day or every other day, but even every 2 days or once a week treatment is possible. Try to treat patients at the same hour and situation for the entire course. Paroxysm-type disorders are treated by relieving each case of paroxysm and by conducting prophylactic therapy courses planned in between paroxysms. It is recommended to conduct 3-4 therapy courses a year, each one consisting of 7-15 sessions. If you are able to determine the paroxysm recurrence rate, it is advisable to conduct prophylactic therapy courses 10 – 14 days prior to paroxysm.

SCENAR effects selectively, i.e. only on pathological systems (organs and tissues), and does not affect healthy ones. SCENAR features are as follows:

Try to initiate therapy when there is an active complaint from patient.

SCENAR quickly restores functional disorders in the body. Organic disorders take more time to treat.

Repeat SCENAR course if there are new complaints from patient. For instance, patient took treatment course for hypertension, and later on he caught cold and began coughing. In this case, treatment for his new complaints must be repeated. Due to no adaptation to treatment, there is no need to continuously increase power level during each SCENAR session.

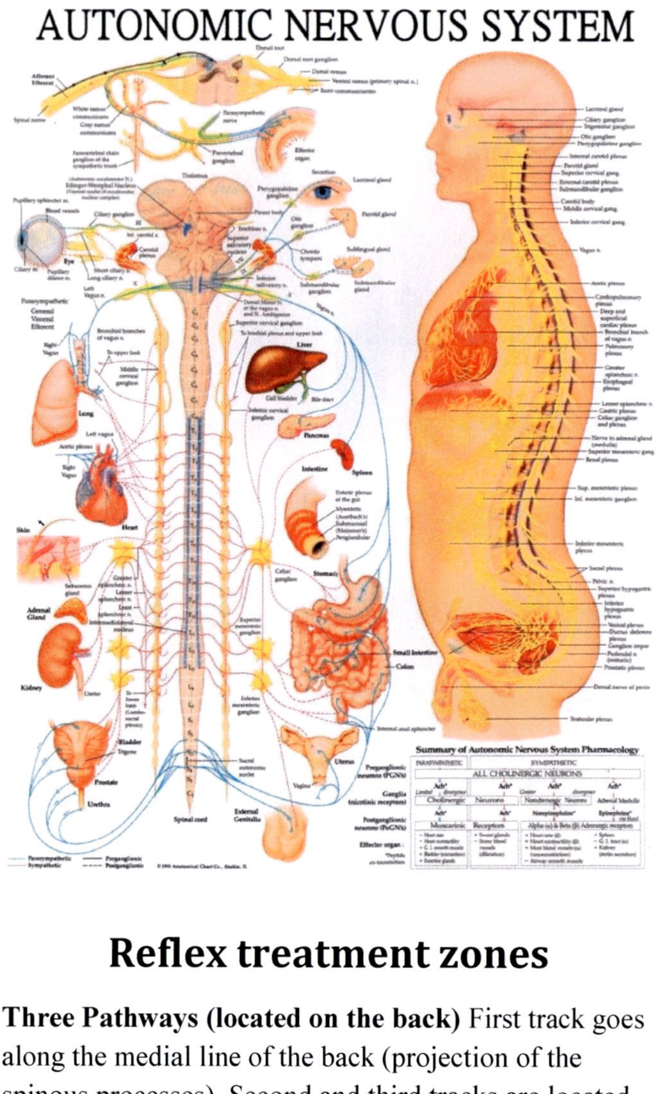
AUTONOMIC NERVOUS SYSTEM
Summary of Autonomic Nervous System Pharmacology
ALL CHOLINERGIC NEURONS

Reflex treatment zones

Three Pathways (located on the back) First track goes along the medial line of the back (projection of the spinous processes). Second and third tracks are located 2.5 – 3 cm to the right and to the left from the medial line of the back (projection of the paravertebral points).

Six points (facial exit projections of trigeminal nerve) Outlet points of trifacial nerve branches called **Six-point zone** and located: on both sides of under-the-inner eyebrow edges by the nose bridge, at both wings of nostril, and slightly below of both angles of the mouth.

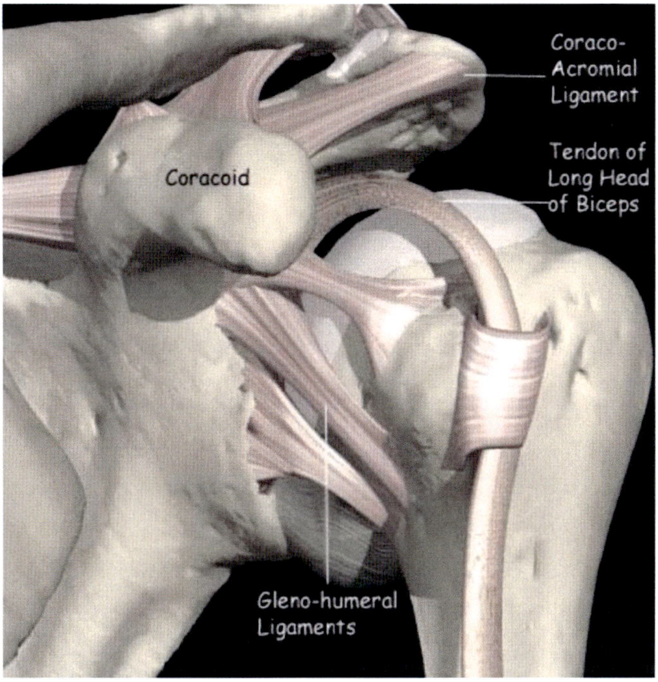
Coraco-
Acromial
Ligament
Tendon of
Long Head
of Biceps
Coracoid
Gleno-humeral
Ligaments

Cervico-occipital area. It is located to the right and to the left from the spinous processes and below the haired edge at a distance of about three longer sides of the electrode.

Forehead area. It includes the entire forehead, but its medial line at the electrode width.

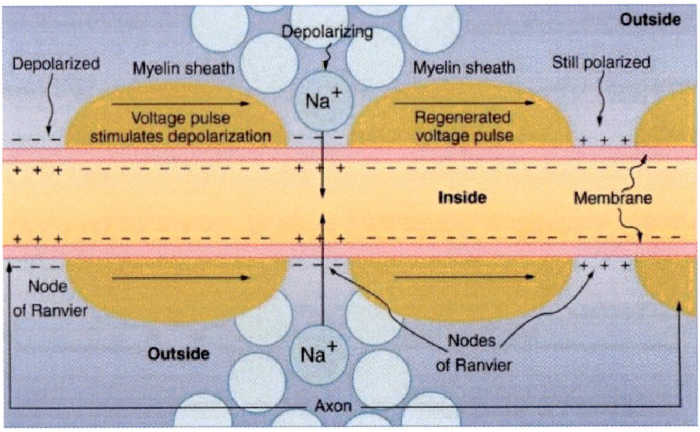
Outside
Depolarizing
Depolarized
Myelin sheath
Myelin sheath
Still polarized
Na+
Voltage pulse
stimulates depolarization
Regenerated
voltage pulse
Inside
Membrane
Node
of Ranvier
Outside
Na+
Nodes
of Ranvier
Axon

Adrenal area. Adrenal projection is on the back in the middle of the 12th rib and occupies the area under the electrode.

Lower part of the abdomen. Its treatment area can be defined in the following way: put patient's palm on the lower part of abdomen (mid-pubis), palm edges of rectangular form comply with the area to be treated.

Coccyx-sacral area. Put patient's palm on the projection of spinous processes at the coccyx area, palm edges of rectangular form comply with the area to be treated.

Abdomen. Draw vertical and horizontal lines across the umbilicus to divide the abdomen into four parts.

Spinous process of the 7th cervical vertebra. Apply device electrodes to the spinous process of the 7th cervical vertebra.

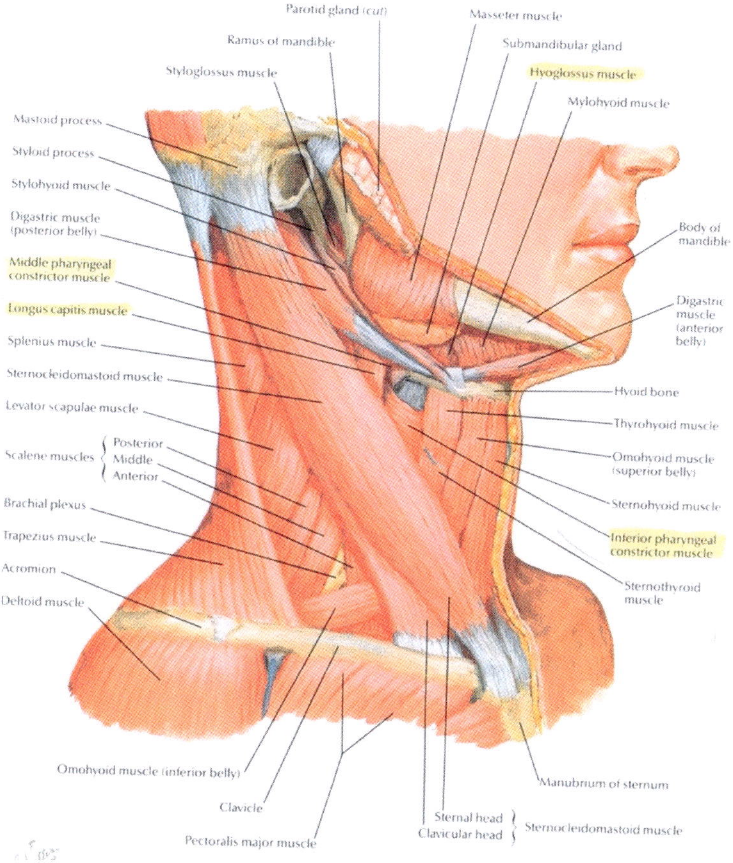
Parotid gland (cut)
Masseter muscle
Ramus of mandible
Submandibular gland
Styloglossus muscle
Hyoglossus muscle
Mylohyoid muscle
Mastoid process
Styloid process
Stylohyoid muscle
Digastric muscle (posterior belly)
Middle pharyngeal constrictor muscle
Longus capitis muscle
Splenius muscle
Sternocleidomastoid muscle
Levator scapulae muscle
Scalene muscles
Posterior
Middle
Anterior
Brachial plexus
Trapezius muscle
Acromion
Deltoid muscle
Body of mandible
Digastric muscle (anterior belly)
Hyoid bone
Thyrohyoid muscle
Omohyoid muscle (superior belly)
Sternohyoid muscle
Inferior pharyngeal constrictor muscle
Sternothyroid muscle
Omohyoid muscle (inferior belly)
Manubrium of sternum
Clavicle
Sternal head
Clavicular head
Sternocleidomastoid muscle
Pectoralis major muscle

Jugular fossa. It is located in the sternum area (fossa between clavicles and sternum).

Buttocks (anatomic area of buttocks and their folds).

Solar plexus zone - located at stomach projection region. This is a roundish zone of about 10 cm in diameter.

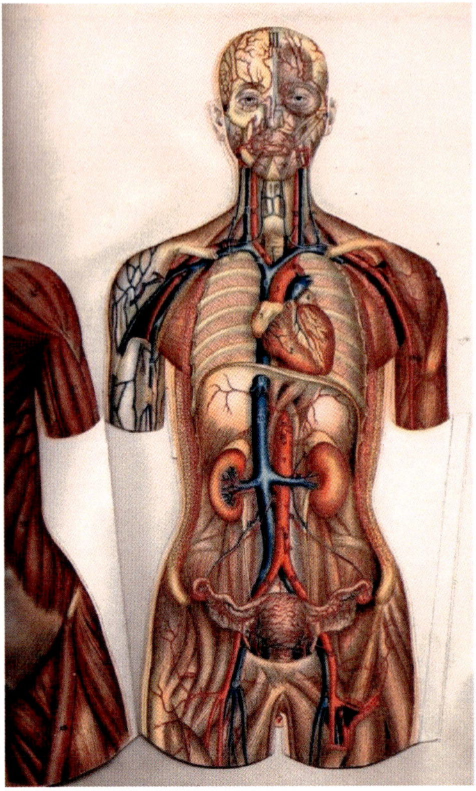

Sino carotid node zone – is located at the carotid and sternocleidomastoid muscle intersection on the front surface of a neck. There are two such zones (left and right). They are one of the smallest zones in their size, have a round form and each are up to 2cm in diameter.

Zone of "100 diseases" is located on an upper third of the shin's outer surface. There are two such zones (left and right). They are oviform zones, each of about 4cm in diameter.

The Pain direct projection zone should be marked out separately. It is located over the area of painful sensations or discomfort phenomena as well as over a sick organ (liver, gall-bladder, etc.).

Extra treatment zones. Along with general reflex zones usage, extra treatment zones should be widely used, too.

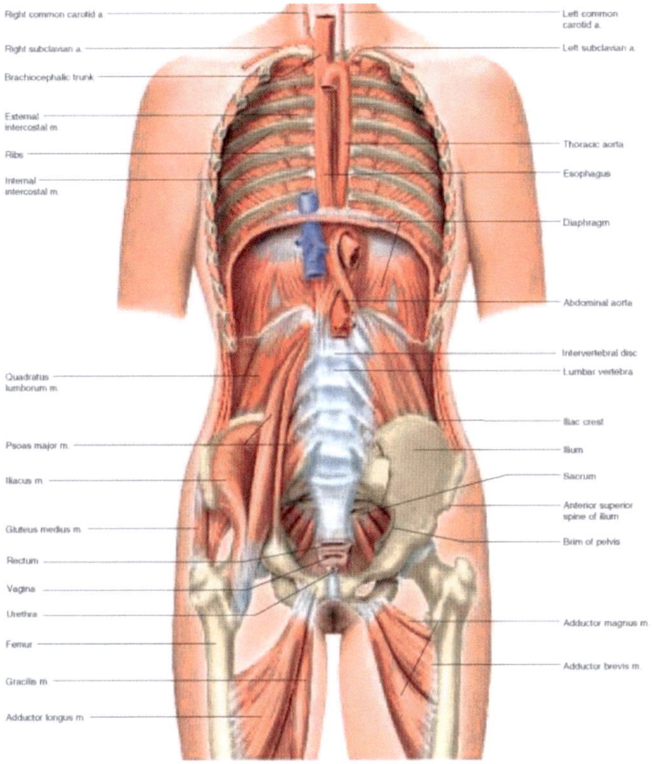

Right common carotid a.
Right subclavian a.
Brachiocephalic trunk
External intercostal m.
Ribs
Internal intercostal m.
Quadratus lumborum m.
Psoas major m.
Iliacus m.
Gluteus medius m.
Rectum
Vagina
Urethra
Femur
Gracilis m.
Adductor longus m.
Left common carotid a.
Left subclavian a.
Thoracic aorta
Esophagus
Diaphragm
Abdominal aorta
Intervertebral disc
Lumbar vertebra
Iliac crest
Ilium
Sacrum
Anterior superior spine of ilium
Brim of pelvis
Adductor magnus m.
Adductor brevis m.

Reflexogenic zones, i.e. the body regions with a certain reflex caused by adequate receptors stimulation. **Reflexogenic zones** take an active part in the regulation of the body's vital functions and allow the use of various effects on them for treatment purposes. Projection zones, i.e. the zones projected by internal organs, blood and lymphatic vessels, nerves and nerve plexuses. Anatomic regions receive their names depending on their disposition on the human body, and there are a lot of them. Special attention should be paid to the distal parts of extremities taking into account their abundant neurotropic innervation as well as the fact that the majority of meridians (energy channels) are originating and ending over there.

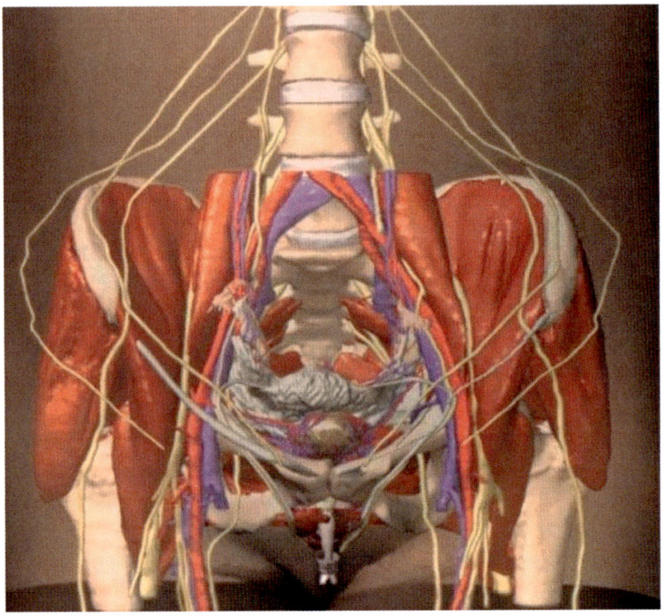

Zakharyin-Ghed zones, i.e. the zones that are closely bound up with various internal organs, but their dispositions do not coincide with the projections of these organs. Segmental zones play an important role in the innervation of various organs and systems and so they may be used for various diseases. Effect upon the skin is followed by functional changes in organs and tissues which belong to the same segment of a spinal cord to which effected skin surface belongs, too. Changes of vessels' tone, muscles, secretive and motor activity of organs take place at the same time, as far as microcirculation and cell metabolism of tissues and organs are changing, too.

General treatment zones

While using SCENAR-devices for many years specialists have come to conclusion that the five zones of general reflex application have to be necessarily marked. The given zones may be used for any pathology.

Facial Nerve (VII): Schema

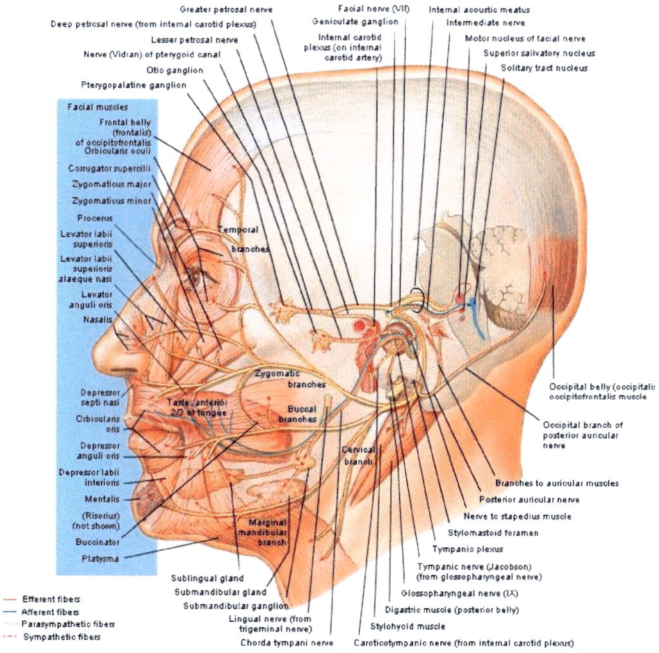

Greater petrosal nerve
Deep petrosal nerve (from internal carotid plexus)
Lesser petrosal nerve
Nerve (Vidian) of pterygoid canal
Otic ganglion
Pterygopalatine ganglion
Facial nerve (VII)
Geniculate ganglion
Internal carotid plexus (on internal carotid artery)
Internal acoustic meatus
Intermediate nerve
Motor nucleus of facial nerve
Superior salivatory nucleus
Solitary tract nucleus
Facial muscles
Frontal belly (frontalis) of occipitofrontalis
Orbicularis oculi
Corrugator supercilii
Zygomaticus major
Zygomaticus minor
Procerus
Levator labii superioris
Levator labii superioris alaeque nasi
Levator anguli oris
Nasalis
Depressor septi nasi
Orbicularis oris
Depressor anguli oris
Depressor labii inferioris
Mentalis
(Risorius) (not shown)
Buccinator
Platysma
Temporal branches
Zygomatic branches
Taste: anterior 2/3 of tongue
Buccal branches
Cervical branch
Marginal mandibular branch
Occipital branch of posterior auricular nerve
Branches to auricular muscles
Posterior auricular nerve
Nerve to stapedius muscle
Stylomastoid foramen
Tympanic plexus
Tympanic nerve (Jacobson) (from glossopharyngeal nerve)
Glossopharyngeal nerve (IX)
Digastric muscle (posterior belly)
Stylohyoid muscle
Caroticotympanic nerve (from internal carotid plexus)
Chorda tympani nerve
Lingual nerve (from trigeminal nerve)
Submandibular ganglion
Submandibular gland
Sublingual gland
Efferent fibers
Afferent fibers
Parasympathetic fibers
Sympathetic fibers

Treatment methods are as follows:

- **Pain location;**
- **Circular segment treatment on a claimed complaint level,**

- **Follow-the-pain treatment;**
- **Distal parts of extremities treatment method;**
- **Pirogov's ring treatment method;**
- **Cross-treatment method.**

Pain location treatment method. Pain location and its borders have to be determined at first. Then treatment effect is carried out by applying the device to the local skin area or by making massage movements in continuous treatment mode. Effective treatment duration is defined by the state-of-health improvement or pain relief.

Circular segment treatment method on the claimed complaint level. The skin should be treated beginning with the backbone's spinous processes at the level of the sick organ disposition towards its upright projection followed by the organ's projection treatment and then again towards the backbone, thus ending the circle.

"Follow-the-pain" method, i.e. device treatment over the area of the painful sensations symptom or discomfort phenomena as well as over a sick organ (liver, gall-bladder, etc.). These areas may be treated in continuous treatment mode by applying the device to a local skin area or by making massage motions. If painful sensations are not caused by calculus motion (urolithiasis, cholelithic disease), then individually dosed treatment mode is used. If there is a pain translocation, the device should be Trans located in the same direction. It will take about 15 – 40 minutes to get some positive effect (state-of-health improvement, pains relief).

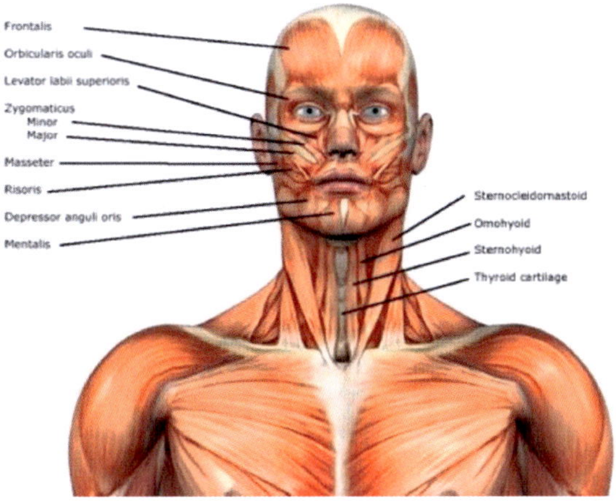
Frontalis
Orbicularis oculi
Levator labii superioris
Zygomaticus
Minor
Major
Masseter
Risoris
Depressor anguli oris
Mentalis
Sternocleidomastoid
Omohyoid
Sternohyoid
Thyroid cartilage

Distal parts of extremities treatment method. The skin of hands and feet should be treated "gloves" and "socks" likewise. There are energy channels and the main microcirculatory bed originating and ending on hands and feet. Treatment should be initiated with the palmar surface of the left hand beginning with the little finger first and ending with the thumb, then continued with the palm and then transferred to the back of the hand which should be treated using same-as-above procedure sequence. Feet are treated in the same order as hands.

Cross-treatment method. It is applied in cases of pathologies accompanied with paresis and paralyses (insult, for example). Treatment should be initiated with a healthy arm followed by a sick leg, while next procedure should be done vice versa, i.e. a healthy leg - sick arm. Device treatment should be aimed at getting muscular fascicles contraction by means of energy level selection (the higher is the energy level, the higher will be the muscle contraction rate).

Zones of general reflex treatment are parts of the skin which stimulation results in simultaneous and successive activation of body functions and systems. In case of patient complaint variety and complexity of their differentiation the course of therapy should be started with general reflex zones.

Facial Nerve Branches and Parotid Gland in Situ

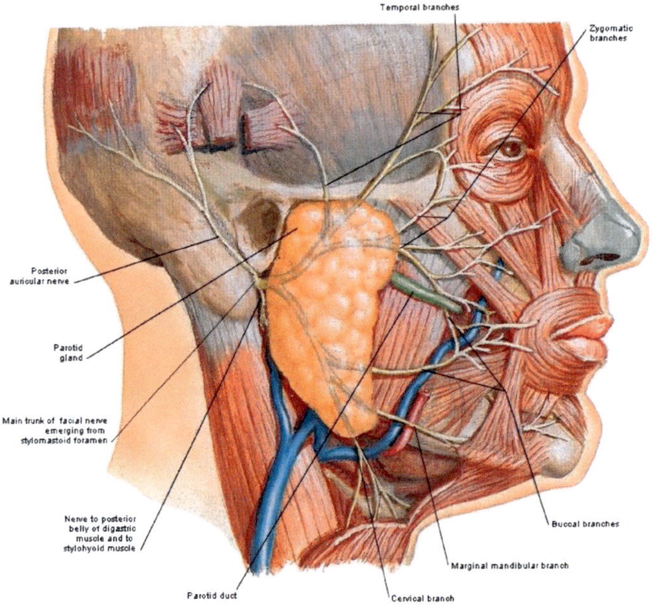

Temporal branches
Zygomatic branches
Posterior auricular nerve
Parotid gland
Main trunk of facial nerve emerging from stylomastoid foramen
Nerve to posterior belly of digastric muscle and to stylohyoid muscle
Parotid duct
Cervical branch
Marginal mandibular branch
Buccal branches

occipital region

part of the forehead between eyes ("the third eye")

projection of frontal sinus

projection of maxillary sinus

nostrils and bridge of the nose

facial exit points of trigeminal (eyebrows medial line, next to bridge of the nose, outside mouth angle)

cervical zone;

region of the 7-th & 8-th cervical vertebra;

paravertebral zones to the left & to the right of vertebral column

scapula region

region over thoracic vertebra

lumbosacral segment of the spine

outward area of forearm;

region of left elbow joint

region of liver and pancreas (treated in the presence of marked intoxication)

adrenal region (treated if patient is calm and not in excited state)

front surface of thigh lower third

surface of sural muscle

front and outer surface of the shank

Front and outer surface of feet

Place the electrode on the area under investigation.

Remain in skin contact without moving.

Measure the Initial Reaction (IR) and compare measurements

Look for highest of the initial reactions

Replace the Machine on the area with the highest IR number and treat until the light and audio signal comes ON, Hold still for 3 seconds before removing from skin. This is called a Dose (Dose 1).

Compare areas that have had a Dose (Dose 1). The one with the highest dose is treated again until the relative speed of the reaction becomes 0. This is also indicated with light and audio signals and is called a Zero (Dose 2), compare areas that have been taken to Zero and choose the highest to set FM.

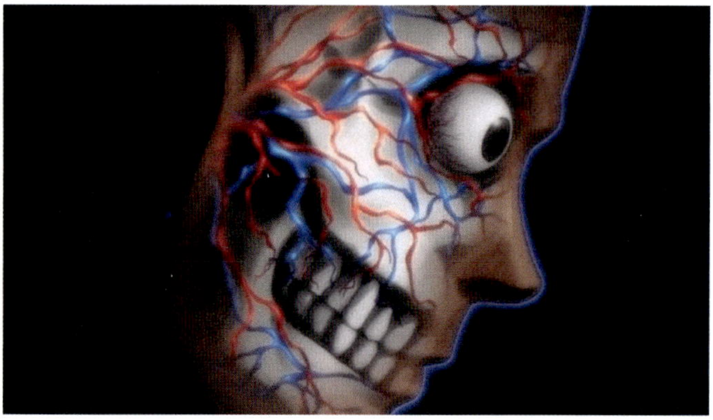

When to use:

- **To localize symptoms**
- **To save time when looking for asymmetry**

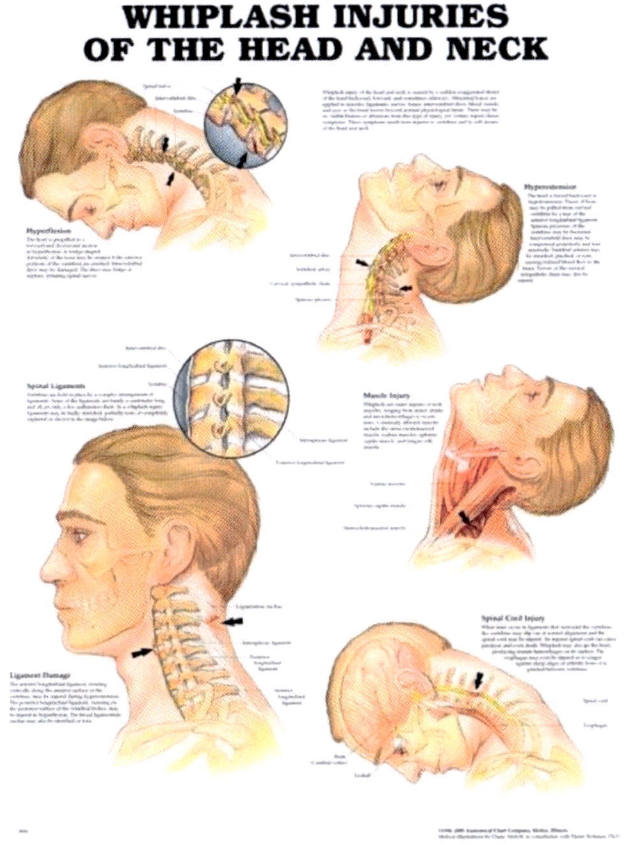
WHIPLASH INJURIES
OF THE HEAD AND NECK
Hyperflexion
Hyperextension
Spinal Ligaments
Muscle Injury
Ligament Damage
Spinal Cord Injury

- **To avoid healing crisis.**
- **To optimize the action time.**

If areas of small asymmetry have been revealed during the treatment in Subjectively Dosed (continuous, constant) mode, you may work on them again in Diagnostic (Individually Dosed) mode.

The electrode is placed lengthways at any of the general zones (normally start with Three Pathways)

When placing the electrode, do not leave gaps between positions of the electrode along the route.

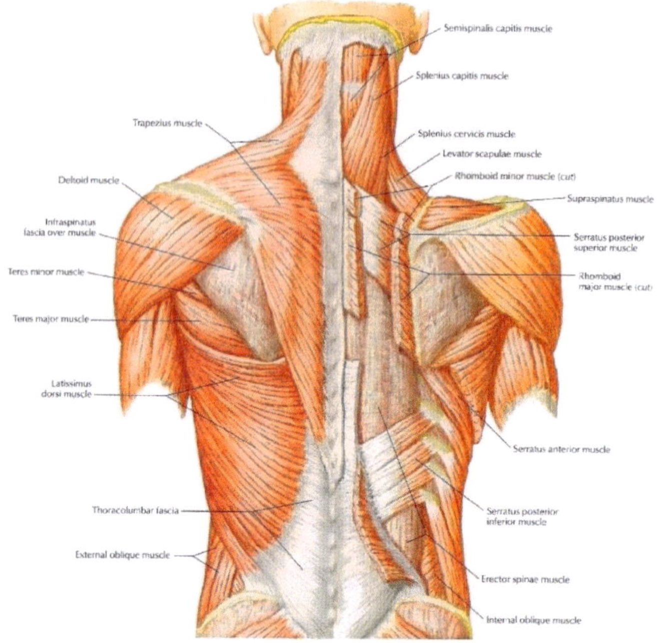
Semispinalis capitis muscle
Splenius capitis muscle
Trapezius muscle
Splenius cervicis muscle
Levator scapulae muscle
Rhomboid minor muscle (cut)
Deltoid muscle
Supraspinatus muscle
Infraspinatus fascia over muscle
Serratus posterior superior muscle
Teres minor muscle
Rhomboid major muscle (cut)
Teres major muscle
Latissimus dorsi muscle
Serratus anterior muscle
Thoracolumbar fascia
Serratus posterior inferior muscle
External oblique muscle
Erector spinae muscle
Internal oblique muscle

Before performing any diagnostic technique, place the electrode at 45 degree angle on the shoulder blade and increase the power. Choose an above-threshold power level to work with. With children, the power used can be minimum.

Before placing the device on skin and taking IR readings, ensure the screen shows 'Nobody' (in some models).

Inside a Muscle

The muscles that make your body move are linked to bones by strong tendons, made of tough material. Each muscle is made up of many cells, called fibers. When you want to move, your brain sends a message, which is carried to the muscle by nerves. Every single muscle fiber receives the message and contracts at the same time. This causes the muscle to pull on the bone it is attached to. Look inside this muscle to see more closely how this works.

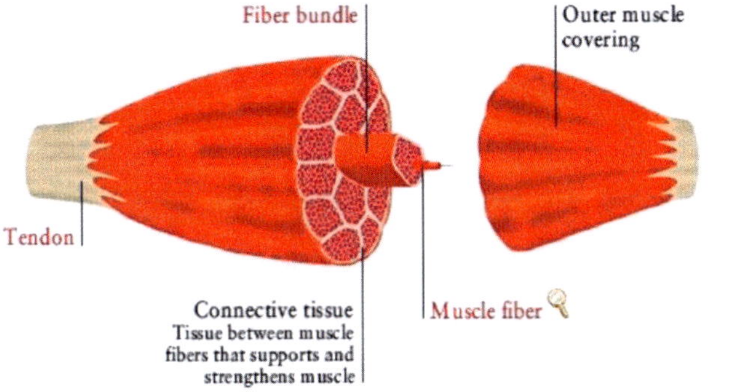

Fiber bundle
Outer muscle covering
Tendon
Connective tissue
Tissue between muscle fibers that supports and strengthens muscle
Muscle fiber

If "Nobody" is displayed on screen for 5-6 sec, provided the device is in good skin contact, take it off the skin, register this point as "N" and move on.

If you are treating to dose and the screen reads "Nobody", wait until the device switches itself off or until it starts reading the body reaction.

Fiber Bundle

YOUR MUSCLE FIBERS can measure as much as 12 inches (30 cm) in length. They run along the muscle in parallel bundles. Each bundle is encased in a tough connective tissue, which supports and reinforces the muscle. Connective tissue is also wrapped around the whole muscle. A further layer of tissue, with a much finer texture, surrounds each separate fiber.

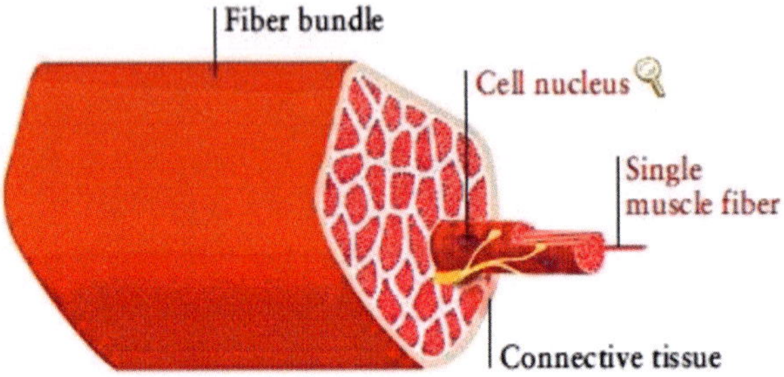
Fiber bundle
Cell nucleus
Single muscle fiber
Connective tissue

If "**Nobody**" appears three times subsequently on the route, place the electrode on each position again and wait until the device switches itself off or wait for a Dose (Dose 1).

Minimum action time is essential when taking **Initial Reaction** (IR) readings, i.e., remove the electrode from the skin as soon as the first two numbers have appeared on the display.

Inside a Nerve

INDIVIDUAL NERVE FIBERS, or axons, are held together in parallel bundles. Each fiber carries nerve impulses from the nucleus of a nerve cell. Most have a white outer layer, called myelin, that allows impulses to travel quickly. Each fiber bundle is held together by a protective sheath, and joins with other bundles to form a nerve.

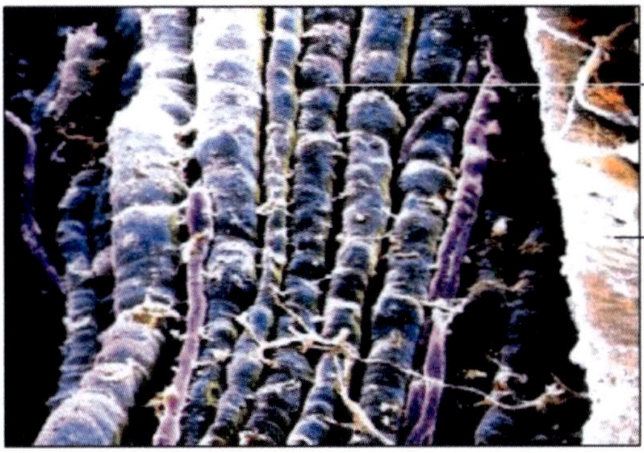

Nerve fiber (axon)
Outer sheath of bundle

Compare IR measurements to give a Dose (Dose 1) with the difference of +4 or greater on the Vertical and +1 or greater on the Horizontal.

Note: For the first dose, the IR should be +4 (more or less) or greater than the following (preceding) IR. After this, any IR higher by 4 or greater should only be dosed.

Compare Doses and Zeros (Doses 1 & 2) with the difference of +1 or greater.

On the last point of the route we always dose.

If you wait for a Zero (Dose 2) longer than two minutes, you can leave this position and move on.

X-Ray of the Spine

An X-RAY of the spine, or backbone, shows that it is made up of lots of small bones called vertebrae (one is called a vertebra.) Between pairs of vertebrae are thick disks make of a tough, flexible material called cartilage, which enable you to bend your spine. The bony processes that project from the sides of the vertebrae are just visible in this image.

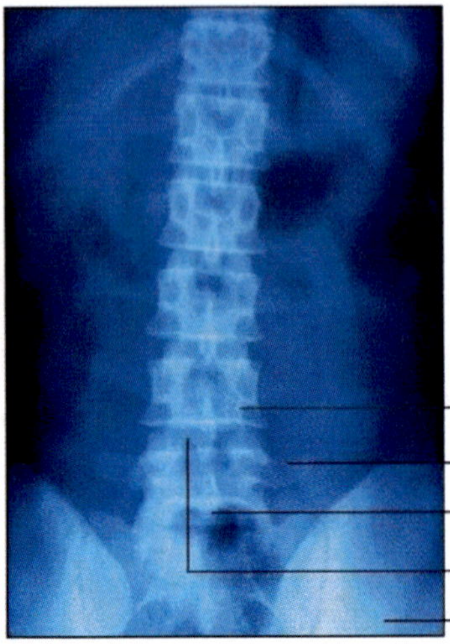
Vertebra
Bony process
Spine
Disk between vertebrae
Pelvis

If the speed of reaction does not change for two minutes, stop treating this position and move on.

Chapter 10. Three Pathways

The **first path** passes along the **spinal column** from the second cervical vertebra to the coccyx inclusive. Initiate it's treatment from the lower edge of the seventh cervical vertebra and shift the device along the spinous processes downward to the coccyx, and then from the second to the seventh cervical vertebrae inclusive.

The **second and third paths** are located **paravertebrally**, some 3-5cm to the left (2nd path) and to the right (3rd path) from the spinal median. Treat them by alternately applying device to the symmetrical areas: first of the 2nd path, then of the 3-rd one, again of the 2nd path, and so on, beginning from the lower edge of the seventh cervical vertebra till the coccyx.

Be aware of correct position of the device electrodes during treatment: their longer sides should be parallel to the spinal median.

INSIDE A CELL

YOUR BODY is made up of billions of microscopic cells. There are lots of different types of cell, but they all have a similar basic structure. The nucleus governs the cell, controlling all its activities. The cell membrane is the thin outer layer that surrounds and protects the cell. The liquid cytoplasm contains an array of specialized cell structures that each have their own function. All these parts work together to maintain the living cell.

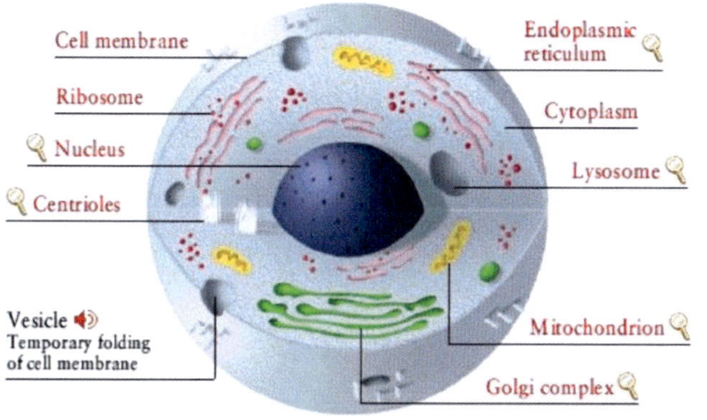
Cell membrane
Ribosome
Nucleus
Centrioles
Vesicle
Temporary folding of cell membrane
Endoplasmic reticulum
Cytoplasm
Lysosome
Mitochondrion
Golgi complex

SCENAR application to the **Three Pathways** activates trophic influence of the vegetative nervous system, restores dysfunction of the spinal inhibition system, stimulates hormones production, activates metabolism in tissues, improves excitability and conductivity of the nervous fibers.

SCENAR application to any segment of the spinal cord intensifies blood flow and improves metabolism in the entire body due to the reflex character of regulation improvement of the blood flow and metabolism thanks to effect of SCENAR on a segment of the spinal column takes place in all areas of the body, enervated from the given segment.

SINGLE MUSCLE FIBER

EACH SINGLE MUSCLE FIBER contains a bundle of tiny, banded rods called fibrils. The bands on these fibrils give this type of muscle another name: "striped muscle". When the muscle fiber receives a signal from the brain (sent through the nervous system) its fibrils contract all together, making the fiber shorter. This, in turn, causes the pulling action of the whole muscle on the bone.

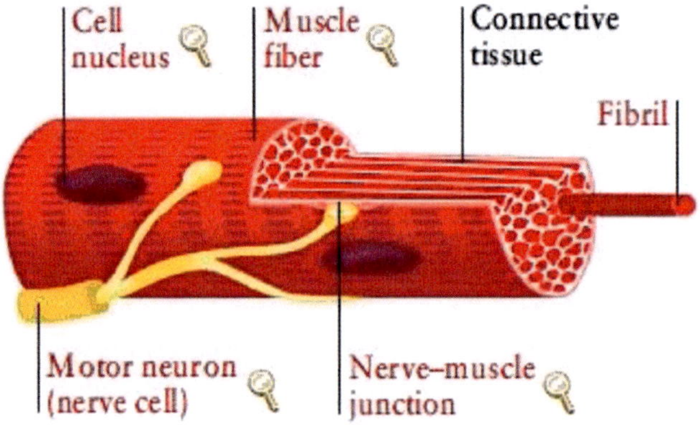

Cell nucleus
Muscle fiber
Connective tissue
Fibril
Motor neuron (nerve cell)
Nerve–muscle junction

The **frequency** is constant, 60 or 90 Hz, comfortable stimulation. A comfortable threshold of stimulation should be selected near the zone to be treated. One of the patterns of moving the electrode along the lines is given in the explaining scheme.

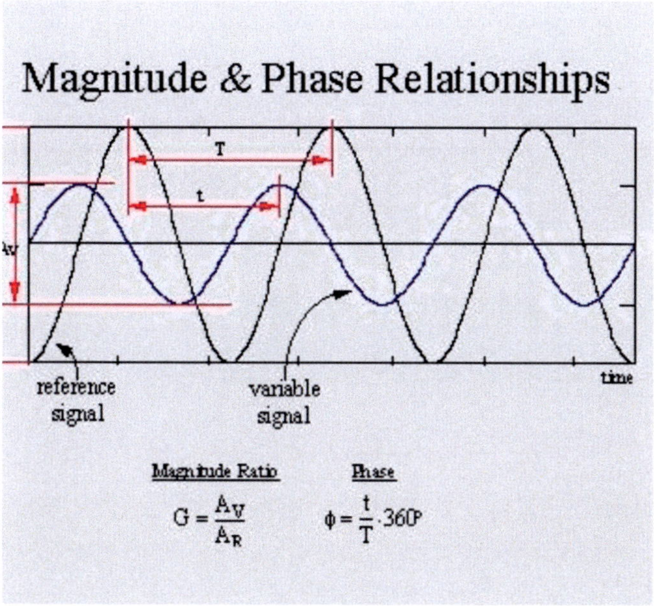
Magnitude & Phase Relationships
T
t
Av
reference
signal
variable
signal
time
Magnitude Ratio
Phase
G = Av / AR
ϕ = t / T · 360°

Put the device below the **spinous process** of the VII cervical vertebra; locate the longer part of the electrode along the body (cephalocaudal) axis.

Do not take the electrode away until light-sound dose signal.

Move the electrode down along the backbone (along the arrow direction) for one length of the electrode.

After each dose signal move the device down along the backbone till the skin fold.

Put the electrode to the hair border along the medium line and treat the cervical part of the backbone (1-2 positions) in the same way.

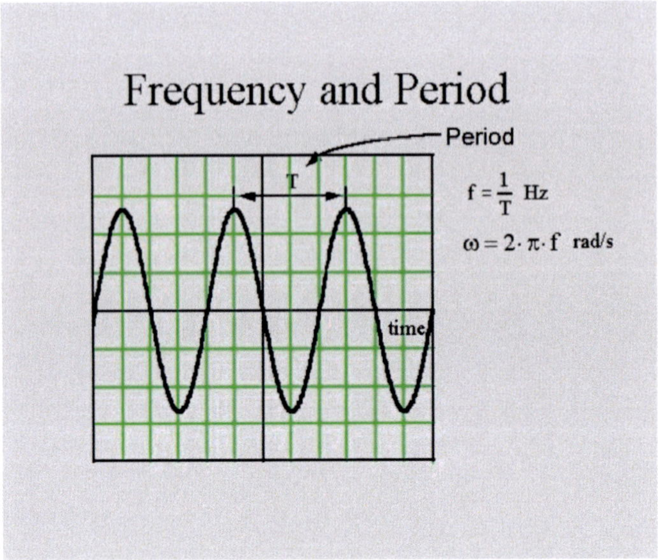
Frequency and Period
Period
T
time
$f = \frac{1}{T}$ Hz
$\omega = 2 \cdot \pi \cdot f$ rad/s

Return to the beginning of the thoracic part and put the device on the paravertebral line (to the left from the backbone) on the level of the spinous process of the VII cervical vertebra.

The first path passes along the spinal column from the second cervical vertebra to the coccyx inclusive. Initiate its treatment from the lower edge of the seventh cervical vertebra and shift the device along the spinous processes downward to the coccyx, and then from the second to the seventh cervical vertebrae inclusive.

The second and third paths are located paravertebral, some 3-5cm to the left (2nd path) and to the right (3rd path) from the spinal median. Treat them by alternately applying device to the symmetrical areas: first of the 2nd path, then of the 3rd one, again of the 2nd path, and so on, beginning from the lower edge of the seventh cervical vertebra till the **coccyx**. Be aware of correct position of the device electrodes during treatment: their longer sides should be parallel to the spinal median. SCENAR application to the "Three paths" activates trophic influence of the vegetative nervous system, restores dysfunction of the spinal inhibition system, stimulates hormones production, activates metabolism in tissues, and improves excitability and conductivity of the nervous fibers. SCENAR application to any segment of the spinal cord intensifies blood flow and improves metabolism in the entire body Due to the reflex character of regulation improvement of the blood flow and metabolism thanks to effect of SCENAR on a segment of the spinal column takes place in all areas of the body, innervated from the given segment.

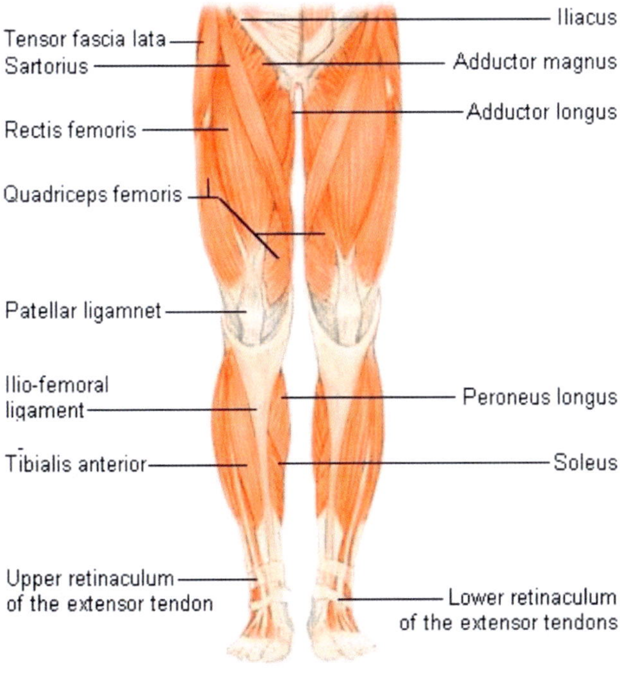
Iliacus
Tensor fascia lata
Sartorius
Adductor magnus
Adductor longus
Rectis femoris
Quadriceps femoris
Patellar ligamnet
Ilio-femoral ligament
Peroneus longus
Tibialis anterior
Soleus
Upper retinaculum of the extensor tendon
Lower retinaculum of the extensor tendons

After dose signals put the device on the symmetrical zone on the other side of the backbone (according to the scheme).

Treat all the zones of thoracic, lumbar and sacral parts in the same way.

Be aware of correct position of the device electrodes during treatment: their longer sides should be parallel to the spinal median.

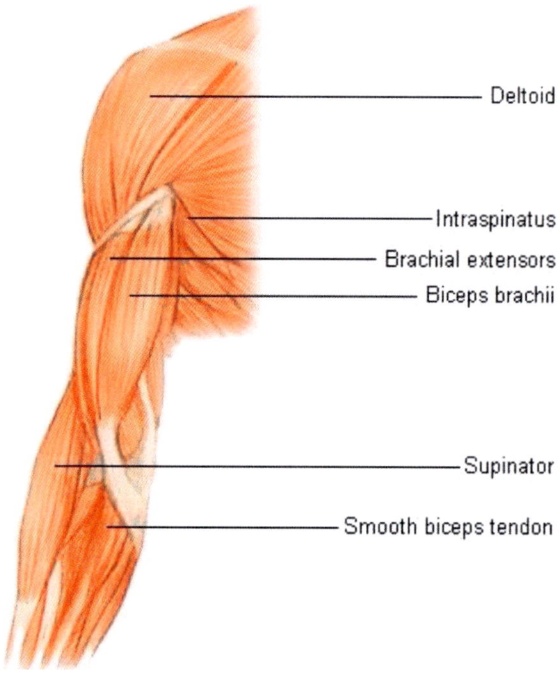
Deltoid
Intraspinatus
Brachial extensors
Biceps brachii
Supinator
Smooth biceps tendon

SCENAR application to the "Three paths" activates trophic influence of the vegetative nervous system, restores dysfunction of the spinal inhibition system, stimulates hormones production, activates metabolism in tissues, and improves excitability and conductivity of the nervous fibers.

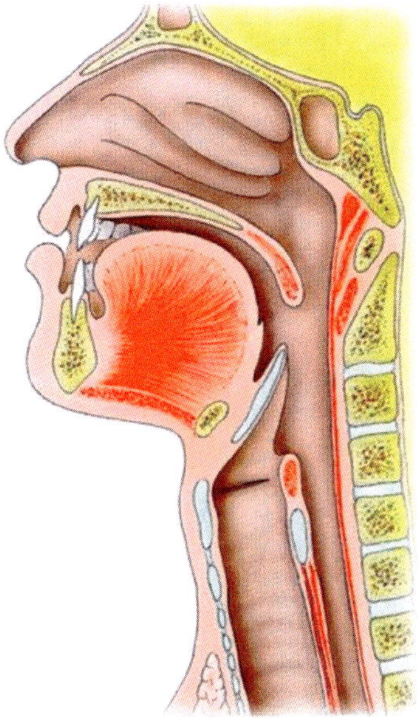

SCENAR application to any segment of the spinal cord intensifies blood flow and improves metabolism in the entire body due to the reflex character of regulation improvement of the blood flow and metabolism, thanks to the effect that SCENAR on a segment of the spinal column takes place in all areas of the body, enervated from the given segment.

Chapter 11.
Six Points

The treatment algorithm of the trigeminal nerve's outlets is carried out in the following way: initiate treatment with the left upper point, then proceed with symmetric point to the right, then midpoint to the left followed by symmetric point to the right. Next is the left lower point to the left followed by symmetric one to the right. By affecting the ending points of one of the 12-paired craniocerebral nerves, we thereby dispatch neuropulses throughout the tregeminal nerve fibers directly to the Central Nervous System.

Solar plexus zone - located at stomach projection region. This is a roundish zone of about 10 mm in diameter.

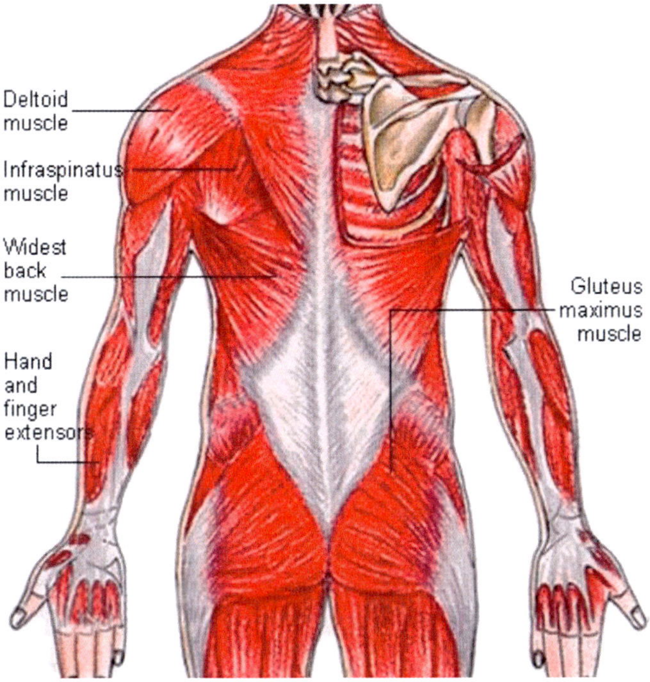
Deltoid
muscle
Infraspinatus
muscle
Widest
back
muscle
Hand
and
finger
extensors
Gluteus
maximus
muscle

Sinocarotid node zone - is located at the carotid and sternocleidomastoid muscle intersection on the front surface of a neck. There are two such zones (left and right).

Cutaneous Nerves of Head and Neck

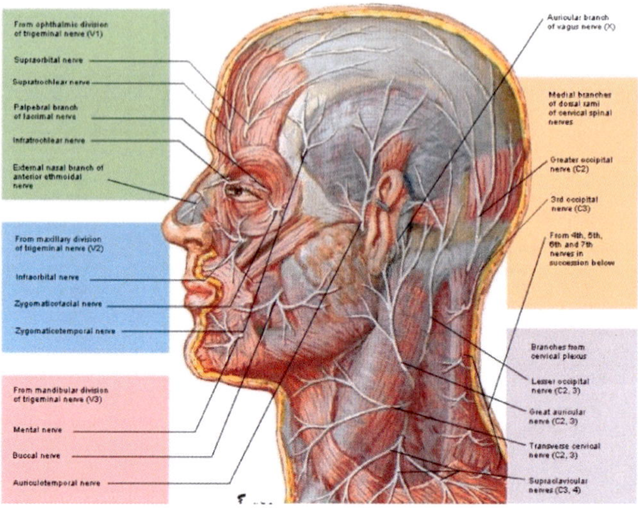
From ophthalmic division of trigeminal nerve (V1)
Supraorbital nerve
Supratrochlear nerve
Palpebral branch of lacrimal nerve
Infratrochlear nerve
External nasal branch of anterior ethmoidal nerve
From maxillary division of trigeminal nerve (V2)
Infraorbital nerve
Zygomaticofacial nerve
Zygomaticotemporal nerve
From mandibular division of trigeminal nerve (V3)
Mental nerve
Buccal nerve
Auriculotemporal nerve
Auricular branch of vagus nerve (X)
Medial branches of dorsal rami of cervical spinal nerves
Greater occipital nerve (C2)
3rd occipital nerve (C3)
From 4th, 5th, 6th and 7th nerves in succession below
Branches from cervical plexus
Lesser occipital nerve (C2, 3)
Great auricular nerve (C2, 3)
Transverse cervical nerve (C2, 3)
Supraclavicular nerves (C3, 4)

They are one of the smallest zones in their size, have a round form, and each are up to 2cm in diameter.

The points are the outputs of the tri-facial nerve branches.

The points are located on the face as follows:

The first pair is located in the area of the eyebrows close to the bridge of the nose.

The second pair is located on the outskirts of the wings of the nostrils.

The third pair is located slightly lower than the mouth angles.

The operation is performed in the metered mode, while moving the probes along the horizontal line (in this order - Right eyebrow, Left eyebrow, Right outskirt, Left outskirt, Right lower mouth angle, Left lower angle) when the light and sound signals appear.

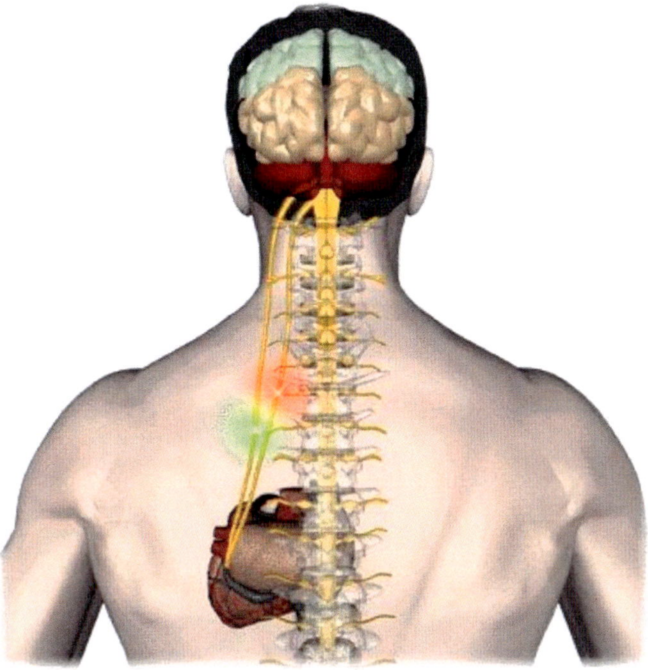

Treatment methods

- **Pain location;**
- **Circular segment treatment on a claimed complaint level,**
- **Follow-the-pain treatment;**
- **Distal parts of extremities treatment method;**
- **Pirogov's ring treatment method;**
- **Cross-treatment method.**

Specific Areas:

First branch: above the eyebrows, around the nose, at the point where the nerve leaves the cranium, internal canthus of the eye, bridge of the nose and the eyebrow area.

Second branch: at the wing of the nose, the fold between the nose and lip, above the lip, inside the mouth (use a probe).

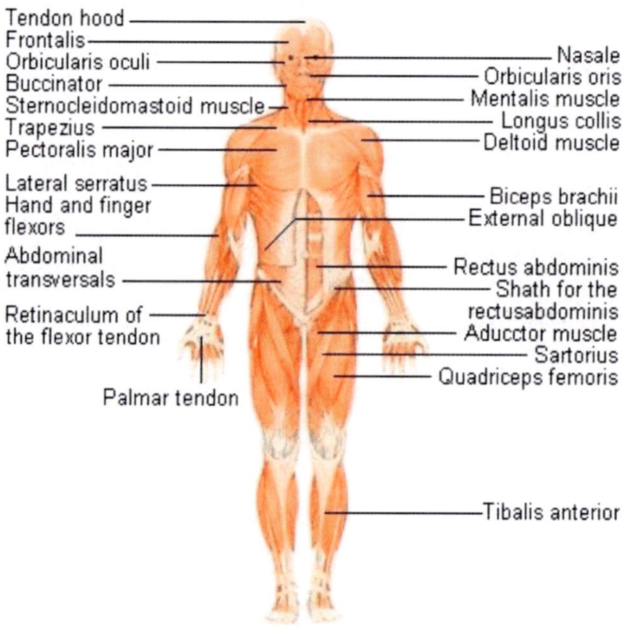
Tendon hood
Frontalis
Orbicularis oculi
Buccinator
Sternocleidomastoid muscle
Trapezius
Pectoralis major
Lateral serratus
Hand and finger flexors
Abdominal transversals
Retinaculum of the flexor tendon
Palmar tendon
Nasale
Orbicularis oris
Mentalis muscle
Longus collis
Deltoid muscle
Biceps brachii
External oblique
Rectus abdominis
Shath for the rectusabdominis
Aducctor muscle
Sartorius
Quadriceps femoris
Tibalis anterior

Third branch: at the chin where the nerve leaves the mandible, inside the mouth in the lower jaw (use a probe), underneath and behind the ear.

Chapter 12.
Pirogov's Ring

The **Pirogov's ring** is **treated on the neck beginning with spinous processes of the cervical vertebras**. The device is rearranged stepwise or moved without taking it off the skin toward the front surface of the neck and then again toward the spinous processes of the cervical vertebras, thus ending the circle. This treatment zone contains large blood vessels, lymph nodes, nerve trunks, thyroid and parathyroid glands. This zone is liable to treatment if there is a nasopharyngeal pathology (rhinitis, sinusitis, laryngitis, and tonsillitis), stomatology or brain pathologies.

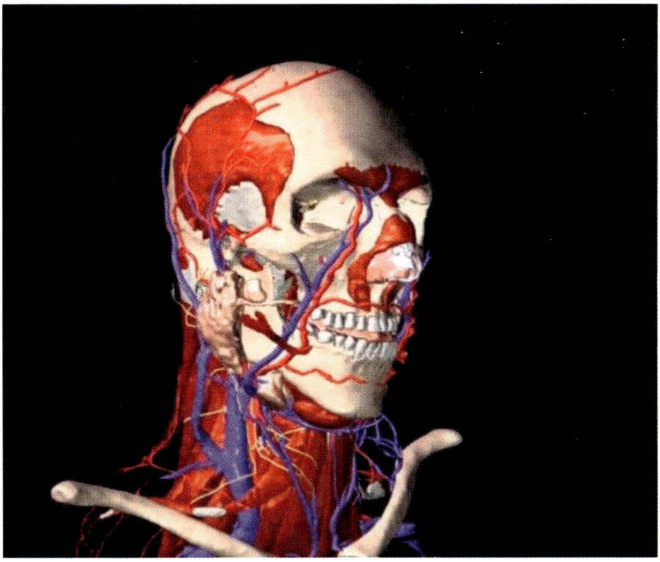

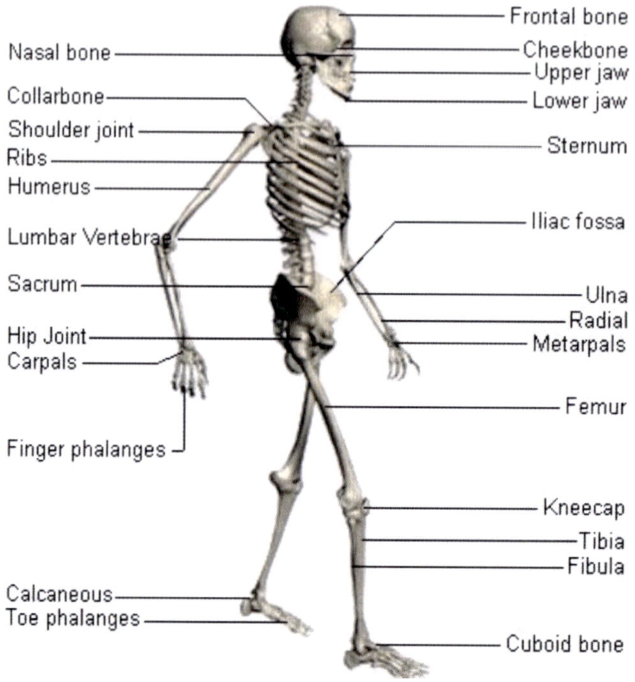
Frontal bone
Nasal bone
Cheekbone
Upper jaw
Collarbone
Lower jaw
Shoulder joint
Sternum
Ribs
Humerus
Iliac fossa
Lumbar Vertebrae
Sacrum
Ulna
Radial
Hip Joint
Metarpals
Carpals
Femur
Finger phalanges
Kneecap
Tibia
Fibula
Calcaneous
Toe phalanges
Cuboid bone

It is applied in cases of pathologies accompanied with pareses and paralyses (insult, for example). Treatment should be initiated with a healthy arm followed by a sick leg, while next procedure should be done vice versa, i.e. a healthy leg - sick arm. Device treatment should be aimed at getting muscular fascicles contraction by means of energy level selection (the higher is the energy level, the higher will be the muscle contraction rate).

Lymph Vessels and Nodes of Head and Neck

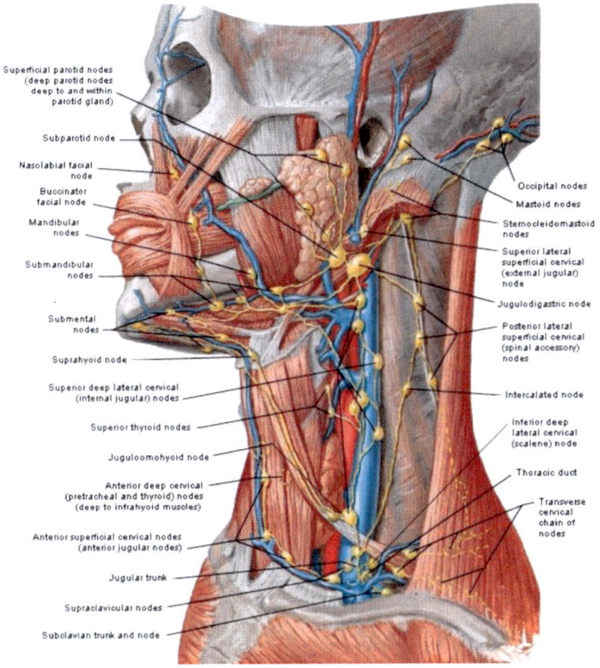

Superficial parotid nodes (deep parotid nodes deep to and within parotid gland)
Subparotid node
Nasolabial facial node
Buccinator facial node
Mandibular nodes
Submandibular nodes
Submental nodes
Suprahyoid node
Superior deep lateral cervical (internal jugular) nodes
Superior thyroid nodes
Juguloomohyoid node
Anterior deep cervical (pretracheal and thyroid) nodes (deep to infrahyoid muscles)
Anterior superficial cervical nodes (anterior jugular nodes)
Jugular trunk
Supraclavicular nodes
Subclavian trunk and node
Occipital nodes
Mastoid nodes
Sternocleidomastoid nodes
Superior lateral superficial cervical (external jugular) node
Jugulodigastric node
Posterior lateral superficial cervical (spinal accessory) nodes
Intercalated node
Inferior deep lateral cervical (scalene) node
Thoracic duct
Transverse cervical chain of nodes

Chapter 13. Treatment Protocols for Three Pathways and Six Points

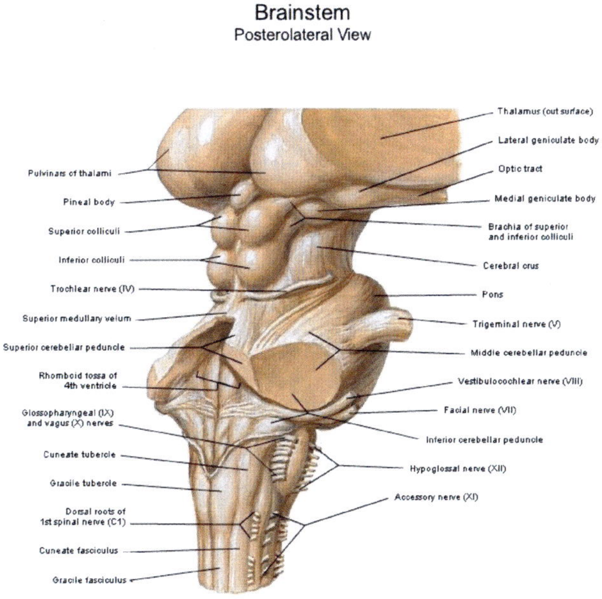
Brainstem
Posterolateral View
Thalamus (cut surface)
Lateral geniculate body
Optic tract
Medial geniculate body
Brachia of superior and inferior colliculi
Cerebral crus
Pons
Trigeminal nerve (V)
Middle cerebellar peduncle
Vestibulocochlear nerve (VIII)
Facial nerve (VII)
Inferior cerebellar peduncle
Hypoglossal nerve (XII)
Accessory nerve (XI)
Pulvinars of thalami
Pineal body
Superior colliculi
Inferior colliculi
Trochlear nerve (IV)
Superior medullary velum
Superior cerebellar peduncle
Rhomboid fossa of 4th ventricle
Glossopharyngeal (IX) and vagus (X) nerves
Cuneate tubercle
Gracile tubercle
Dorsal roots of 1st spinal nerve (C1)
Cuneate fasciculus
Gracile fasciculus

By convention, **the route starts from below C7 down the spinal column to the tip of the coccyx**, finishing up on the neck. **On the neck, go from the hairline down to C7**. Usually there is only room for one electrode length. In bald people, start from the position of the third eye (eyebrows for paravertebral route) and work to C7. Always make a dose at the last point of the route. The **electrode should be placed overlapping or abutted, down to the coccyx**. Six points on the face. The sites used are the exit points of the trigeminal nerve from the skull. Start from the left to the right (relative to the therapist). Always make a dose on the last point.

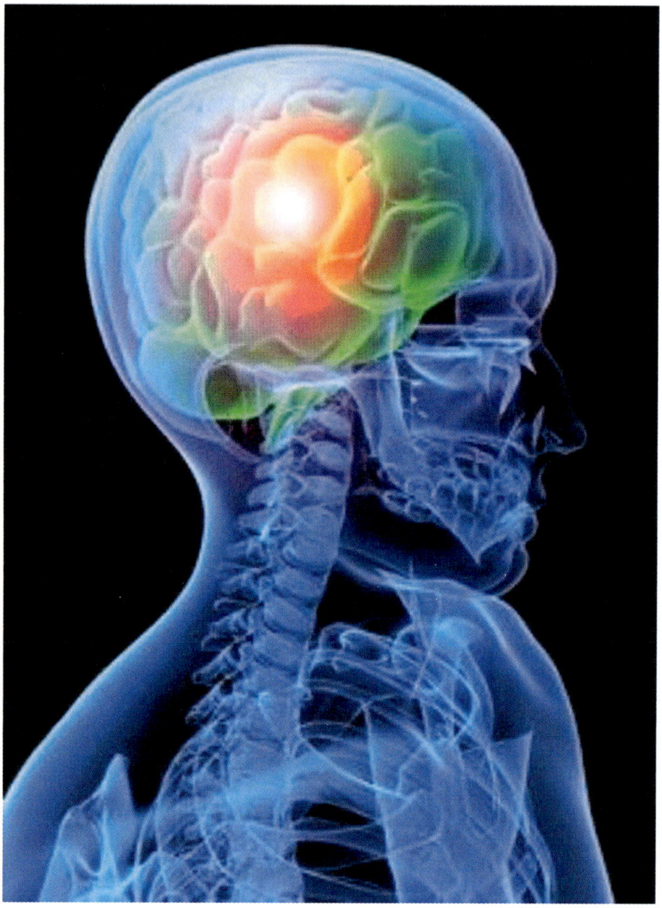

Rules in Scenar Therapy

First rule: Work according to a complaint

Second rule: Work on three pathways and six points

Third rule: Work on the horizontals and segments/dermatomes

Reciprocal principles:

- Upper/Lower
- External / internal
- Top / bottom
- Left / right
- Front/back

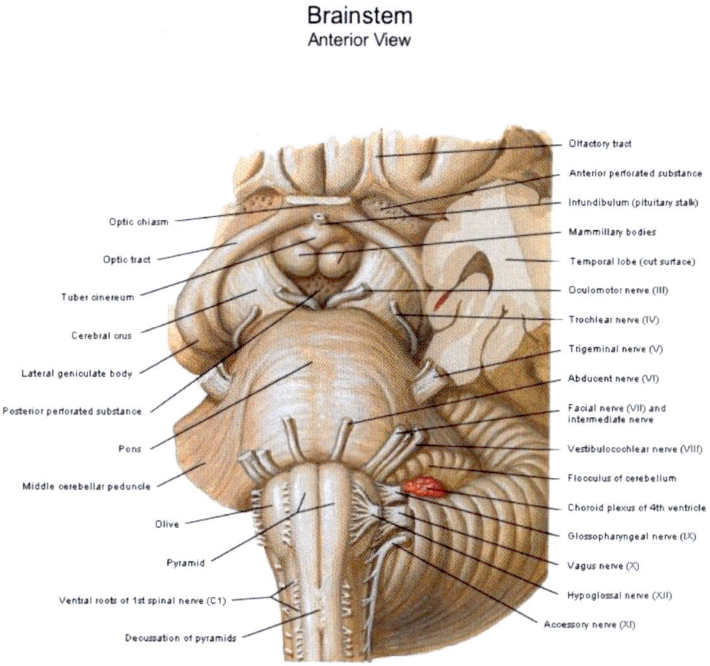
Brainstem
Anterior View
Olfactory tract
Anterior perforated substance
Infundibulum (pituitary stalk)
Mammillary bodies
Temporal lobe (cut surface)
Oculomotor nerve (III)
Trochlear nerve (IV)
Trigeminal nerve (V)
Abducent nerve (VI)
Facial nerve (VII) and intermediate nerve
Vestibulocochlear nerve (VIII)
Flocculus of cerebellum
Choroid plexus of 4th ventricle
Glossopharyngeal nerve (IX)
Vagus nerve (X)
Hypoglossal nerve (XII)
Accessory nerve (XI)
Optic chiasm
Optic tract
Tuber cinereum
Cerebral crus
Lateral geniculate body
Posterior perforated substance
Pons
Middle cerebellar peduncle
Olive
Pyramid
Ventral roots of 1st spinal nerve (C1)
Decussation of pyramids

High amplitude impulses are non-damaging.

Bio-feedback and an ever -changing input signal prevent habituation of the patient to the treatment.

Treat when the client has active complaints, at any stage of exacerbation.

Start the next course of treatment if the complaints reappear or new complaints are presented.

Results may be delayed.

A therapist develops an expertise as experience with the SCENAR increases.

There are no strict rules. The treatment can be a creative process. Be different, change the settings frequently

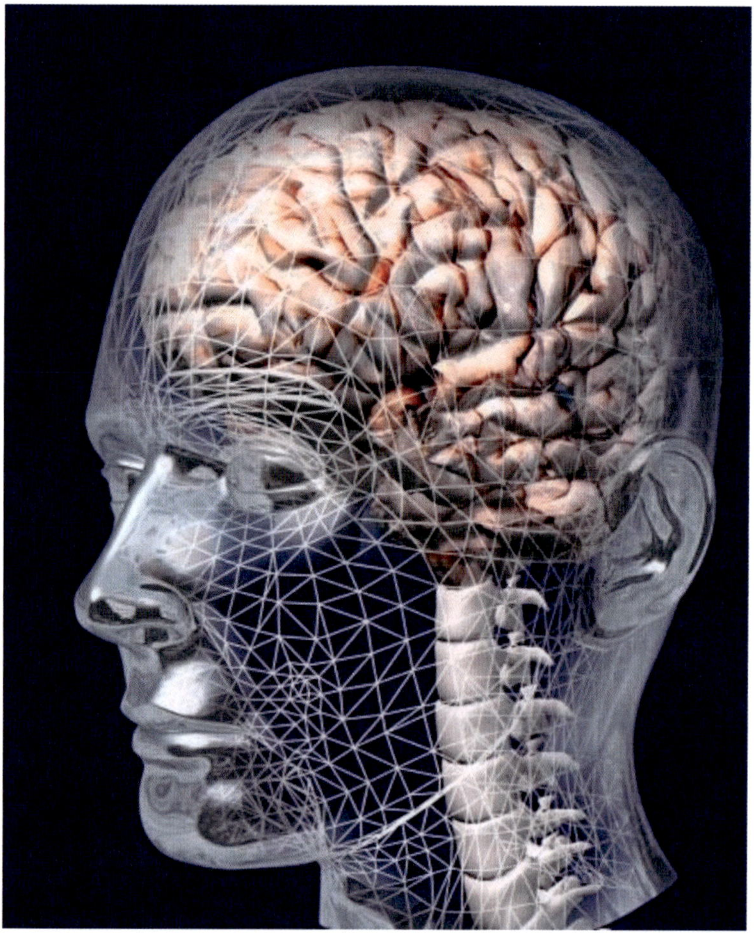

The General Rules

The electrode is placed lengthways at any of the general zones (normally start with three pathways).

When placing the electrode do not leave a gap between positions of the electrode along the route.

For diagnostic purposes, place the electrode at 45° angle on the shoulder and increase the power. Choose an above-threshold power level to work with. In children, the power used can be minimum.

Before putting the device on the skin and taking IR readings, ensure the screen shows ‘Nobody’.

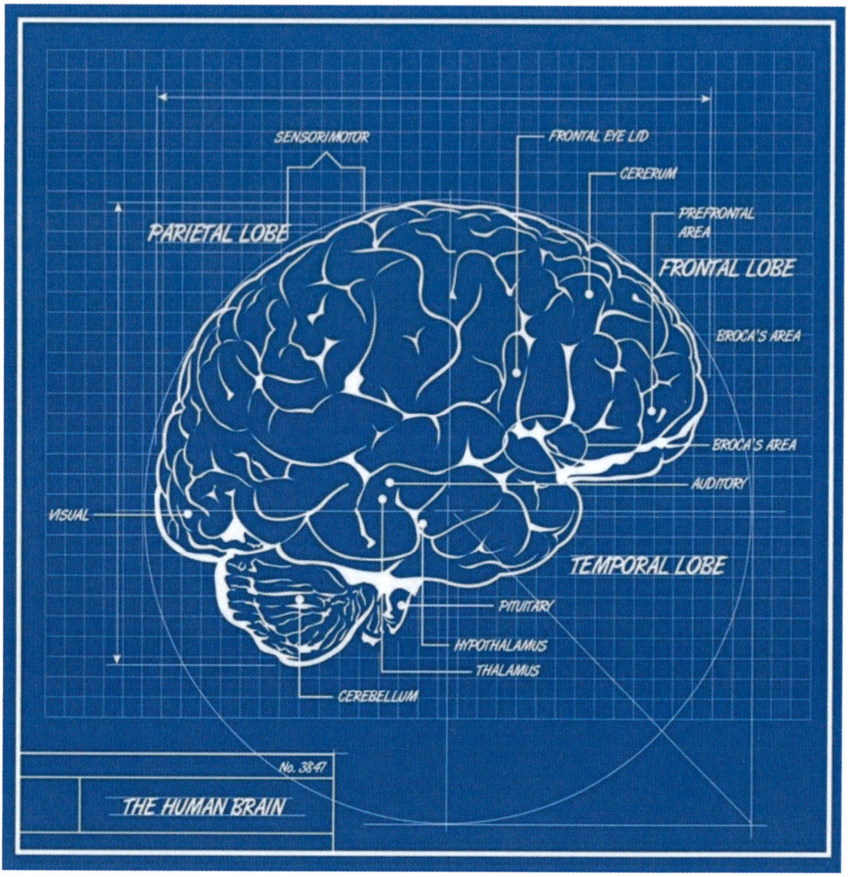
SENSORIMOTOR
FRONTAL EYE LID
CERERUM
PREFRONTAL AREA
PARIETAL LOBE
FRONTAL LOBE
BROCA'S AREA
BROCA'S AREA
AUDITORY
VISUAL
TEMPORAL LOBE
PITUITARY
HYPOTHALAMUS
THALAMUS
CEREBELLUM
No. 3847
THE HUMAN BRAIN

If "Nobody" stays on the screen for 5-6 sec when the device is in contact with the skin, take the device off the skin and move on.

Minimum action time is essential when taking Initial Reaction (IR) readings, i.e., remove the electrode from the skin as soon as the first two numbers on the display appear, even if you have to replace the device in the same position to give a "dose" or "0".

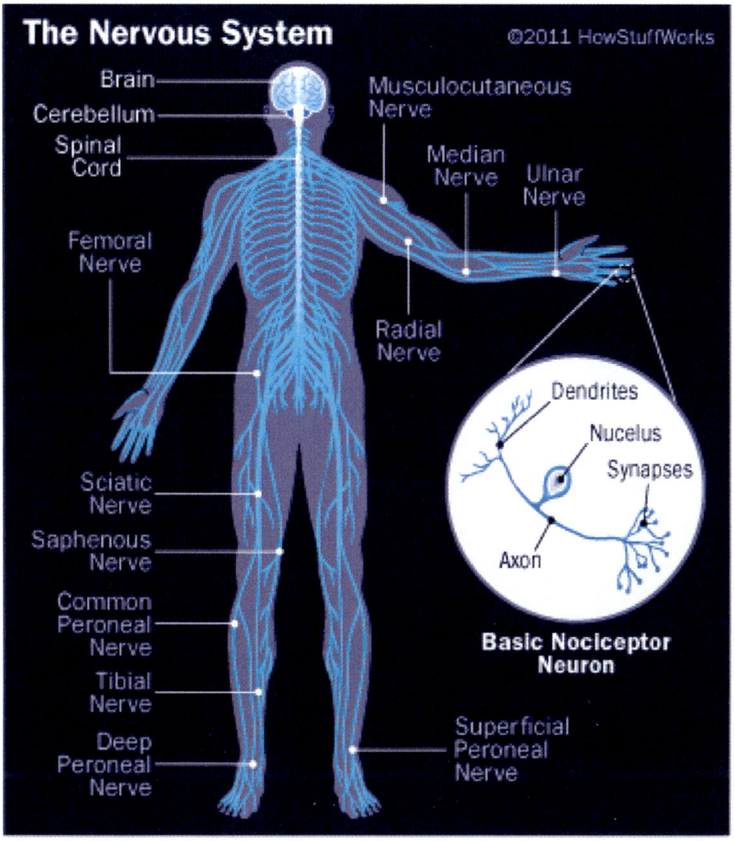

The Nervous System
©2011 HowStuffWorks
Brain
Cerebellum
Spinal Cord
Femoral Nerve
Musculocutaneous Nerve
Median Nerve
Ulnar Nerve
Radial Nerve
Dendrites
Nucelus
Synapses
Axon
Basic Nociceptor Neuron
Sciatic Nerve
Saphenous Nerve
Common Peroneal Nerve
Tibial Nerve
Deep Peroneal Nerve
Superficial Peroneal Nerve

When comparing IR's to give a dose, look for a difference of +4 or greater, when working along the vertical and +1, when working along the horizontal. When comparing doses or 0's, treat again if there is a difference of +1 or greater.

On the last point on the route only, because we usually dose, if "Nobody" appears wait for 5-6 seconds and register as "N". Then carry on. If you are awaiting for a dose take device off the skin and place it again, waiting for the dose or until the device switches itself off (30 seconds) or shows any numbers.

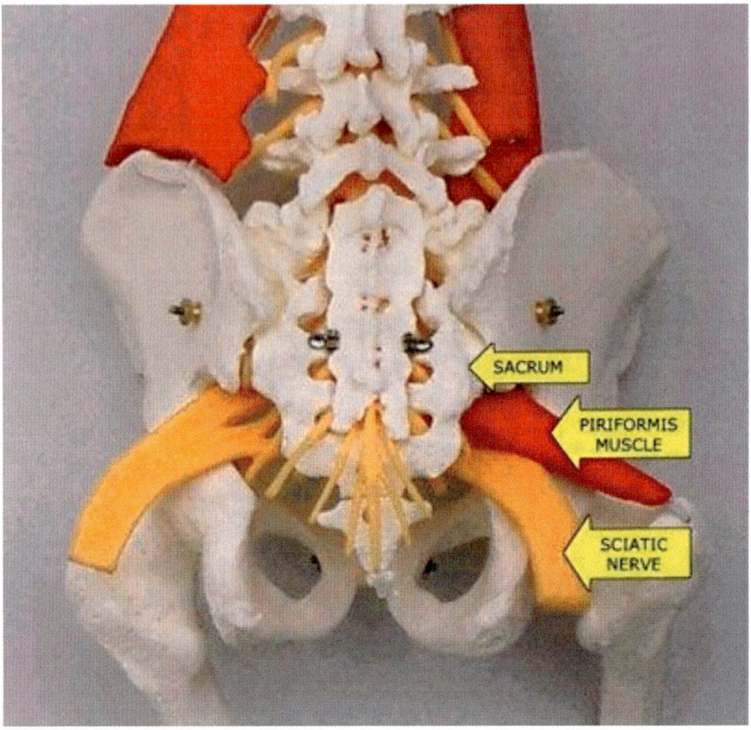
SACRUM
PIRIFORMIS MUSCLE
SCIATIC NERVE

If **"Nobody"** appears three times subsequently on the route, place the electrode on each position again and wait for another 30 seconds (until the device switches itself off again) or wait for a dose.

If you need to wait more than 2 minutes for the speed of the reaction to go down to "0", you can leave it and move on.

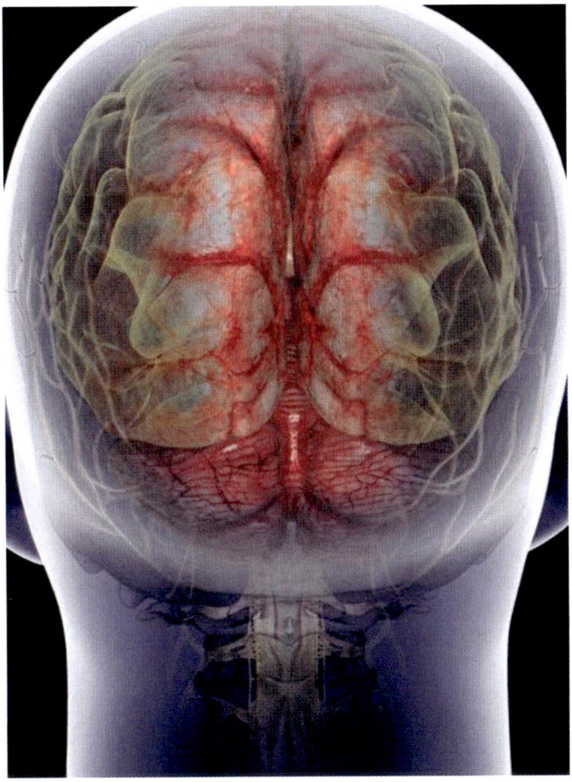

If speed of the reaction goes to 0 before the dose is given, the prognosis is good.

If the procedure is interrupted and you have to stop, you should start from the beginning again.

You should conduct the whole procedure at the same power level. If the patient cannot bear the pain from the impulse at any point during the procedure, take the electrode off the skin, reset the power and start from the beginning.

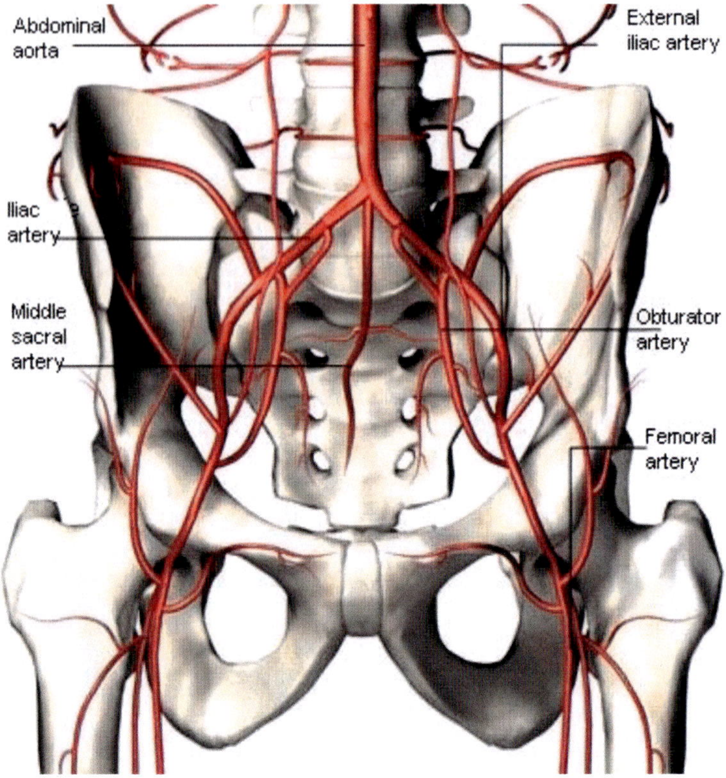
Abdominal aorta
External iliac artery
Iliac artery
Middle sacral artery
Obturator artery
Femoral artery

If speed is visible for 2 minutes you should leave and move on.

When treating zones, you should use a pen to draw zones on the patient's skin as this will reinforce the treatment effect.

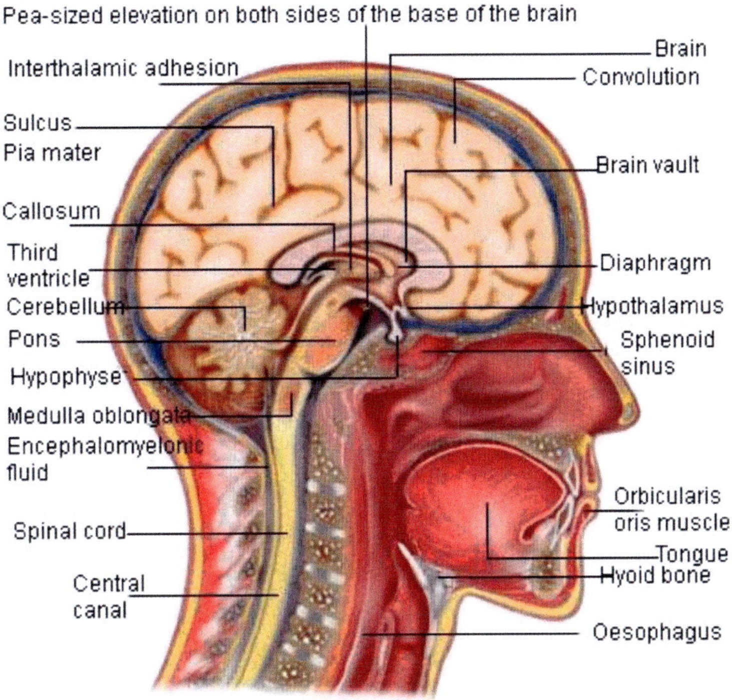
Pea-sized elevation on both sides of the base of the brain
Interthalamic adhesion
Sulcus
Pia mater
Callosum
Third ventricle
Cerebellum
Pons
Hypophyse
Medulla oblongata
Encephalomyelonic fluid
Spinal cord
Central canal
Brain
Convolution
Brain vault
Diaphragm
Hypothalamus
Sphenoid sinus
Orbicularis oris muscle
Tongue
Hyoid bone
Oesophagus

It is important to be exact in replacing the SCENAR to give a dose or set FM Var etc. Turn off the machine and use the electrode itself to measure distances. Turning it off and then back on to treat an area also reminds the organism where to put its attention.

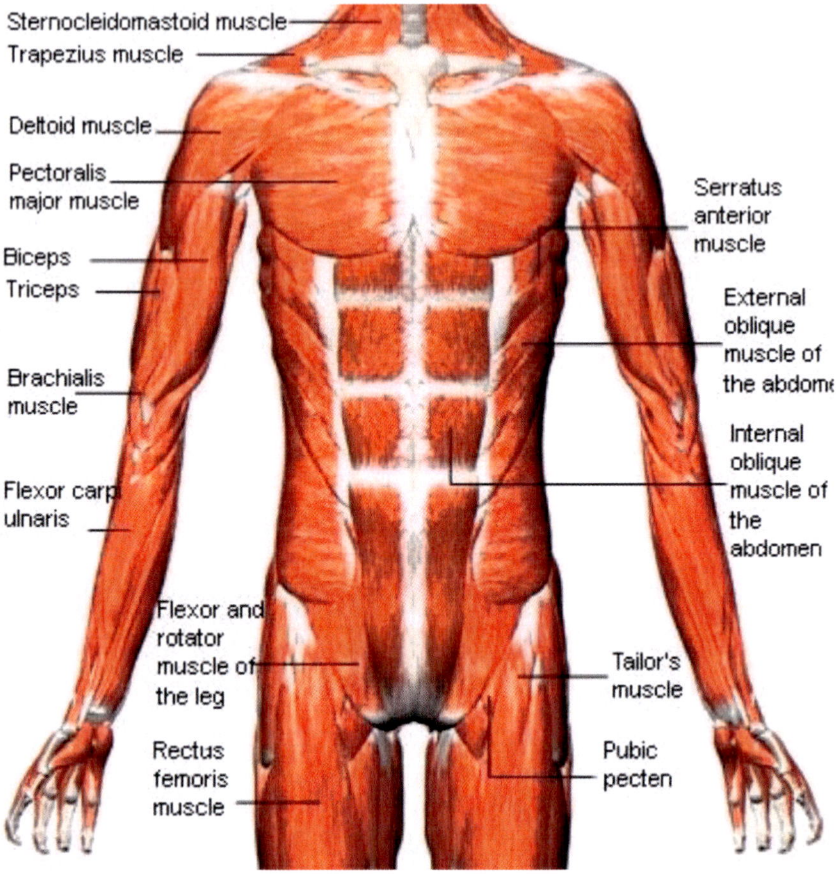
Sternocleidomastoid muscle
Trapezius muscle
Deltoid muscle
Pectoralis major muscle
Biceps
Triceps
Brachialis muscle
Flexor carpi ulnaris
Flexor and rotator muscle of the leg
Rectus femoris muscle
Serratus anterior muscle
External oblique muscle of the abdome
Internal oblique muscle of the abdomen
Tailor's muscle
Pubic pecten

If you have not set any Fm (has not formed a function) you will have to carry on treating secondary signs or asymmetry in corresponding zones in Diag 0.

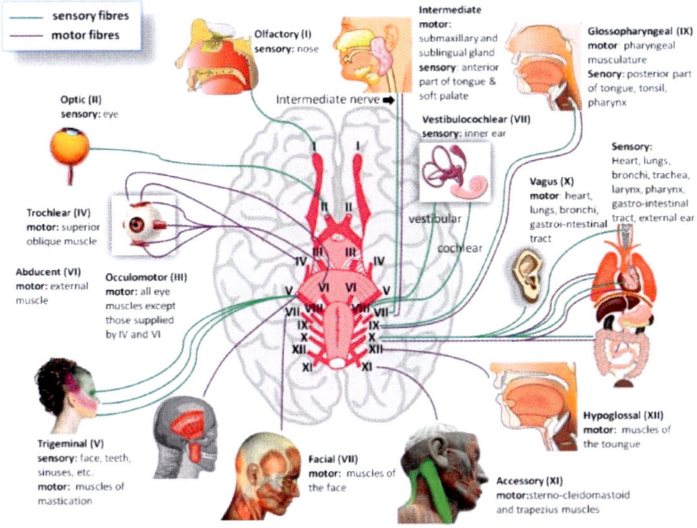
sensory fibres
motor fibres
Olfactory (I)
sensory: nose
Intermediate
motor:
submaxillary and
sublingual gland
sensory: anterior
part of tongue &
soft palate
Intermediate nerve
Glossopharyngeal (IX)
motor: pharyngeal
musculature
Senory: posterior part
of tongue, tonsil,
pharynx
Optic (II)
sensory: eye
Vestibulocochlear (VII)
sensory: inner ear
Sensory:
Heart, lungs,
bronchi, trachea,
larynx, pharynx,
gastro-intestinal
tract, external ear
Vagus (X)
motor: heart,
lungs, bronchi,
gastroi-ntestinal
tract
Trochlear (IV)
motor: superior
oblique muscle
vestibular
cochlear
Abducent (VI)
motor: external
muscle
Occulomotor (III)
motor: all eye
muscles except
those supplied
by IV and VI
I
II
III
IV
V
VI
VII
VIII
IX
X
XII
XI
Hypoglossal (XII)
motor: muscles of
the toungue
Trigeminal (V)
sensory: face, teeth,
sinuses, etc.
motor: muscles of
mastication
Facial (VII)
motor: muscles of
the face
Accessory (XI)
motor:sterno-cleidomastoid
and trapezius muscles

The neck is defined as the region from the hairline down to C7 level. In patients with a long neck it will be possible to take IR readings from 2 vertical positions, starting from the level of eyes on the forehead. In patients with a shaved skull, start IR readings from the point PC3 (third eye) all the way over the skull and down to C7.

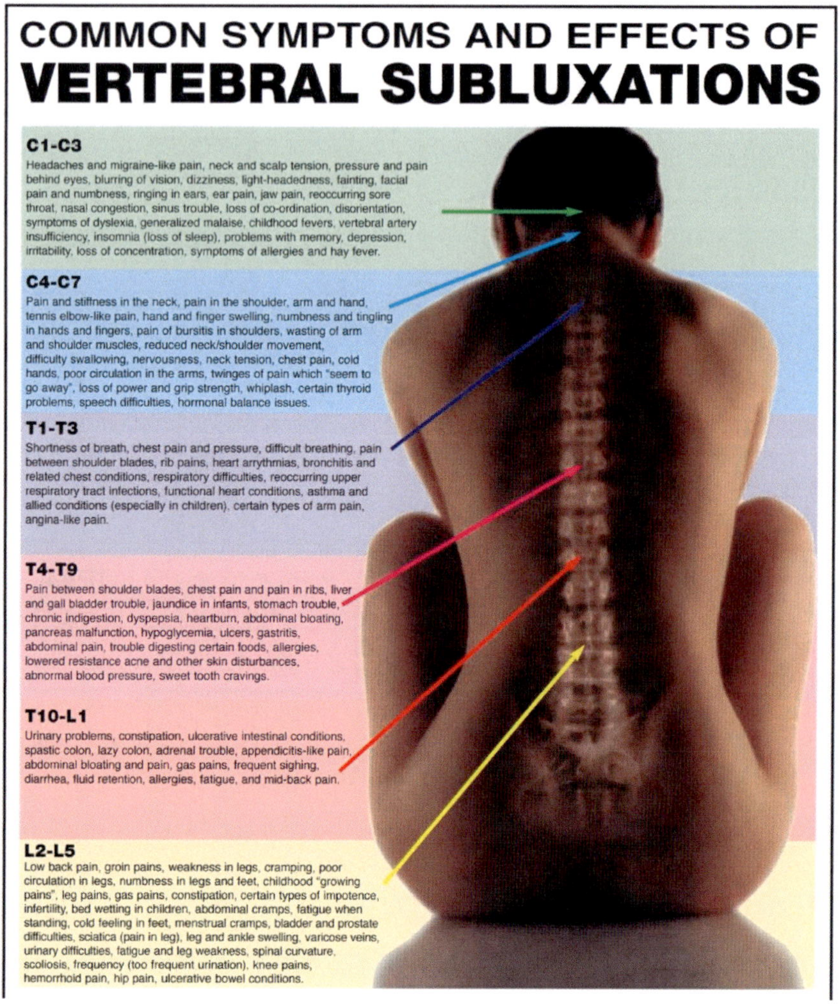
COMMON SYMPTOMS AND EFFECTS OF
VERTEBRAL SUBLUXATIONS
C1-C3
Headaches and migraine-like pain, neck and scalp tension, pressure and pain behind eyes, blurring of vision, dizziness, light-headedness, fainting, facial pain and numbness, ringing in ears, ear pain, jaw pain, reoccurring sore throat, nasal congestion, sinus trouble, loss of co-ordination, disorientation, symptoms of dyslexia, generalized malaise, childhood fevers, vertebral artery insufficiency, insomnia (loss of sleep), problems with memory, depression, irritability, loss of concentration, symptoms of allergies and hay fever.
C4-C7
Pain and stiffness in the neck, pain in the shoulder, arm and hand, tennis elbow-like pain, hand and finger swelling, numbness and tingling in hands and fingers, pain of bursitis in shoulders, wasting of arm and shoulder muscles, reduced neck/shoulder movement, difficulty swallowing, nervousness, neck tension, chest pain, cold hands, poor circulation in the arms, twinges of pain which "seem to go away", loss of power and grip strength, whiplash, certain thyroid problems, speech difficulties, hormonal balance issues.
T1-T3
Shortness of breath, chest pain and pressure, difficult breathing, pain between shoulder blades, rib pains, heart arrythmias, bronchitis and related chest conditions, respiratory difficulties, reoccurring upper respiratory tract infections, functional heart conditions, asthma and allied conditions (especially in children), certain types of arm pain, angina-like pain.
T4-T9
Pain between shoulder blades, chest pain and pain in ribs, liver and gall bladder trouble, jaundice in infants, stomach trouble, chronic indigestion, dyspepsia, heartburn, abdominal bloating, pancreas malfunction, hypoglycemia, ulcers, gastritis, abdominal pain, trouble digesting certain foods, allergies, lowered resistance acne and other skin disturbances, abnormal blood pressure, sweet tooth cravings.
T10-L1
Urinary problems, constipation, ulcerative intestinal conditions, spastic colon, lazy colon, adrenal trouble, appendicitis-like pain, abdominal bloating and pain, gas pains, frequent sighing, diarrhea, fluid retention, allergies, fatigue, and mid-back pain.
L2-L5
Low back pain, groin pains, weakness in legs, cramping, poor circulation in legs, numbness in legs and feet, childhood "growing pains", leg pains, gas pains, constipation, certain types of impotence, infertility, bed wetting in children, abdominal cramps, fatigue when standing, cold feeling in feet, menstrual cramps, bladder and prostate difficulties, sciatica (pain in leg), leg and ankle swelling, varicose veins, urinary difficulties, fatigue and leg weakness, spinal curvature, scoliosis, frequency (too frequent urination), knee pains, hemorrhoid pain, hip pain, ulcerative bowel conditions.

When you are making a dose, if the readings on the screen are turning into 'Nobody', consider the IR on this dose as 'Nobody'. If the same situation happens when you were making "0", consider this IR and dose at this area as "Nobody".

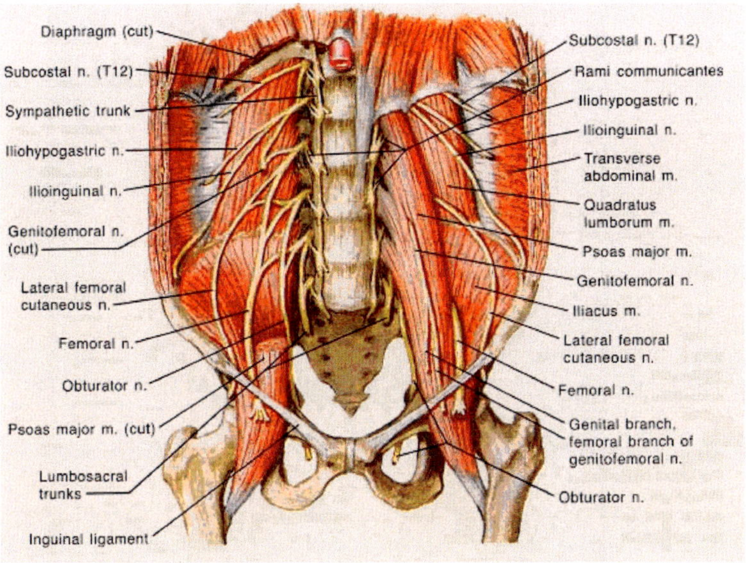
Diaphragm (cut)
Subcostal n. (T12)
Sympathetic trunk
Iliohypogastric n.
Ilioinguinal n.
Genitofemoral n. (cut)
Lateral femoral cutaneous n.
Femoral n.
Obturator n.
Psoas major m. (cut)
Lumbosacral trunks
Inguinal ligament
Subcostal n. (T12)
Rami communicantes
Iliohypogastric n.
Ilioinguinal n.
Transverse abdominal m.
Quadratus lumborum m.
Psoas major m.
Genitofemoral n.
Iliacus m.
Lateral femoral cutaneous n.
Femoral n.
Genital branch, femoral branch of genitofemoral n.
Obturator n.

When comparing IR's we need a difference of +4 or higher. When comparing doses and '0's we work on a difference of +1 or higher.

If first IR is higher by +4 than second IR, you can go back to first position and dose. Normally we go forward only.

If you did not get any "0"s, move onto the next zone.

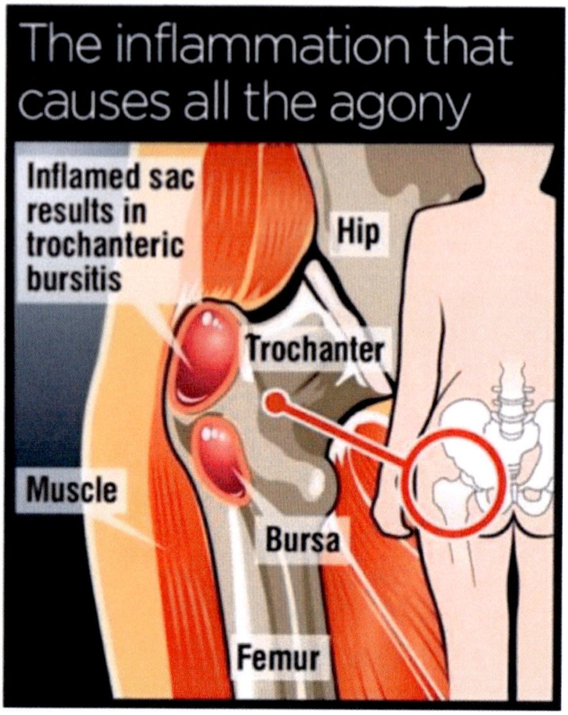
The inflammation that causes all the agony
Inflamed sac results in trochanteric bursitis
Hip
Trochanter
Muscle
Bursa
Femur

Get three different "0" positions along the spinal column and then, at the position which has the highest reading, then treat by setting Fm for 2 minutes. Complete the procedure with "0" on the face and possibly set Fm. Place the electrode vertically along the central route starting from C7. Measure the IR^1. Take the electrode off the skin and place it on the second position. Measure IR^2. If the difference is higher by 4 or more units, replace the device and wait for a dose. If not, continue taking IR's down the spinal column, looking for a difference of + 4 units and making doses where necessary. A second dose is needed for comparison. Compare the following readings: one IR will be higher than the last IR which was given a dose by 4 units.

IR > IRx by + 4 Dose *

IR > IRx[1] following*** + 4 Dose*

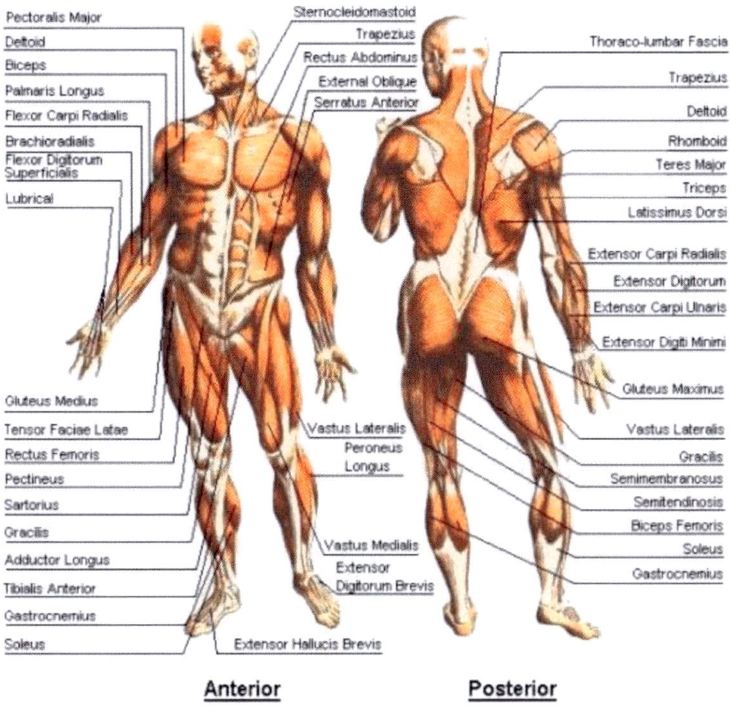
Pectoralis Major
Deltoid
Biceps
Palmaris Longus
Flexor Carpi Radialis
Brachioradialis
Flexor Digitorum Superficialis
Lubrical
Gluteus Medius
Tensor Faciae Latae
Rectus Femoris
Pectineus
Sartorius
Gracilis
Adductor Longus
Tibialis Anterior
Gastrocnemius
Soleus
Sternocleidomastoid
Trapezius
Rectus Abdominus
External Oblique
Serratus Anterior
Vastus Lateralis
Peroneus Longus
Vastus Medialis
Extensor Digitorum Brevis
Extensor Hallucis Brevis
Thoraco-lumbar Fascia
Trapezius
Deltoid
Rhomboid
Teres Major
Triceps
Latissimus Dorsi
Extensor Carpi Radialis
Extensor Digitorum
Extensor Carpi Ulnaris
Extensor Digiti Minimi
Gluteus Maximus
Vastus Lateralis
Gracilis
Semimembranosus
Semitendinosis
Biceps Femoris
Soleus
Gastrocnemius
Anterior
Posterior

Always make a dose on the last point on the route. Compare readings at all the points where a dose was given. At the position where the highest ongoing reaction value was obtained replace the device and bring the speed of the reaction down to “0”. Note the final reaction value at the moment when speed of the reaction hits “0” (it is essential to wait for the multi-tone bell) Dose* > Dose* then “0” Work on the paravertebral route, first left, then right, then left, measuring IR’s as before and dosing when there is a difference of +4. On each side, bring to zero the highest threshold of reaction i.e., one on the left and one on the right. Step 6 Set FmVar Compare "0"s on each of the pathways. Where the highest reading was obtained at "0" in one of the pathways (central, left or right) change the action regime to Diag 0, FmVar and treat for 2 minutes.

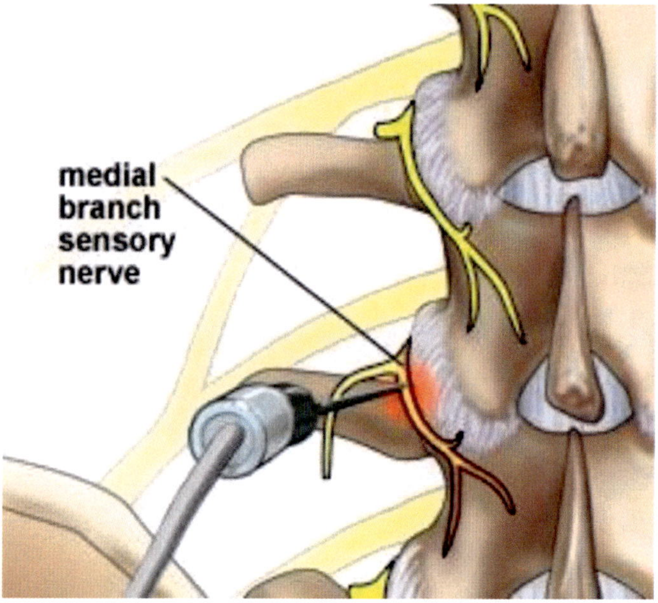
medial
branch
sensory
nerve

Find the position where the highest reading was obtained at "0". If the reading at "0" is higher on the face then on the back, treat at that position on FmVar. If the reading of "0" is less on the face, do not set Fm.

When: At the beginning of the course of treatment if there are many complaints. Whenever a patient presents a lot of complaints or many diagnoses you need to find a zone of small asymmetry.

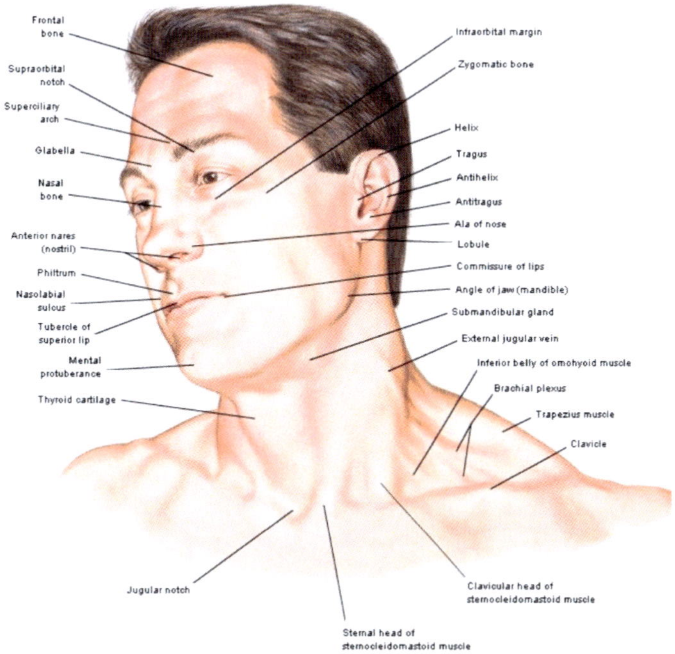

Frontal bone
Supraorbital notch
Superciliary arch
Glabella
Nasal bone
Anterior nares (nostril)
Philtrum
Nasolabial sulcus
Tubercle of superior lip
Mental protuberance
Thyroid cartilage
Infraorbital margin
Zygomatic bone
Helix
Tragus
Antihelix
Antitragus
Ala of nose
Lobule
Commissure of lips
Angle of jaw (mandible)
Submandibular gland
External jugular vein
Inferior belly of omohyoid muscle
Brachial plexus
Trapezius muscle
Clavicle
Jugular notch
Clavicular head of sternocleidomastoid muscle
Sternal head of sternocleidomastoid muscle

The method allows you to

- get a picture of how to work with a patient.
- discover the optimal direction for work (shows which part of the spinal column corresponding to an area of the body has the highest reading). This area of the body will need further treatment.
- choose a horizontal (i.e., where there are more doses, either on the right or on the left, top or bottom of the body).
- stimulate change in the organism and localize the focus of complaint.
- determine a prognosis.

When comparing IR's we need a difference of +4 or higher. When comparing doses and '0's we work on a difference of +1 or higher.

If first IR is higher by +4 than second IR, you can go back to first position and dose. After this: every 4 higher Initial Reaction should only be dosed.

Only subsequently higher by +4 IR should be dosed, only subsequently higher by +1 doses* should be "0"Ed and only subsequently higher by +1 "0"s should be FmVar'd. Set FmVar for 2 minutes.

After Setting Fm, start as from the beginning. Place the electrode vertically along the central route starting from C7. Measure the IR^1. Take the electrode off the skin and place it on the second position. Measure IR^2. If the difference is higher by 4 or more units, replace the device and wait for a dose. If not, continue taking IR's down the spinal column, looking for a difference of + 4 units and making doses where necessary. You are only setting the doses, "0"s and FmVars on higher values.

NERVOUS SYSTEM OF THORAX AND UPPER LIMB (ANTERIOR VIEW)

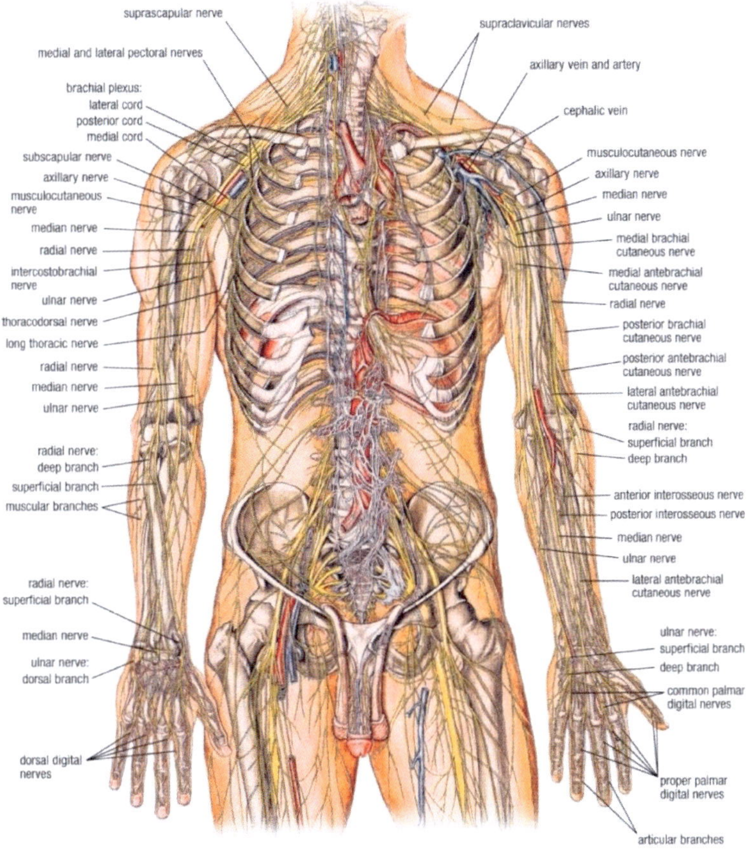

suprascapular nerve
medial and lateral pectoral nerves
brachial plexus:
lateral cord
posterior cord
medial cord
subscapular nerve
axillary nerve
musculocutaneous nerve
median nerve
radial nerve
intercostobrachial nerve
ulnar nerve
thoracodorsal nerve
long thoracic nerve
radial nerve
median nerve
ulnar nerve
radial nerve:
deep branch
superficial branch
muscular branches
radial nerve:
superficial branch
median nerve
ulnar nerve:
dorsal branch
dorsal digital nerves
supraclavicular nerves
axillary vein and artery
cephalic vein
musculocutaneous nerve
axillary nerve
median nerve
ulnar nerve
medial brachial cutaneous nerve
medial antebrachial cutaneous nerve
radial nerve
posterior brachial cutaneous nerve
posterior antebrachial cutaneous nerve
lateral antebrachial cutaneous nerve
radial nerve:
superficial branch
deep branch
anterior interosseous nerve
posterior interosseous nerve
median nerve
ulnar nerve
lateral antebrachial cutaneous nerve
ulnar nerve:
superficial branch
deep branch
common palmar digital nerves
proper palmar digital nerves
articular branches

Detect another position

A second dose is needed for comparison. Compare the following readings: one IR will be higher than the last IR which was given a dose by 4 units. IR > IRx by + 4? Dose * IR IR IR > IRx^1 following*** + 4? Dose*

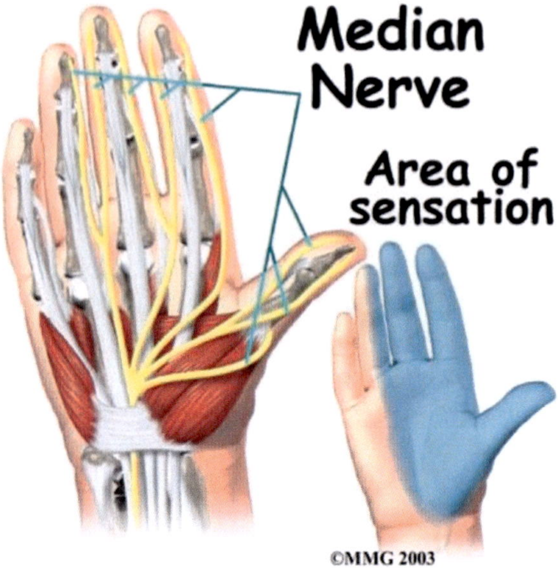
Median
Nerve
Area of
sensation
©MMG 2003

Bring to “0”

On any subsequent “dose” set “0”, if the dose is higher by +1 and on any subsequent “0”, if higher, set FmVar.

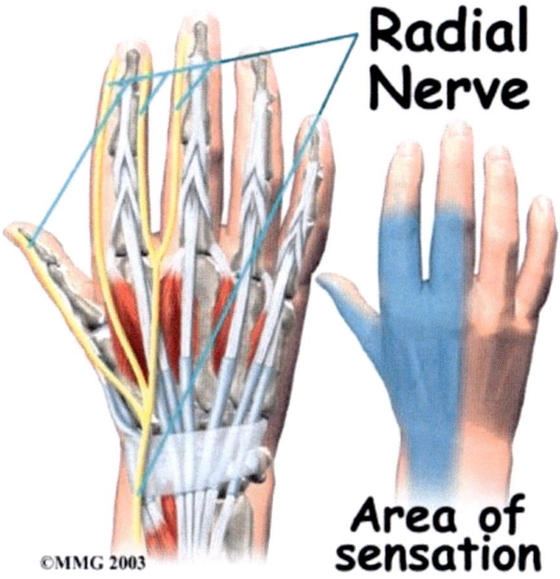
Radial
Nerve
Area of
sensation
©MMG 2003

After setting Fm

Start as you are starting a new route, looking for difference between IR's of +4 and higher. Always make a dose on the last point on the route.

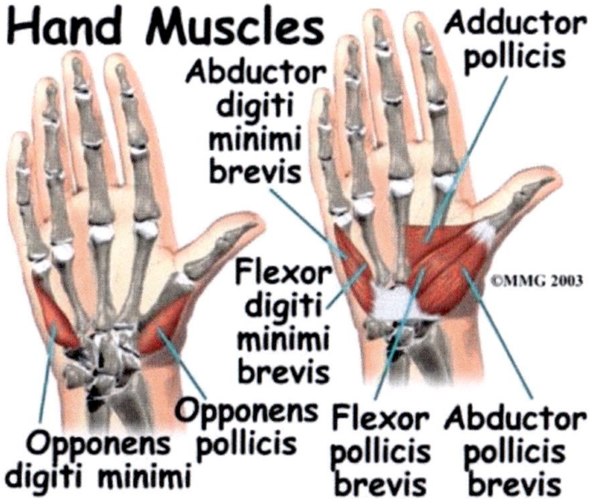
Hand Muscles
Adductor
pollicis
Abductor
digiti
minimi
brevis
Flexor
digiti
minimi
brevis
©MMG 2003
Opponens
pollicis
Flexor
pollicis
brevis
Abductor
pollicis
brevis
Opponens
digiti minimi

Paravertebral route

Work on the paravertebral route, first left, then right, then left, measuring IR's as before and dosing on subsequent IR which is higher by +4. Then follow the routine as for the central route.

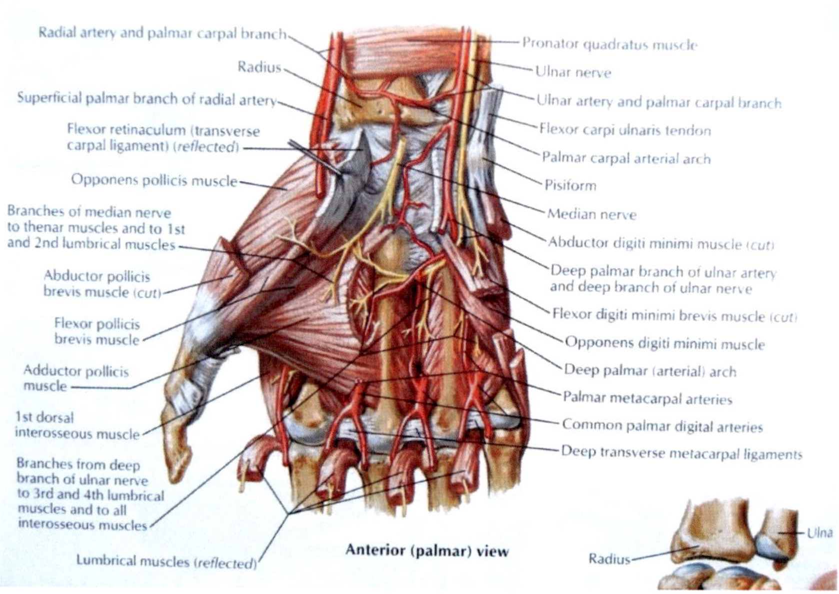

Radial artery and palmar carpal branch
Radius
Superficial palmar branch of radial artery
Flexor retinaculum (transverse carpal ligament) (*reflected*)
Opponens pollicis muscle
Branches of median nerve to thenar muscles and to 1st and 2nd lumbrical muscles
Abductor pollicis brevis muscle (*cut*)
Flexor pollicis brevis muscle
Adductor pollicis muscle
1st dorsal interosseous muscle
Branches from deep branch of ulnar nerve to 3rd and 4th lumbrical muscles and to all interosseous muscles
Lumbrical muscles (*reflected*)
Pronator quadratus muscle
Ulnar nerve
Ulnar artery and palmar carpal branch
Flexor carpi ulnaris tendon
Palmar carpal arterial arch
Pisiform
Median nerve
Abductor digiti minimi muscle (*cut*)
Deep palmar branch of ulnar artery and deep branch of ulnar nerve
Flexor digiti minimi brevis muscle (*cut*)
Opponens digiti minimi muscle
Deep palmar (arterial) arch
Palmar metacarpal arteries
Common palmar digital arteries
Deep transverse metacarpal ligaments
Anterior (palmar) view
Radius
Ulna

Face route

Start from the bottom left position on the face, measure the IR's and dose when there is a difference of +4. Follow the same routine as for St 3 or St 5.

Main Factors of acupressure on the human body

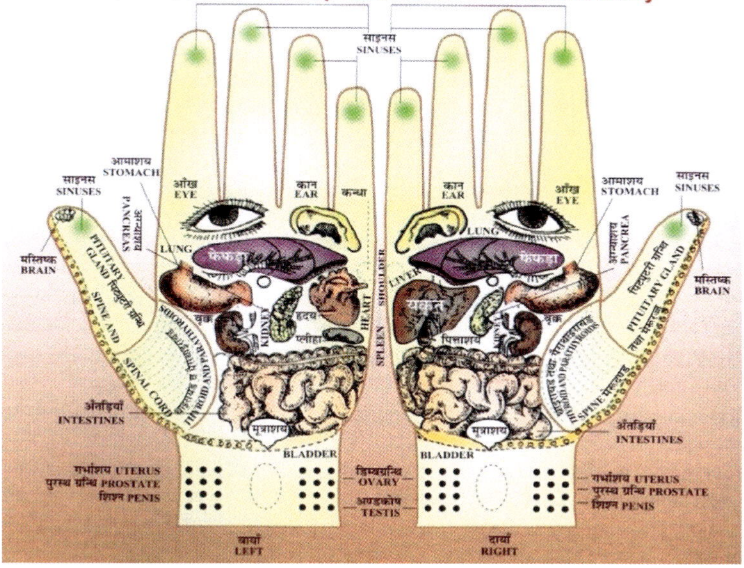
SINUSES
STOMACH
SINUSES
EYE
EAR
BRAIN
PANCREAS
PITUITARY GLAND
LUNG
SPINE AND SPINAL CORD
THYROID AND PARATHYROID
KIDNEY
HEART
SHOULDER
SPLEEN
LIVER
INTESTINES
BLADDER
UTERUS
PROSTATE
PENIS
OVARY
TESTIS
LEFT
RIGHT

Last point on the route

Make a dose on the last point on the face route.

Set "0": Set '0' on the highest dose*.

Start from C7 along the central route. Measure IR, note the reading and place your finger on the area after you take the device off the skin.

Keep your finger on the skin while you continue to measure other IR's. When an IR is found that is higher by +1, place your finger on the new position. Keep your finger in place until you detect a reading that is higher again by +1, and move your finger there. Carry on this routine along the central route, placing finger as above until the end of the central route. Do not make a dose on the last point of the route.

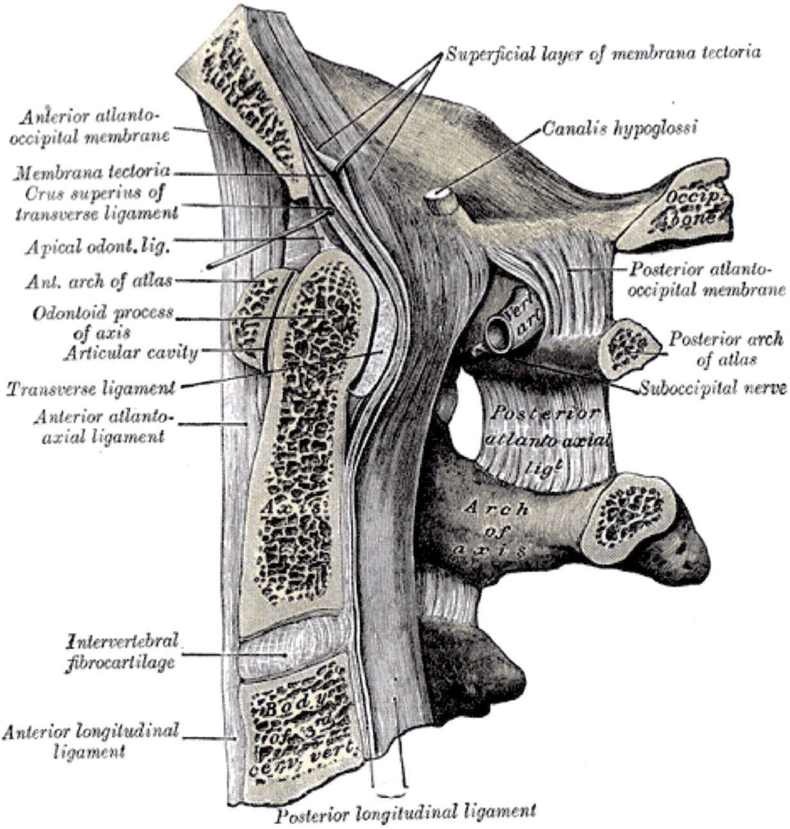
Superficial layer of membrana tectoria
Canalis hypoglossi
Occip. bone
Anterior atlanto-occipital membrane
Membrana tectoria
Crus superius of transverse ligament
Apical odont. lig.
Ant. arch of atlas
Odontoid process of axis
Articular cavity
Transverse ligament
Anterior atlanto-axial ligament
Posterior atlanto-occipital membrane
Vert. art.
Posterior arch of atlas
Suboccipital nerve
Posterior atlanto-axial ligt
Arch of axis
Axis
Intervertebral fibrocartilage
Body of 3rd cerv. vert.
Anterior longitudinal ligament
Posterior longitudinal ligament

Make a dose on the **highest IR,** and then point with a finger at this spot.

Also make a dose on the lowest reading of IR, but not pointing with a finger (as you are not encouraging the brain to focus on the area of small reading).

The same routine applies to the paravertebral route. Carry on the routine, placing the finger on IR's which are higher by +1, and not making a dose on the last point of the route. On the highest IR make a dose. Make a dose on the lowest as well, but not pointing with the finger.

SPINAL AND CRANIAL NERVES

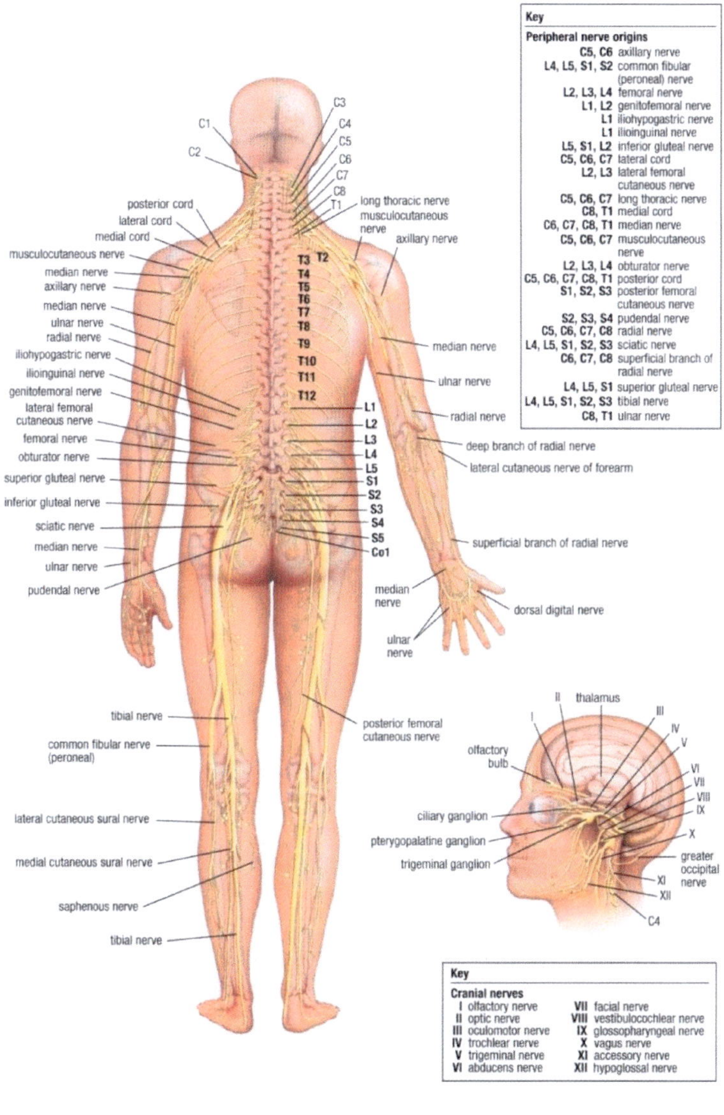
Key
Peripheral nerve origins
C5, C6 axillary nerve
L4, L5, S1, S2 common fibular (peroneal) nerve
L2, L3, L4 femoral nerve
L1, L2 genitofemoral nerve
L1 iliohypogastric nerve
L1 ilioinguinal nerve
L5, S1, L2 inferior gluteal nerve
C5, C6, C7 lateral cord
L2, L3 lateral femoral cutaneous nerve
C5, C6, C7 long thoracic nerve
C8, T1 medial cord
C6, C7, C8, T1 median nerve
C5, C6, C7 musculocutaneous nerve
L2, L3, L4 obturator nerve
C5, C6, C7, C8, T1 posterior cord
S1, S2, S3 posterior femoral cutaneous nerve
S2, S3, S4 pudendal nerve
C5, C6, C7, C8 radial nerve
L4, L5, S1, S2, S3 sciatic nerve
C6, C7, C8 superficial branch of radial nerve
L4, L5, S1 superior gluteal nerve
L4, L5, S1, S2, S3 tibial nerve
C8, T1 ulnar nerve
C1
C2
C3
C4
C5
C6
C7
C8
T1
T2
T3
T4
T5
T6
T7
T8
T9
T10
T11
T12
L1
L2
L3
L4
L5
S1
S2
S3
S4
S5
Co1
posterior cord
lateral cord
medial cord
musculocutaneous nerve
median nerve
axillary nerve
median nerve
ulnar nerve
radial nerve
iliohypogastric nerve
ilioinguinal nerve
genitofemoral nerve
lateral femoral cutaneous nerve
femoral nerve
obturator nerve
superior gluteal nerve
inferior gluteal nerve
sciatic nerve
median nerve
ulnar nerve
pudendal nerve
long thoracic nerve
musculocutaneous nerve
axillary nerve
median nerve
ulnar nerve
radial nerve
deep branch of radial nerve
lateral cutaneous nerve of forearm
superficial branch of radial nerve
median nerve
dorsal digital nerve
ulnar nerve
tibial nerve
common fibular nerve (peroneal)
posterior femoral cutaneous nerve
lateral cutaneous sural nerve
medial cutaneous sural nerve
saphenous nerve
tibial nerve
I
II
thalamus
III
IV
V
VI
VII
VIII
IX
X
olfactory bulb
ciliary ganglion
pterygopalatine ganglion
trigeminal ganglion
greater occipital nerve
XI
XII
C4
Key
Cranial nerves
I olfactory nerve
II optic nerve
III oculomotor nerve
IV trochlear nerve
V trigeminal nerve
VI abducens nerve
VII facial nerve
VIII vestibulocochlear nerve
IX glossopharyngeal nerve
X vagus nerve
XI accessory nerve
XII hypoglossal nerve

The same routine applies on the face route: measure the first IR, place your finger, next – with difference of +1 move your finger there, and carry on in the same fashion until the last point. Do not make a dose on the last point. On the highest IR make a dose. Make a dose on the lowest as well, but not pointing with the finger.

Compare all doses on the central route, paravertebral route and facial route; where highest, make “0”.

Great Vessels of Superior Mediastinum

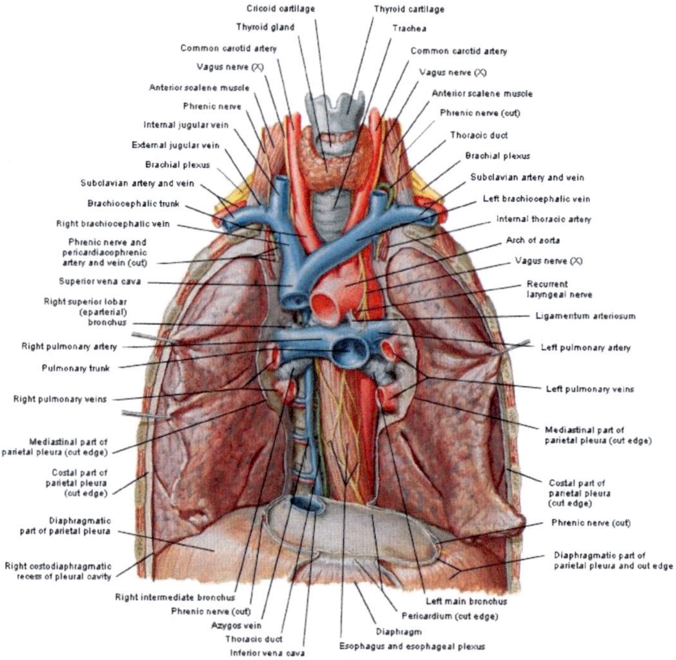

Cricoid cartilage
Thyroid cartilage
Thyroid gland
Trachea
Common carotid artery
Common carotid artery
Vagus nerve (X)
Vagus nerve (X)
Anterior scalene muscle
Anterior scalene muscle
Phrenic nerve
Phrenic nerve (cut)
Internal jugular vein
Thoracic duct
External jugular vein
Brachial plexus
Brachial plexus
Subclavian artery and vein
Subclavian artery and vein
Left brachiocephalic vein
Brachiocephalic trunk
Internal thoracic artery
Right brachiocephalic vein
Arch of aorta
Phrenic nerve and pericardiacophrenic artery and vein (cut)
Vagus nerve (X)
Superior vena cava
Recurrent laryngeal nerve
Right superior lobar (eparterial) bronchus
Ligamentum arteriosum
Right pulmonary artery
Left pulmonary artery
Pulmonary trunk
Right pulmonary veins
Left pulmonary veins
Mediastinal part of parietal pleura (cut edge)
Mediastinal part of parietal pleura (cut edge)
Costal part of parietal pleura (cut edge)
Costal part of parietal pleura (cut edge)
Diaphragmatic part of parietal pleura
Phrenic nerve (cut)
Right costodiaphragmatic recess of pleural cavity
Diaphragmatic part of parietal pleura and cut edge
Right intermediate bronchus
Left main bronchus
Phrenic nerve (cut)
Pericardium (cut edge)
Azygos vein
Diaphragm
Thoracic duct
Esophagus and esophageal plexus
Inferior vena cava

These numbers will help to estimate the success of the treatment with SCENAR, i.e. whether it is going to be quick recovery or slow progress in recovery. In any Functional System, the different organs are united by any different regulatory pathways. Even parts of the membrane of one nerve cell can be serviced by various functional systems. For example, impulses from a membrane in one system can be transferred to another, e.g., from the heart to the lung cells. It is known that the skin is closely interconnected with all functional systems and organs and it takes part in all bodily reactions, i.e., the skin reflects the internal medium of the organism. All Functional Systems are linked through their common blood and lymph supply which themselves exchange substrates with intra-cellular fluid. In addition, any Functional System has a simpler organization, which can be represented as a self-organizing closed cyclical structure.

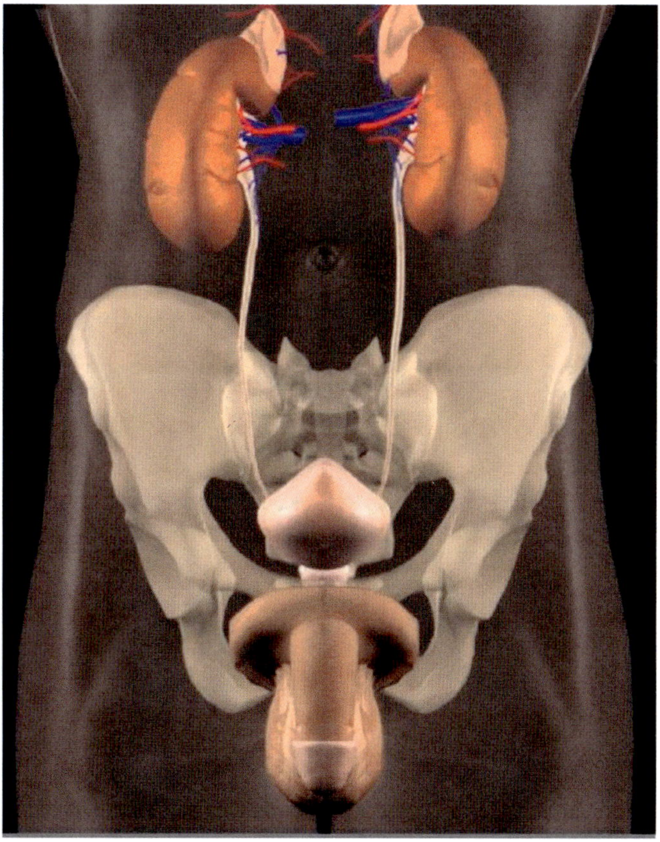

Regulation of the functions and measurement of the reaction (e.g., what quantity of gastric juice to release or to pick up a pencil without missing it) both have an adaptive meaning. The measurement of the reaction is what differentiates the Functional System from the Pathological one. When the measurement of reaction is correct the system is Functional; if not it is a Pathological system. The more perfect a mechanism of the regulation needs to be, the more precise is the measurement of the reaction. Inadequate reactions of the organism are always a pathogenic factor for the organism.

ADDUCTOR MAGNUS

YOUR ADDUCTOR MAGNUS muscles are found in the upper parts of both your legs. They pull each leg inward toward the other one. Each adductor magnus muscle is attached at one end to the pelvis, or hip, and at the lower end to the upper leg bone.

When to use:

- In the presence of clearly defined local symptoms.

- In an emergency - for achieving functional changes in organs/systems.
- When large surfaces are being treated.

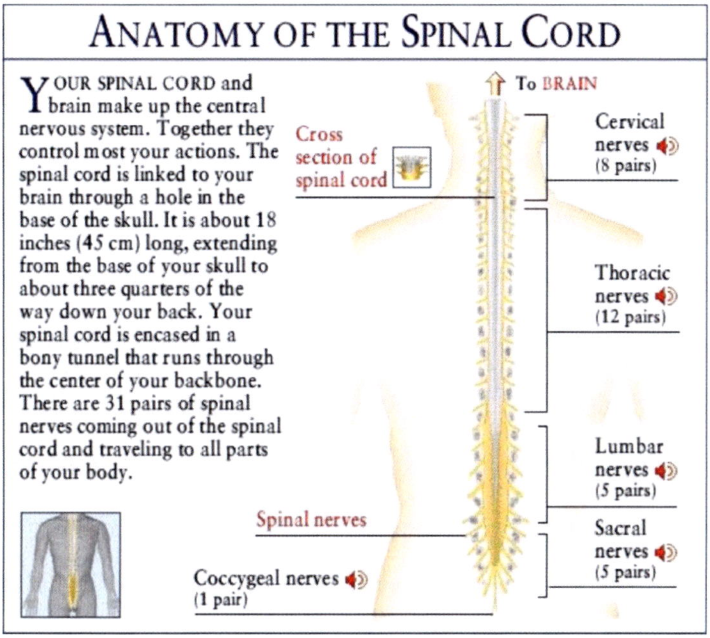
ANATOMY OF THE SPINAL CORD
YOUR SPINAL CORD and brain make up the central nervous system. Together they control most your actions. The spinal cord is linked to your brain through a hole in the base of the skull. It is about 18 inches (45 cm) long, extending from the base of your skull to about three quarters of the way down your back. Your spinal cord is encased in a bony tunnel that runs through the center of your backbone. There are 31 pairs of spinal nerves coming out of the spinal cord and traveling to all parts of your body.
To BRAIN
Cross section of spinal cord
Cervical nerves (8 pairs)
Thoracic nerves (12 pairs)
Lumbar nerves (5 pairs)
Sacral nerves (5 pairs)
Spinal nerves
Coccygeal nerves (1 pair)

Move the device steadily (speed) and firmly (pressure) in one direction. Start treatment at any presenting primary signs. In the presence of active complaints (especially in combination with primary signs) start treating here.

Treat one site at a time, until any small asymmetry (or secondary sign) appears. When you have achieved an asymmetry, change the action regime (Freq, Mod, z, Dmpf, Intensity or any combination of these). Work, looking for a small asymmetry.

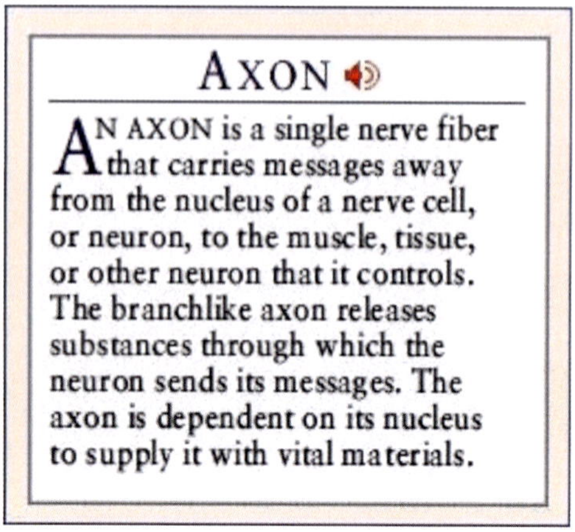

AXON

AN AXON is a single nerve fiber that carries messages away from the nucleus of a nerve cell, or neuron, to the muscle, tissue, or other neuron that it controls. The branchlike axon releases substances through which the neuron sends its messages. The axon is dependent on its nucleus to supply it with vital materials.

Then work on the area of small asymmetry, varying the direction of the electrode (4 directions), attempting to achieve a dynamic change (in the pain, in the color, in stickiness of the electrode, in the local sensation, in the sound from the device). Ideally work until the sign disappears or until an opposite sign appears. Finish the procedure when you have achieved a subjective improvement of the patient's condition.

CARTILAGE

CARTILAGE is a tough material that you can feel supporting your nose and ears. It also occurs between the bones of your spine, over the ends of bones, and in joints, where it gives support and allows movement. Before a baby is born, its skeleton is made entirely of cartilage, which is gradually replaced by the adult skeleton.

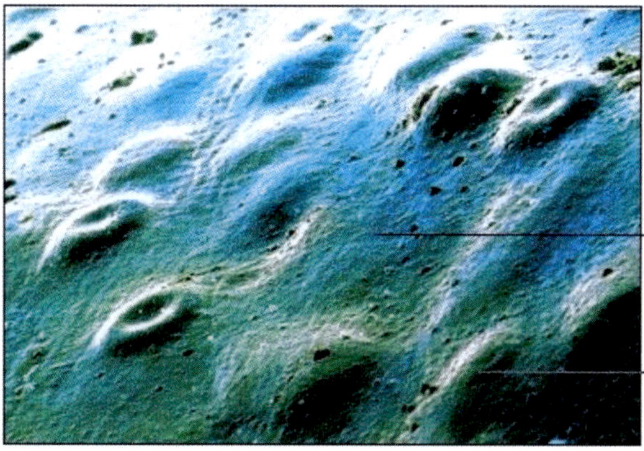
Smooth surface of cartilage
Cartilage-producing cells

When there are no more reactions or there is an insignificant subjective effect:

- Change the action regime and extend the area of action along a horizontal line or along a segment.
- Include the general action area (3 paths).
- Continue to reveal areas of small asymmetry and secondary sign.

Cell Membrane

THE CELL MEMBRANE is a strong, thin, flexible layer that surrounds each cell. It helps a cell to keep its shape and stops its contents spilling out. The cell membrane, however, is much more than a simple barrier: it controls which substances enter or leave a cell, carries identifying chemical markers on its surface (so that cells can recognize each other), and has antennalike receptors that pick up chemical messages and pass them to the inside of the cell.

Always look for dynamic changes: at examination, in complaints, in sensations, skin condition and between treatments. Any change, even a worsening, is regarded as dynamic and useful.

Chapter 14.
Choosing the Area to Treat

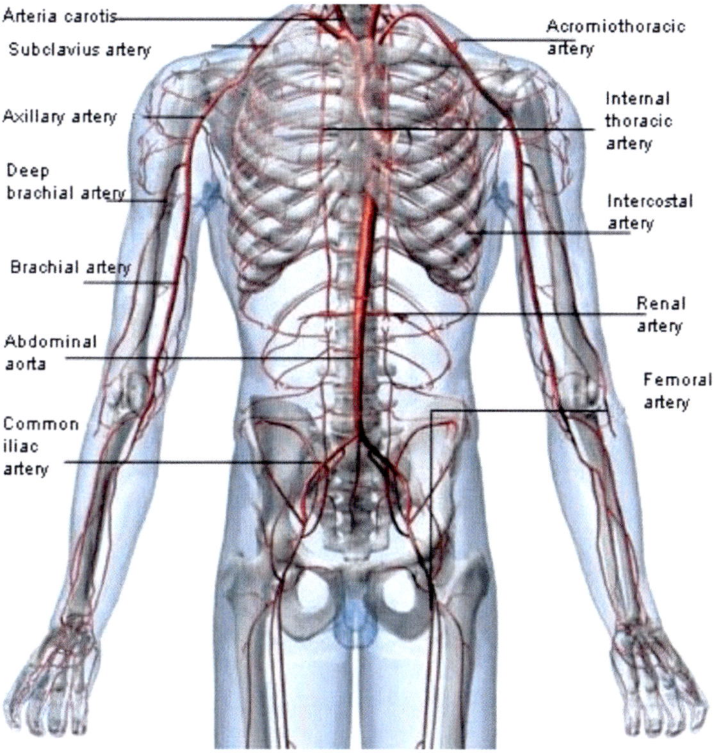
Arteria carotis
Subclavius artery
Axillary artery
Deep
brachial artery
Brachial artery
Abdominal
aorta
Common
iliac
artery
Acromiothoracic
artery
Internal
thoracic
artery
Intercostal
artery
Renal
artery
Femoral
artery

Work according to the first rule, i.e., **work on any complaint (usually pain).**

Determine the pathological focus and the projection of the pain. Work locally and towards any referred pain.

Look for any asymmetry and work on all asymmetries, trying to achieve dynamics, i.e. aiming for disappearance or trying to achieve the opposite sign.

Where there are many complaints, or none - use the second rule i.e., three pathways and six points. The areas that receive doses, “0”’s and Fm will suggest areas that need treatment.

Treat horizontals and segments

At any stage when **Secondary Factors** appear, treat this area.

Work on the symmetrical area.

CEREBRUM

YOUR CEREBRUM is the largest part of your brain and makes up about 80 percent of its mass. It is divided into the left and right halves, or cerebral hemispheres. Each half takes information from, and controls the muscles of, the opposite side of your body. Your cerebrum is also the center of your intelligence, memory, speech, and consciousness. The outer layer, called the cerebral cortex, is folded and grooved, and is made up of billions of nerve cells, known as gray matter. Inside this is the thick, white matter of the cerebrum, made of connecting nerve fibers.

Frequency of Treatment

Emergency and life or death situation – work every 2 hours until a patient is out of danger.

Attacks of acute pain – work until the pain is gone.

Acute illnesses – work three/four times a day if possible, otherwise every day.

Posterior Thoracic Wall

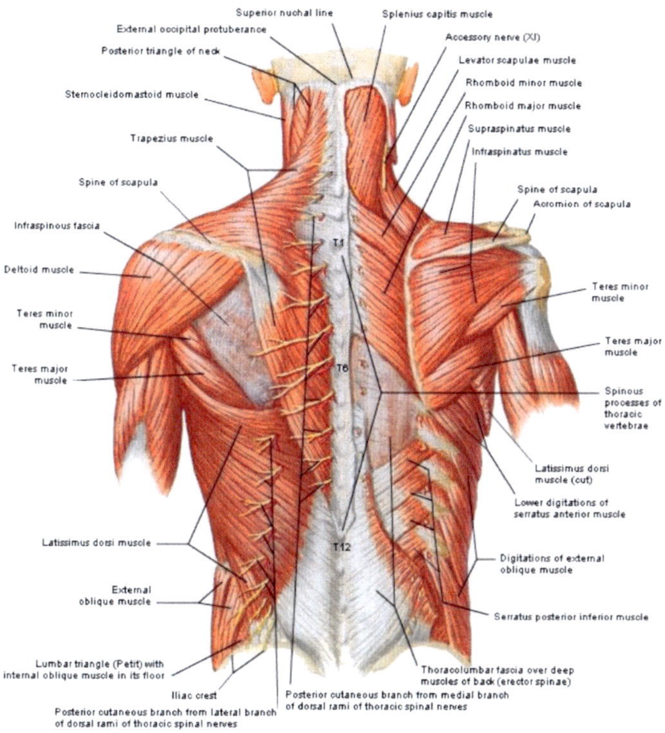
Superior nuchal line
Splenius capitis muscle
External occipital protuberance
Accessory nerve (XI)
Posterior triangle of neck
Levator scapulae muscle
Rhomboid minor muscle
Sternocleidomastoid muscle
Rhomboid major muscle
Supraspinatus muscle
Trapezius muscle
Infraspinatus muscle
Spine of scapula
Spine of scapula
Acromion of scapula
Infraspinous fascia
T1
Deltoid muscle
Teres minor muscle
Teres minor muscle
Teres major muscle
T6
Teres major muscle
Spinous processes of thoracic vertebrae
Latissimus dorsi muscle (cut)
Lower digitations of serratus anterior muscle
Latissimus dorsi muscle
T12
Digitations of external oblique muscle
External oblique muscle
Serratus posterior inferior muscle
Lumbar triangle (Petit) with internal oblique muscle in its floor
Thoracolumbar fascia over deep muscles of back (erector spinae)
Iliac crest
Posterior cutaneous branch from medial branch of dorsal rami of thoracic spinal nerves
Posterior cutaneous branch from lateral branch of dorsal rami of thoracic spinal nerves

Chronic processes – start with a treatment daily and as things progress the interval between treatments can be extended to alternate days, then every third day and so on. A course of treatment is offered, consisting of 10 to 20 treatments. Then take a break. Start a new course of treatment when your patient has got a complaint (any) and begin from treatment of that complaint. (Remember that SCENAR treatments may bring up problems from the past that were inadequately dealt with originally.)

Take readings of the highest dose or "0" on the symmetrical area. If the IR on the symmetrical point is higher make a dose when there is a difference of +1. If the dose is now higher then on the point of pain, bring down to "0". Compare "0"s in both areas. Set FmVar on the higher. Next take readings of IR at the paravertebral position of the corresponding level of the spinal column on the side, where you have set FmVar or where you found the highest readings. If the IR on the paravertebral position is higher than anywhere (point of pain or symmetrical point of pain), make a dose*. If the dose is higher than anywhere – set "0" and if "0" is higher, set FmVar. In this case you are going to start treating a horizontal from the paravertebral point. Otherwise, start treating from the point where you set Fm (could be the point of pain or its' symmetrical point). Work along the horizontal towards the paravertebral point near the spine, treating any asymmetry you have found. **Always work in the direction from the highest number towards the lowest number**, following the corresponding horizontal. Skin reflects the condition of the internal environment of the organism. Be observant and note any changes on the patient's skin. Treat skin spots, bruises, wounds, ulcers, scars, trophic changes, etc., working over the damaged area. If the wound is big, treat the edges of the wound, use different settings on the device. If you work with acute problem use the above threshold level of power, vary the settings. If you work with chronic disturbance on the skin, use threshold level of power and lower frequency, vary the settings. Use the principles of **small asymmetry**.

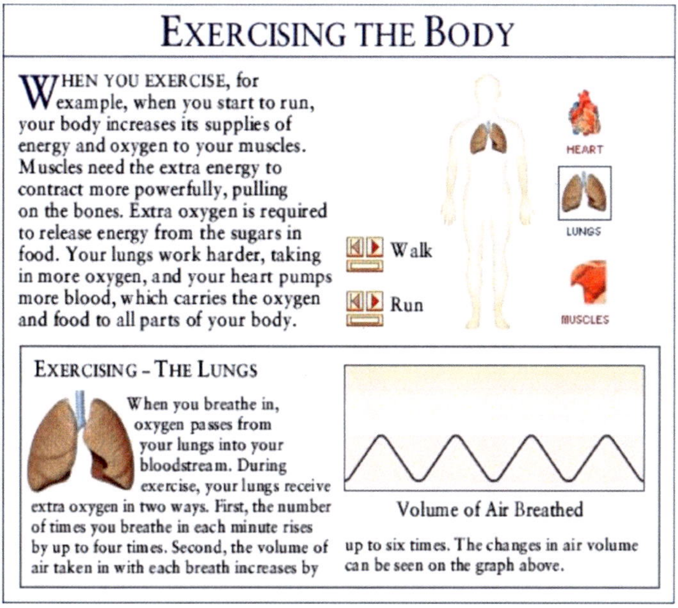
EXERCISING THE BODY
WHEN YOU EXERCISE, for example, when you start to run, your body increases its supplies of energy and oxygen to your muscles. Muscles need the extra energy to contract more powerfully, pulling on the bones. Extra oxygen is required to release energy from the sugars in food. Your lungs work harder, taking in more oxygen, and your heart pumps more blood, which carries the oxygen and food to all parts of your body.
Walk
Run
HEART
LUNGS
MUSCLES
EXERCISING - THE LUNGS
When you breathe in, oxygen passes from your lungs into your bloodstream. During exercise, your lungs receive extra oxygen in two ways. First, the number of times you breathe in each minute rises by up to four times. Second, the volume of air taken in with each breath increases by up to six times. The changes in air volume can be seen on the graph above.
Volume of Air Breathed

Pain location treatment method

Pain location and its borders have to be determined at first. Then treatment effect is carried out by applying the device to the local skin area or by making massage movements in continuous treatment mode. Effective treatment duration is defined by the state-of-health improvement or pain relief.

Circular segment treatment method on the claimed complaint level: The skin should be treated beginning with the backbone's spinous processes at the level of the sick organ disposition towards its upright projection followed by the organ's projection treatment and then again towards the backbone, thus ending the circle.

"Follow-the-pain" method, i.e. device treatment over the area of the painful sensations symptom or discomfort phenomena as well as over a sick organ (liver, gall-bladder, etc.): These areas may be treated in continuous treatment mode by applying the device to a local skin area or by making massage motions. If painful sensations are not caused by calculus motion (urolithiasis, cholelithic disease), then individually dosed treatment mode is used. If there is a pain translocation, the device should be Trans located in the same direction. It will take about 15 – 40 minutes to get some positive effect (state-of-health improvement, pain relief).

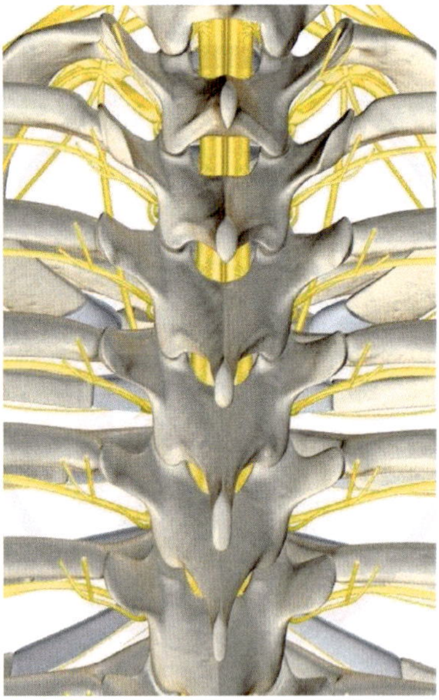

Distal parts of extremities treatment method: The skin of hands and feet should be treated "gloves" and "socks" likewise. There are energy channels and the main microcirculatory bed originating and ending on hands and feet. Treatment should be initiated with the palmar surface of the left hand beginning with the little finger first and ending with the thumb, then continued with the palm and then transferred to the back of the hand which should be treated using same-as-above procedure sequence. Feet are treated in the same order as hands.

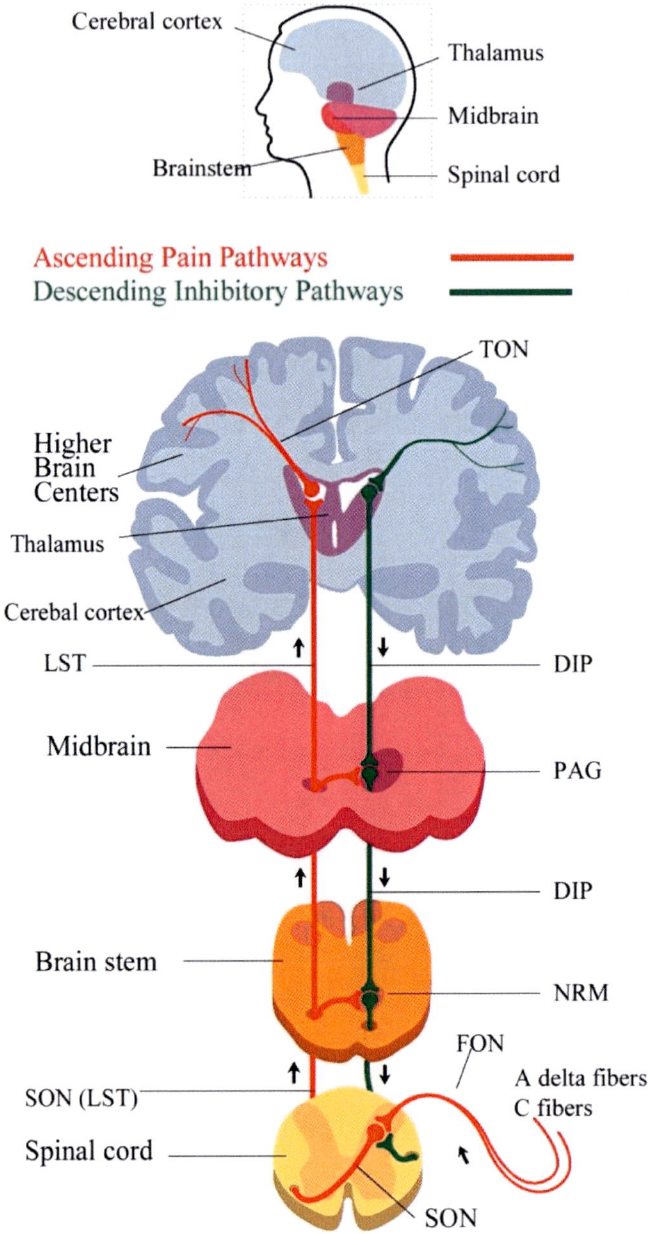

Cerebral cortex
Thalamus
Midbrain
Brainstem
Spinal cord
Ascending Pain Pathways
Descending Inhibitory Pathways
TON
Higher Brain Centers
Thalamus
Cerebal cortex
LST
DIP
Midbrain
PAG
DIP
Brain stem
NRM
FON
A delta fibers
C fibers
SON (LST)
Spinal cord
SON

***Pirogov's ring treatment method*:** The **Pirogov's ring is treated on the neck beginning with spinous processes of the cervical vertebras**. The device is rearranged stepwise or moved without taking it off the skin toward the front surface of the neck and then again toward the spinous processes of the cervical vertebras, thus ending the circle. This treatment zone contains large blood vessels, lymph nodes, nerve trunks, thyroid and parathyroid glands. This zone is liable to treatment if there is a nasopharyngeal pathology (rhinitis, sinusitis, laryngitis, and tonsillitis), stomatology or brain pathologies.

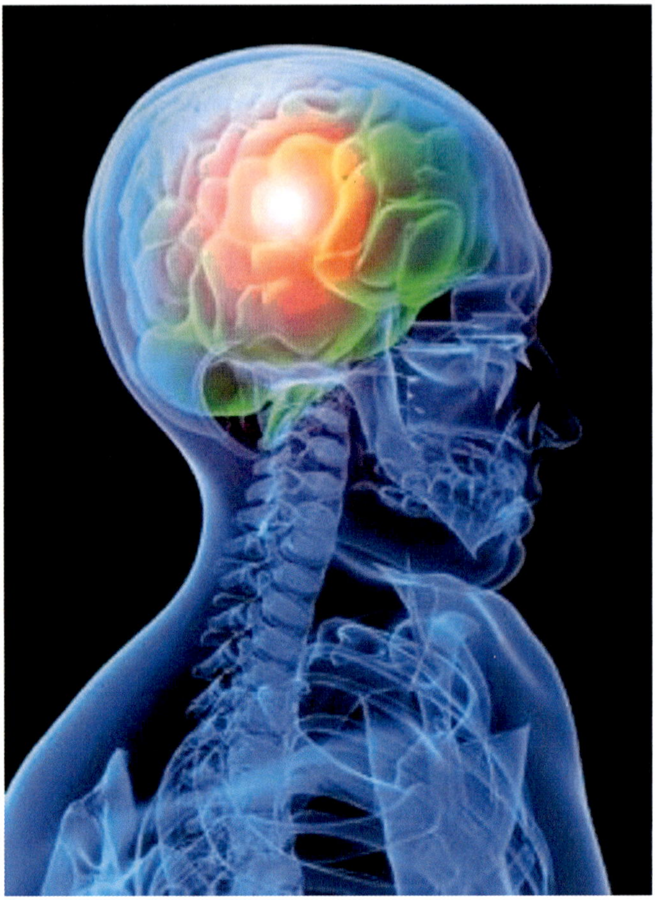

Cross-treatment method: It is applied in cases of pathologies accompanied with paresis and paralyses (insult, for example). Treatment should be initiated with a healthy arm followed by a sick leg, while next procedure should be done vice versa, i.e. a healthy leg - sick arm. Device treatment should be aimed at getting muscular fascicles contraction by means of energy level selection (the higher is the energy level, the higher will be the muscle contraction rate).

How to Treat in DIAG 0 Mode

Turn on the device and reset the defaults by pressing the UP and DOWN buttons together for 3 seconds.

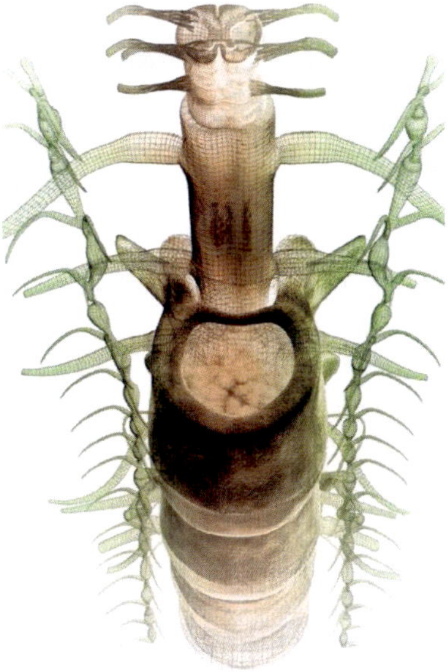

The SCENAR should automatically go into its lowest amplitude setting of (1) on the 97.4+ SCENAR.

Place the SCENAR on the skin outside the area selected for treatment.

Increase the power to a comfortable level of sensation (barely tingling) whilst holding the device on the skin.

Move to the area selected for treatment.

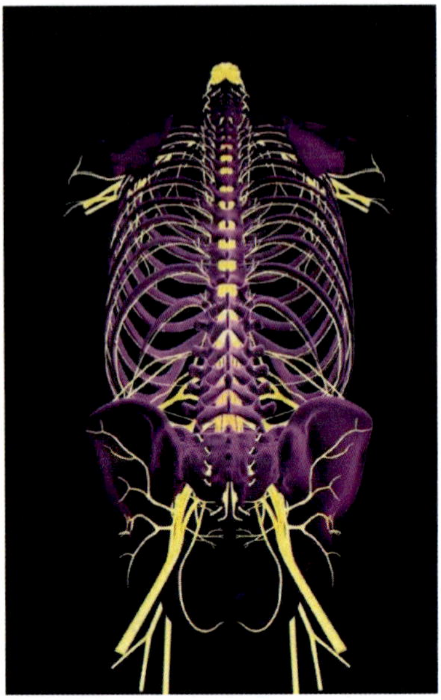

If any topical (recently appeared) primary signs are present start the treatment in the area where they have appeared.

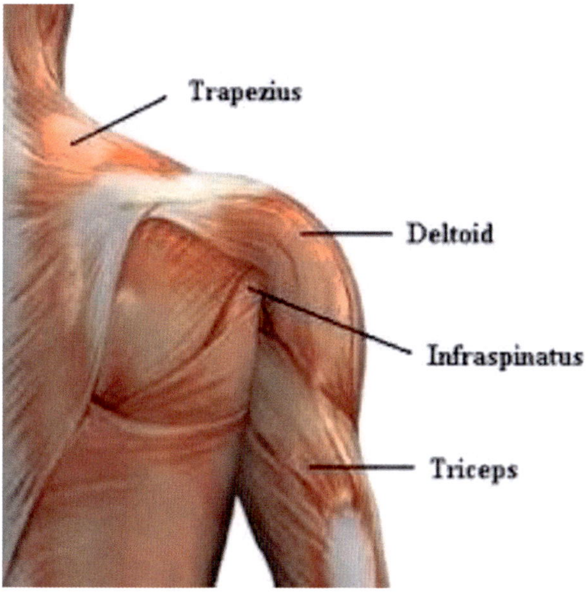
Trapezius
Deltoid
Infraspinatus
Triceps

If active complaints are present, and particularly if there are primary signs at the point of projection (the referenced skin over the affected organ), start the treatment there.

Structure of a Generalized Cell

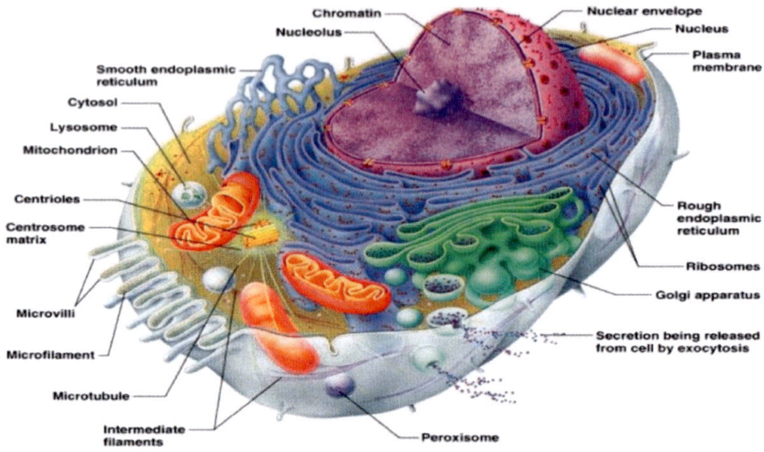

Chromatin
Nucleolus
Nuclear envelope
Nucleus
Plasma membrane
Smooth endoplasmic reticulum
Cytosol
Lysosome
Mitochondrion
Centrioles
Centrosome matrix
Microvilli
Microfilament
Microtubule
Intermediate filaments
Peroxisome
Rough endoplasmic reticulum
Ribosomes
Golgi apparatus
Secretion being released from cell by exocytosis

Apply the SCENAR firmly to the skin and move it over the skin with firm pressure, at a steady speed without changing any of the settings.

Treat one site at a time, varying the direction of the electrode ↕ ↔ (4 directions), until any treatment indicators (secondary signs, small asymmetries) appear. Continue working with the SCENAR, ideally until the redness, stickiness etc. disappears and the area is no different from the surrounding area, or at least until you have achieved a change in the appearance of the area. This is what Russian literature refers to as “**dynamics**”. If secondary signs appear, move to that area and treat until these signs disappear and this area is also no different from its surrounding area. General protocol is to treat the area of complaint in an anti-inflammatory mode as most visits to a practitioner’s office are done for pain, acute or on-going situations, e.g. 148 Hz

Spinal Nerve Function

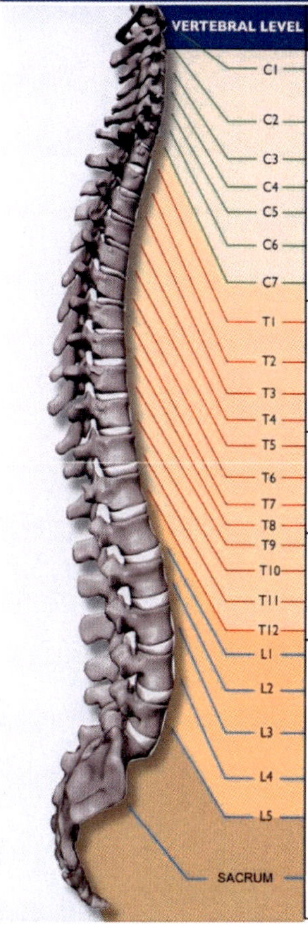

VERTEBRAL LEVEL	AREA OR ORGAN	POSSIBLE SYMPTOMS
C1, C2, C3	MASTER CONTROL FOR ENTIRE NERVOUS SYSTEM BRAIN • PITUITARY • FACE EARS • EYES • NOSE • HEAD • PARATHYROID DIAPHRAGM • NECK MUSCLES SCALP • SINUSES • TONGUE TEETH • JAW • THYROID	HEADACHES • MIGRAINES EARACHES • COLDS/FLU SORE THROAT • SINUSITIS FATIGUE • VERTIGO DIZZINESS • ANXIETY ALLERGIES • MEMORY LOSS VISUAL OR AUDITORY DISTURBANCES
C4, C5, C6, C7	NECK MUSCLES • THYROID SINUSES • MOUTH VOCAL CORDS • TONSILS ARMS • ELBOWS • WRISTS HANDS • FINGERS PARATHYROID • ESOPHAGUS ACROSS SHOULDERS	WEIGHT GAIN • COLD INSOMNIA • FATIGUE COLDS/FLU • SINUSITIS HEADACHES • SORE THROAT VERTIGO • DIZZINESS ALLERGIES • REFLUX NUMBNESS • TINGLING
T1, T2, T3, T4	HEART • LUNGS • THYMUS BRONCHIAL TUBES • TRACHEA CHEST • BREAST • PLEURA GALL BLADDER • ARMS ACROSS SHOULDERS UPPER BACK SHOULDER BLADES	HEART CONDITIONS • ASTHMA BRONCHITIS • INDIGESTION DIFFICULTY SWALLOWING NAUSEA • HEADACHES FATIGUE • PLEURISY CHRONIC COUGHING SHORTNESS OF BREATH BLOATING AFTER EATING
T5, T6, T7, T8	STOMACH • PANCREAS SPLEEN • LIVER DUODENUM PERITONEUM • MIDDLE BACK	GASTRITIS • ULCERS INDIGESTION • CRAVE SWEETS HEADACHES • FATIGUE FEELING TOXIC • RASHES CATCHES COLDS EASILY DIABETES • HYPOGLYCEMIA
T9, T10, T11, T12	ADRENALS SMALL INTESTINE KIDNEYS MIDDLE LOWER BACK	STRESS • FATIGUE IRRITABLE BOWELS • HIVES ECZEMA • RASHES HIGH BLOOD PRESSURE GASSY • BLOATING WATER RETENTION
L1, L2, L3, L4, L5, SACRUM	LARGE INTESTINE SMALL INTESTINE ILEOCECAL VALVE APPENDIX • BLADDER OVARIES • UTERUS PROSTATE • TESTICLES REPRODUCTIVE ORGANS RECTUM • URETHRA LOW BACK • PELVIS BUTTOCKS • GROIN THIGHS • KNEES ANKLES • FEET • TOES SCIATIC NERVE	CONSTIPATION • DIARRHEA GASSY • BLOATING IRRITABLE BOWEL BLADDER INFECTIONS PAINFUL URINATION BED WETTING HEMMORHOIDS MENSTRUAL PROBLEMS PREMENSTRUAL SYNDROME IRREGULAR PERIODS MENOPAUSE INFERTILITY LOW SEX DRIVE NUMBNESS OR TINGLING YEAST INFECTIONS SCIATIC PAIN SPRAINED ANKLES

When you have elicited a small asymmetry (more applicably that of a white spot in a pinkish background or vice versa) change your SCENAR settings back to low frequency. You can change other settings such as modulation, damping, intensity or some combination of these to create dynamics in resistant small asymmetry.

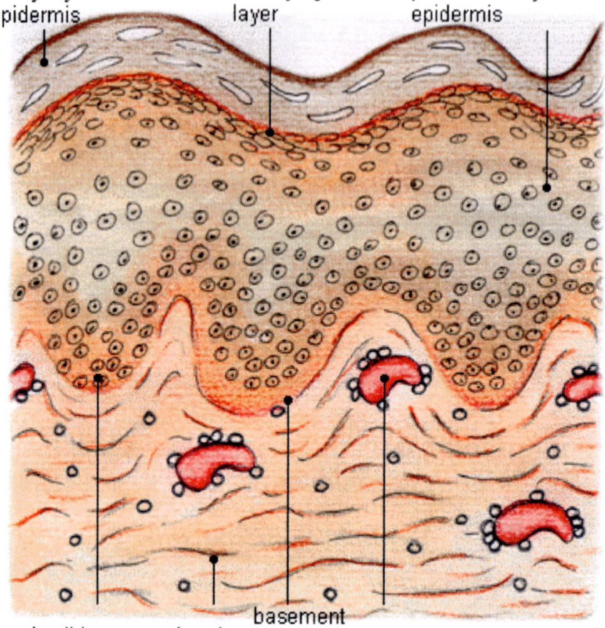
horny layer of the epidermis
cornifying layer
prickle-cell layer of the epidermis
basal-cell layer
dermis
basement mebrane
blood vessel

By continuously verifying any changes in the original vector (pain levels, movement, etc.) with the patient – if they are satisfactory – stop the treatment. If not, check for pain migration or new freedom of movement.

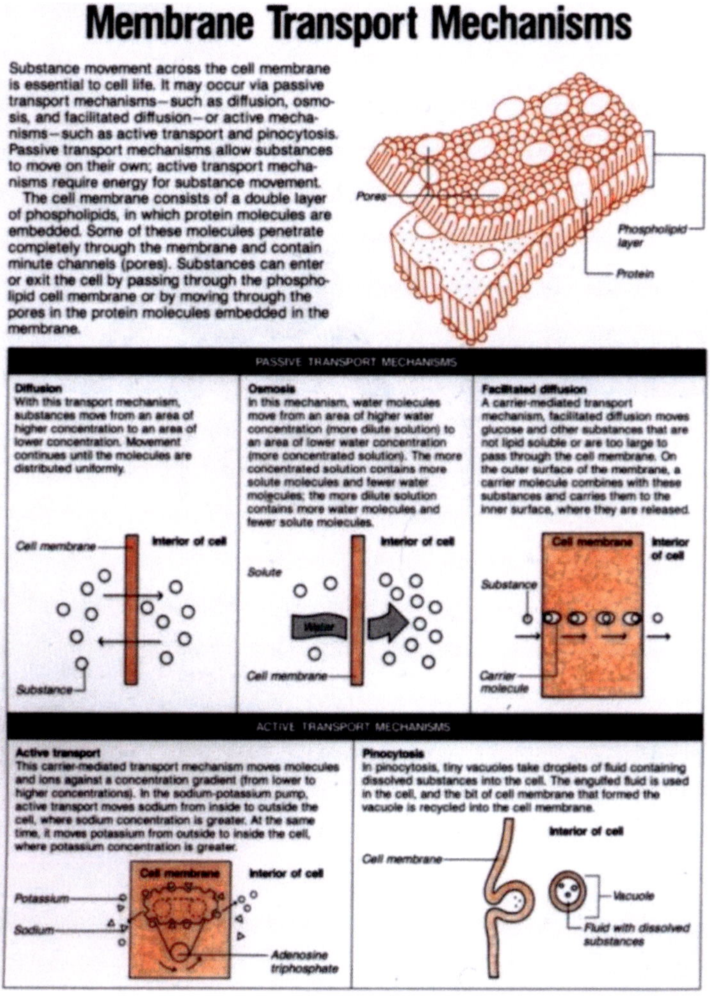
Membrane Transport Mechanisms
Substance movement across the cell membrane is essential to cell life. It may occur via passive transport mechanisms—such as diffusion, osmosis, and facilitated diffusion—or active mechanisms—such as active transport and pinocytosis. Passive transport mechanisms allow substances to move on their own; active transport mechanisms require energy for substance movement.
The cell membrane consists of a double layer of phospholipids, in which protein molecules are embedded. Some of these molecules penetrate completely through the membrane and contain minute channels (pores). Substances can enter or exit the cell by passing through the phospholipid cell membrane or by moving through the pores in the protein molecules embedded in the membrane.
Pores
Phospholipid layer
Protein
PASSIVE TRANSPORT MECHANISMS
Diffusion
With this transport mechanism, substances move from an area of higher concentration to an area of lower concentration. Movement continues until the molecules are distributed uniformly.
Cell membrane
Interior of cell
Substance
Osmosis
In this mechanism, water molecules move from an area of higher water concentration (more dilute solution) to an area of lower water concentration (more concentrated solution). The more concentrated solution contains more solute molecules and fewer water molecules; the more dilute solution contains more water molecules and fewer solute molecules.
Interior of cell
Solute
Water
Cell membrane
Facilitated diffusion
A carrier-mediated transport mechanism, facilitated diffusion moves glucose and other substances that are not lipid soluble or are too large to pass through the cell membrane. On the outer surface of the membrane, a carrier molecule combines with these substances and carries them to the inner surface, where they are released.
Cell membrane
Interior of cell
Substance
Carrier molecule
ACTIVE TRANSPORT MECHANISMS
Active transport
This carrier-mediated transport mechanism moves molecules and ions against a concentration gradient (from lower to higher concentrations). In the sodium-potassium pump, active transport moves sodium from inside to outside the cell, where sodium concentration is greater. At the same time, it moves potassium from outside to inside the cell, where potassium concentration is greater.
Cell membrane
Interior of cell
Potassium
Sodium
Adenosine triphosphate
Pinocytosis
In pinocytosis, tiny vacuoles take droplets of fluid containing dissolved substances into the cell. The engulfed fluid is used in the cell, and the bit of cell membrane that formed the vacuole is recycled into the cell membrane.
Interior of cell
Cell membrane
Vacuole
Fluid with dissolved substances

Regularly monitor the future state of your client, verifying for secondary signs or other treatment indicators.

When to use DIAG=0:

- In the presence of clearly defined local symptoms.
- In an emergency – for achieving rapid functional changes in the body.
- When larger surfaces need to be treated.

Chapter 15. Little Wings and Bowling Ball

The pulsed "Little Wings" technique is well known to directly affect areas as distal as the legs in which "twitches" and other involuntary muscular actions may take place - the singular, short-lived contraction of Bowling Ball undoubtedly must also propagate actions into various local and distal segments of the body - this complex activity is introduced into the facials network as a whole. It is well known that Little Wings stimulates copious neuropeptide secretions and frequently acts as a key to unlock stored emotional trauma.

General Recommendations for **Little Wings**

Technique Suggested Settings: Diag = 0

Mod = 3:1

Dmpf = Sk2

Freq = 121

Increase past 70 until patient feels that it is at the proper intensity. Place the Scenar centered below the ear and hold until the shoulder spasms up. You should be able to feel and hear the noise in the ear and tenseness in the shoulder. Hold for five cycles of the shoulder spasm. You may need to move the Scenar around on the neck and trapezoid to find the right spot. If the patient is particularly stressed or tense, you may not get a reaction on the first try. Patients report an increased relaxation in the neck, pain "melting" away and a sensation of an automatic realignment of the spine. This therapy seems to stimulate the parasympathetic system. There are important differences in the referred pain patterns for the two branches of the SCM muscle; the sternal branch and the clavicle branch. Pain can be sent to the top, sides, back, or front of the head. **A frontal headache is practically a signature of SCM trigger points**. Not shown is an occasional spillover of pain in the sides of the face, which mimics a disorder characterized by brief attacks of pain caused by irritation of the trigeminal nerve. **Pain is also sometimes sent to the back of the neck. SCM trigger points can send pain deep into the ear and to the eye and the sinuses.** They can make the back teeth and the root of the tongue hurt. Sometimes a chronic cough or a sore throat is from trigger points in the lower end of one of the SCM. They can be the source of a painful neck stiffness that keeps your head pulled over to one side.

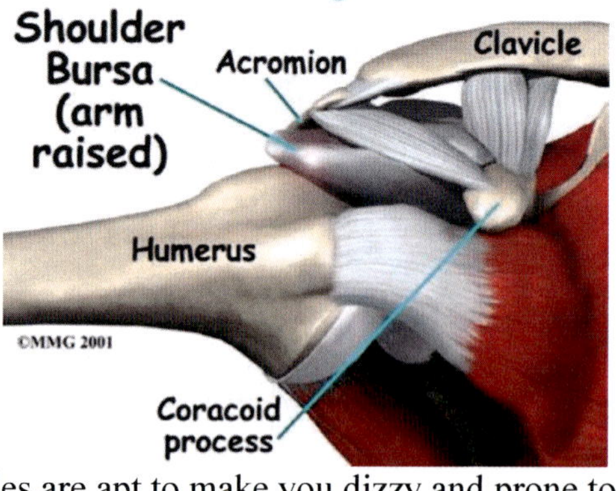
Shoulder
Bursa
(arm
raised)
Acromion
Clavicle
Humerus
©MMG 2001
Coracoid
process

SCM muscles are apt to make you dizzy and prone to lurching or falling unexpectedly. They can also be the cause of unexplained fainting. You can experience a degree of reversible hearing loss on the side where these trigger points exist. Dizziness from trigger points can last for minutes, hours, or days. In some cases, it persists for years, defying all treatments and medical explanations.

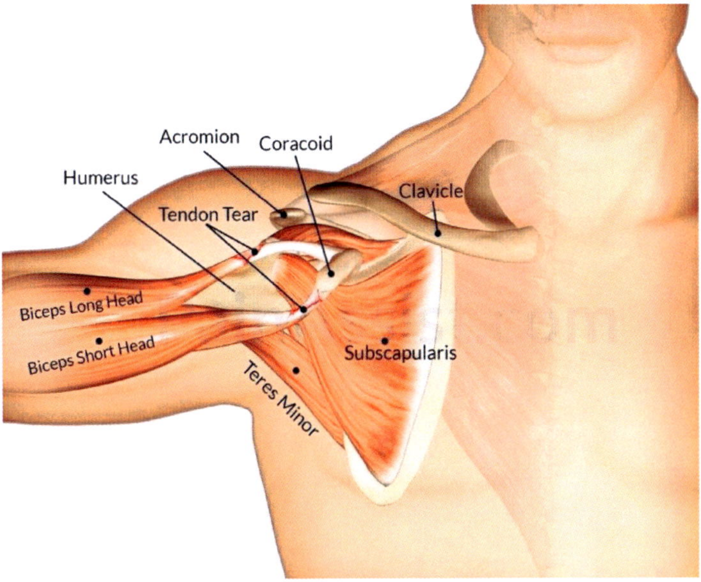
Acromion
Coracoid
Humerus
Clavicle
Tendon Tear
Biceps Long Head
Biceps Short Head
Subscapularis
Teres Minor

SCM trigger points are thought to have a direct effect on the inner ear, thereby affecting your balance. (Travell)

Treatment in Diag. 1

Turn on the device and reset the factory default settings using the UP and DOWN buttons together for 3 seconds. Use the Mode Section (On) button and UP button to select Diag= 1. Increase the Amplitude to a comfortable level of sensation (bearable tingling) whilst holding the SCENAR on the skin and hold it there long enough for the diagnostic assessment to take place (usually less than 2 seconds). Remove it as soon as you have registered the

Initial Reaction (IR) reading, up, remove the SCENAR and try another location until good contact is made and readings appear. If you leave the SCENAR on the skin for longer than 2 seconds, the full set of readings appears and the device begins to treat the area.

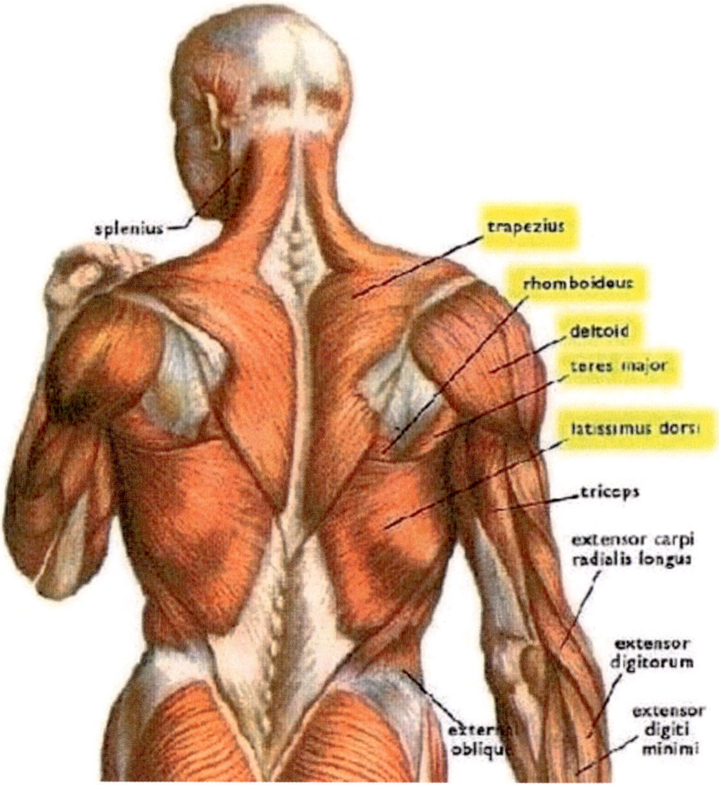

splenius
trapezius
rhomboideus
deltoid
teres major
latissimus dorsi
triceps
extensor carpi radialis longus
extensor digitorum
extensor digiti minimi

Systematically place the SCENAR over the area to be assessed and take initial readings (IR's) and note them down as well as their relative positions. Replace the SCENAR on the position with the highest IR reading and hold the SCENAR still without removing it from the skin until the multi-tone bell goes off and a reading accompanied by an * appears on the lower right hand corner of your screen. SCENAR from the skin and replace it. **Continue doing this until a good contact is established and treat this area until the multi-tone bell sounds as before.**

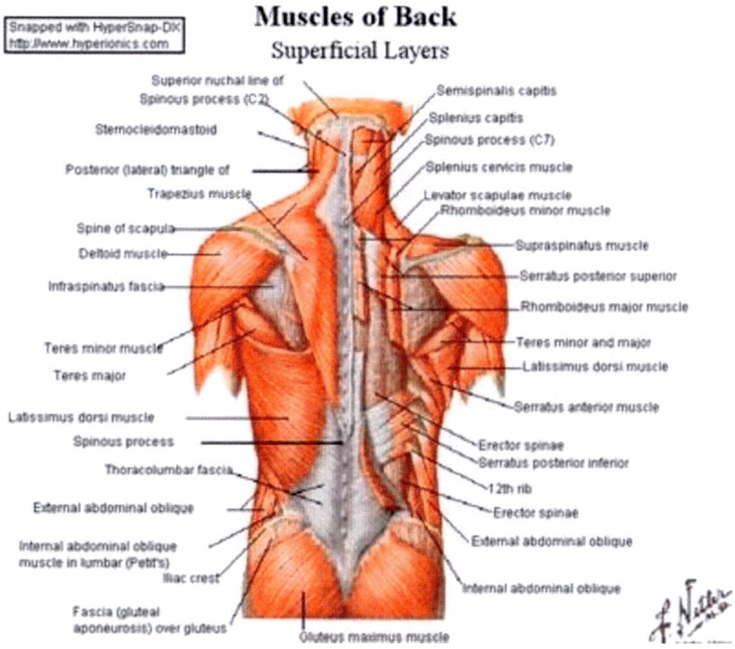

Snapped with HyperSnap-DX
http://www.hyperionics.com
Muscles of Back
Superficial Layers
Superior nuchal line of
Spinous process (C2)
Sternocleidomastoid
Posterior (lateral) triangle of
Trapezius muscle
Spine of scapula
Deltoid muscle
Infraspinatus fascia
Teres minor muscle
Teres major
Latissimus dorsi muscle
Spinous process
Thoracolumbar fascia
External abdominal oblique
Internal abdominal oblique
muscle in lumbar (Petit's)
Iliac crest
Fascia (gluteal
aponeurosis) over gluteus
Gluteus maximus muscle
Semispinalis capitis
Splenius capitis
Spinous process (C7)
Splenius cervicis muscle
Levator scapulae muscle
Rhomboideus minor muscle
Supraspinatus muscle
Serratus posterior superior
Rhomboideus major muscle
Teres minor and major
Latissimus dorsi muscle
Serratus anterior muscle
Erector spinae
Serratus posterior inferior
12th rib
Erector spinae
External abdominal oblique
Internal abdominal oblique

Make a note of the number and indicate the value as a "dosage*). Repeat the above steps looking for another position to give a dose* and make a note of that along with the new value. Now, compare each of the readings for each of the areas that have had a "**dose***". On the area with the highest "dose" reading, replace the SCENAR on the skin in exactly the same area and treat again until V-he relative speed of the reaction (which is the second reading from the left on the top line) reads "0". This may take several minutes and you should wait, holding the SCENAR still until the "0" appears. The

97.4+ should give you an indication by a bell tone and a @symbol with the asterisk. Take a note of the Ongoing Reaction value at the bottom right hand corner of your screen. FM is a technique that uses a combination of **Frequency Modulation to be found in the modulation mode and a Variation of Damping called simply VAR, which is in the Damping Mode**. This treatment mode should be used once a comparison of all the "0's" reveals the highest 0 value. Place the SCENAR on the area of choice in FM for two minutes.

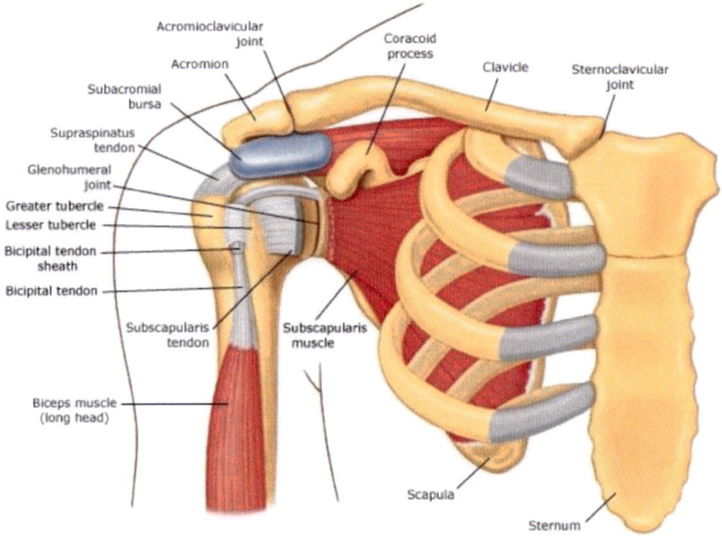

Acromioclavicular joint
Coracoid process
Acromion
Clavicle
Sternoclavicular joint
Subacromial bursa
Supraspinatus tendon
Glenohumeral joint
Greater tubercle
Lesser tubercle
Bicipital tendon sheath
Bicipital tendon
Subscapularis tendon
Subscapularis muscle
Biceps muscle (long head)
Scapula
Sternum

When areas of small asymmetries have been revealed during the treatment in DIAG0, you may work on them again in DIAG1.

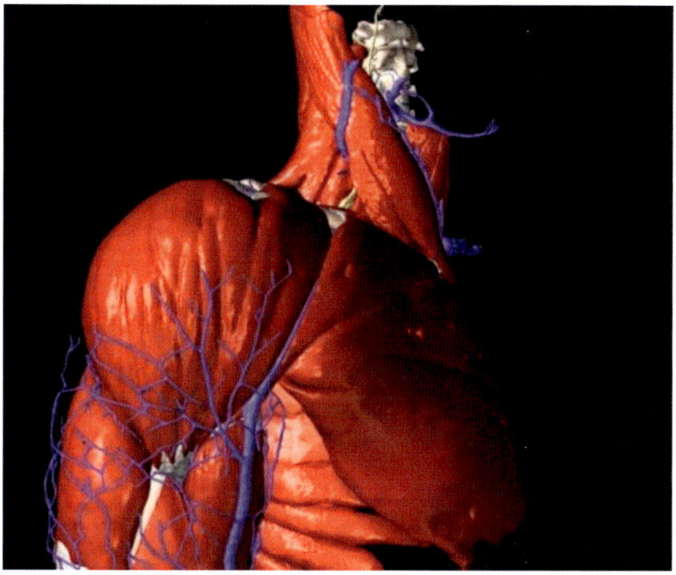

One can observe regional contractions of both extrinsic muscles (such as the **trapezius**, **levator scapula** and **sternocleidomastoid**) and intrinsic muscles (most probably splenius cervicis, spleniuscapitus, semispinales cervicis and semispinales capitus along with others such as scalene on occasion) - these contractions undoubtedly reset resting tonus by way of the gamma gain of the **muscle spindles** (and possibly also the **Golgi tendon** organs.

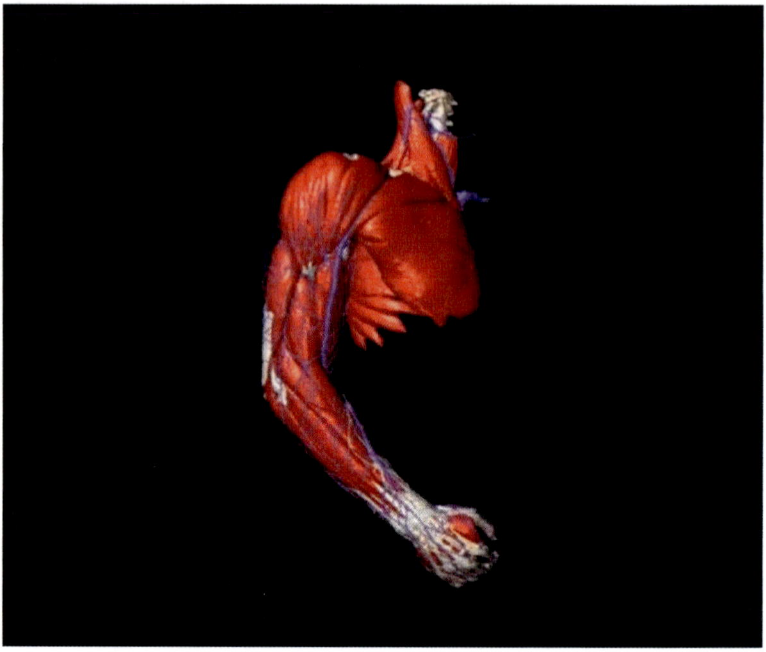

Objective Mode deals with the Diagnostic Mode in more detail but we will learn how to use this function summarily to get feed-back information or Initial Reaction readings (IR) to help you choose where to treat. Systematically place the SCENAR over the area to be assessed and take initial readings (IR's) and note them down as well as their relative positions. **Replace the SCENAR on the position with the highest IR reading and hold the SCENAR still without removing it from the skin until the multi-tone bell goes off and a reading accompanied by an * appears on the lower right hand corner of your screen.** SCENAR from the skin and replace it. Continue doing this until a good contact is established and treat this area until the multi-tone bell sounds as before.

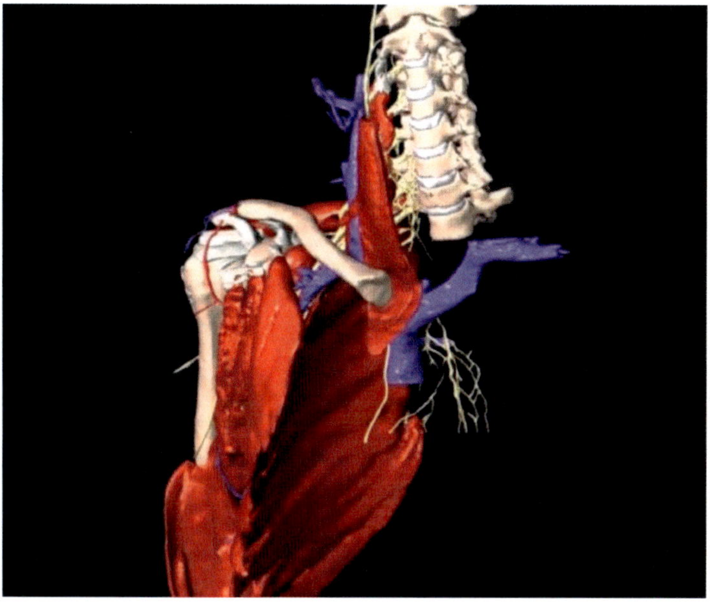

Make a note of the number and indicate the value as a "dosage*). Repeat the above steps looking for another position to give a dose* and make a note of that along with the new value. Now, compare each of the readings for each of the areas that have had a "dose*". On the area with the highest "dose*" reading, replace the SCENAR on the skin in exactly the same area and treat again until the relative speed of the reaction (which is the second reading from the left on the top line) reads "0". This may take several minutes and you should wait, holding the SCENAR still until the "0" appears. The 97.4+ should give you an indication by a bell tone and a @ symbol with the asterisk. Take a note of the Ongoing Reaction value at the bottom right hand corner of your screen. FM/VAR is a technique that uses a combination of Frequency Modulation to be found in the modulation mode and a Variation of Damping called simply VAR, which is in the Damping Mode. This treatment mode should be used once a comparison of all the “0’s” reveals the highest 0 value. Place the SCENAR on the area of choice in FM for two minutes.

When to use DIAG.1

- **To localize symptoms;**
- **To save time when looking for asymmetries;**
- **To optimize the action time;**
- **When areas of small asymmetries have been revealed during the treatment in DIAG0, you may work on them again in DIAG1.**

Chapter 16. Priority Areas for Treatment

Areas and Parts of the Body	Vertebrae	Possible Symptoms
Blood supply to the head, pituitary gland, scalp, bones of the face, brain, inner and middle ear, sympathetic nervous system	C1	Headaches, nervousness, insomnia, head colds, high blood pressure, migraine headaches, nervous breakdowns, chronic tiredness, dizziness
Eyes, optic nerves, auditory nerves, sinuses, mastoid bones, tongue, forehead	C2	Sinus trouble, allergies, pain around the eyes, earache
Cheeks, outer ear, face bones, teeth, trifacial nerve.	C3	Neuralgia, neuritis, acne or pimples, eczema
Nose, lips, mouth, eustachian tube	C4	Hay fever, runny nose, hearing loss, adenoids
Vocal cords, neck glands, pharynx	C5	Laryngitis, hoarseness, throat conditions such as soar throat
Neck muscles, shoulders, tonsils	C6	Stiff neck, pain in upper arm, tonsillitis, chronic cough, croup
Thyroid gland, bursae in the shoulders, elbows	C7	Bursitis, colds, thyroid conditions
Arms from the elbows down, including hands, wrist, and fingers, esophagus and trachea	T1	Asthma, cough, difficult breathing, shortness of breath, pain in lower arms and hands
Heart, including its valves and covering, coronary arteries	T2	Functional heart conditions and certain chest conditions
Lungs, bronchial tubes, pleura, chest, breast	T3	Bronchitis, pleurisy, pneumonia, congestion, influenza
Gall bladder, common duct	T4	Gall bladder conditions, jaundice, congestion
Liver, solar plexus, circulation (general)	T5	Liver conditions, fevers, blood pressure problems, poor circulation, arthritis
Stomach	T6	Stomach troubles, including nervous stomach, indigestion, heart burn, dyspepsia
Pancreas, duodenum	T7	Ulcers, gastritis
Spleen	T8	Lowered resistance
Adrenal and supra-renal glands	T9	Allergies, hives
Kidneys	T10	Kidney troubles, hardening of the arteries, chronic tiredness, nephritis, pyelitis
Kidneys, ureters	T11	Skin conditions such as acne, pimples, eczema, boils
Small intestines, lymph circulation	T12	Rheumatism, gas pains, certain types of sterility
Large intestines, inguinal rings	L1	Constipation, colitis, dysentery, diarrhea, some hernias
Appendix, abdomen, upper leg	L2	Cramps, difficult breathing, minor varicose veins
Sex organs, uterus, bladder, knees	L3	Bladder trouble, , miscarriages, bed wetting, impotency, change of life symptoms, many knee pains
Prostate gland, muscles of the low back, sciatic nerve	L4	Sciatica, lumbago, difficult, painful, too frequent urination, backaches
Lower legs, ankles, feet	L5	Poor circulation in the legs, swollen ankles, weak ankles and arches, cold feet, weakness in the legs, leg cramps
Hip bones, buttocks	Sacrum	Sacro-iliac condition, spinal curvatures
Rectum, anus	Coccyx	Hemorrhoids, pruritus (itching), pain at end of spine on sitting

When the red shaded vertebrae are subluxated they can cause the following health problems, also in red.

Direct projection of the pain.

Primary signs as described in the "Treatment Reaction Indicators" above:

- **Asymmetry**
- **Small Asymmetry**
- **Horizontals**
- **General Zones**
- **Symmetrical Areas**

Figure 1: Hands (Palmar Surface)

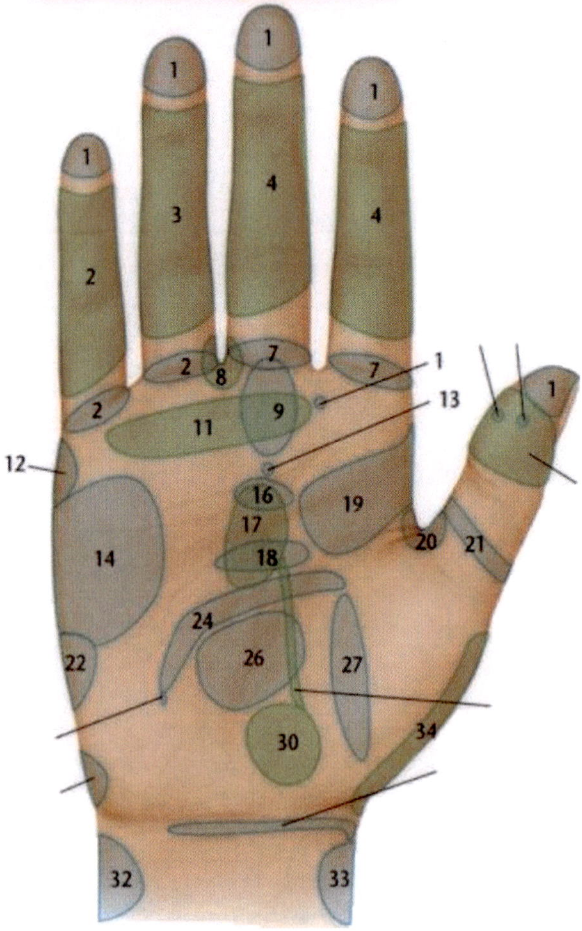

1
1
1
1
2
3
4
4
2
8
7
7
2
1
13
9
11
12
1
16
17
19
14
18
20
21
24
22
26
27
30
34
32
33

Reciprocal areas:

1. Nerves and ears
2. Colds and nerves
3. Pineal gland
4. Pituitary gland
5. Eyes
6. Eustachian tubes
7. Brain
8. Thymus
9. Lungs
10. Shoulders
11. Solar plexus
12. Liver
13. Heart
14. Adrenal glands

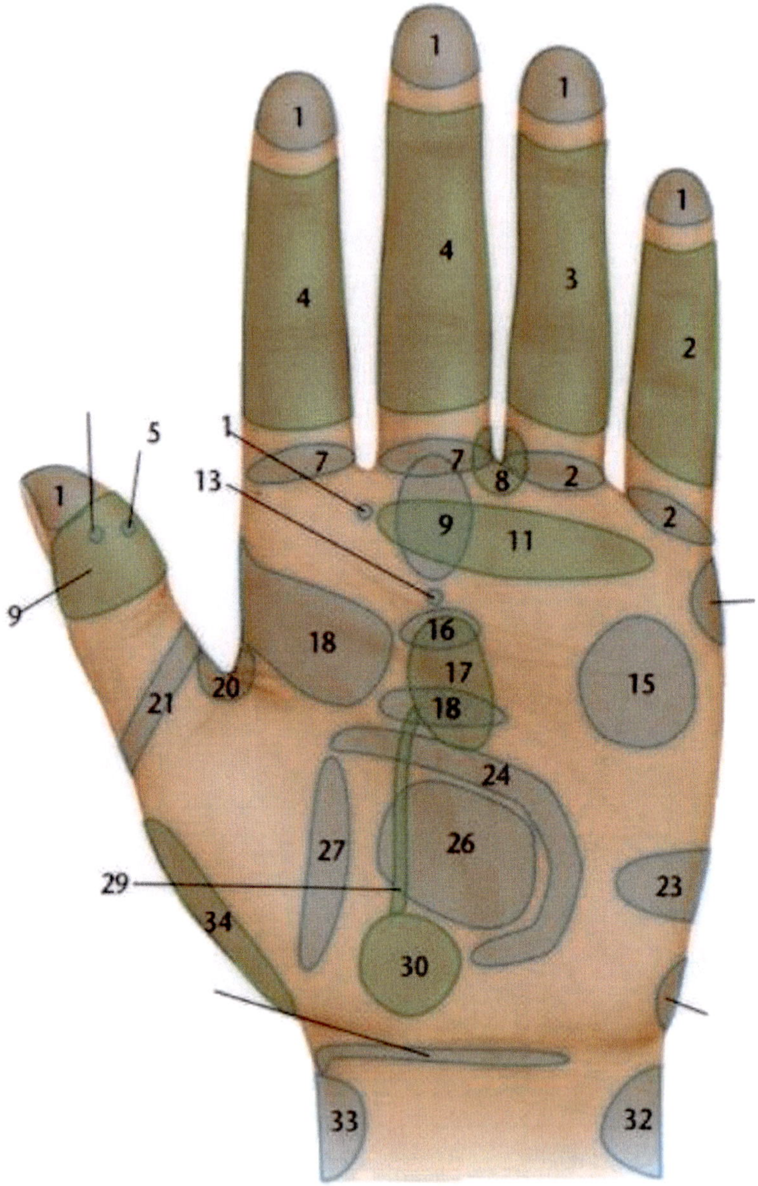
1
1
1
1
1
4
4
3
2
5
1
13
7
7
8
2
2
9
9
11
16
18
17
18
20
21
15
24
26
27
29
23
34
30
33
32

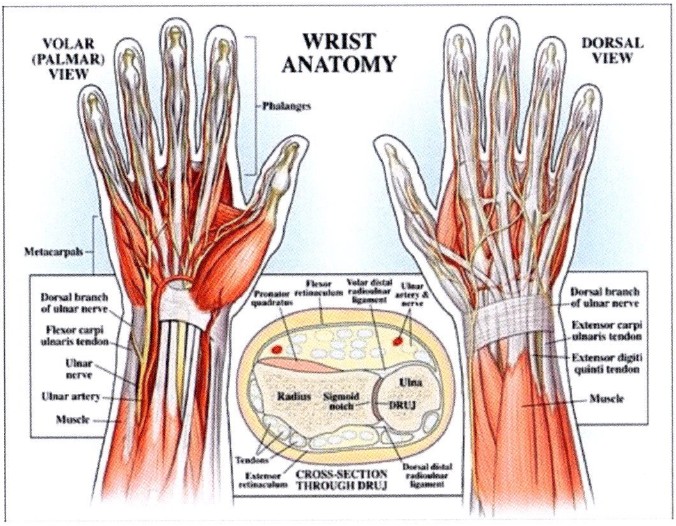
VOLAR (PALMAR) VIEW
WRIST ANATOMY
DORSAL VIEW
Phalanges
Metacarpals
Dorsal branch of ulnar nerve
Flexor carpi ulnaris tendon
Ulnar nerve
Ulnar artery
Muscle
Pronator quadratus
Flexor retinaculum
Volar distal radioulnar ligament
Ulnar artery & nerve
Ulna
Radius
Sigmoid notch
DRUJ
Tendons
Extensor retinaculum
CROSS-SECTION THROUGH DRUJ
Dorsal distal radioulnar ligament
Dorsal branch of ulnar nerve
Extensor carpi ulnaris tendon
Extensor digiti quinti tendon
Muscle

1. Nerves & Ears
2. Kidneys
3. Pancreas
4. Stomach
5. Throat
6. Neck
7. Gall bladder
8. Spleen
9. Colon
10. Appendix
11. Small intestine
12. Thyroid/parathyroid glands

13. Hips

14. Ureter tubes

15. Bladder

16. Hemorrhoids

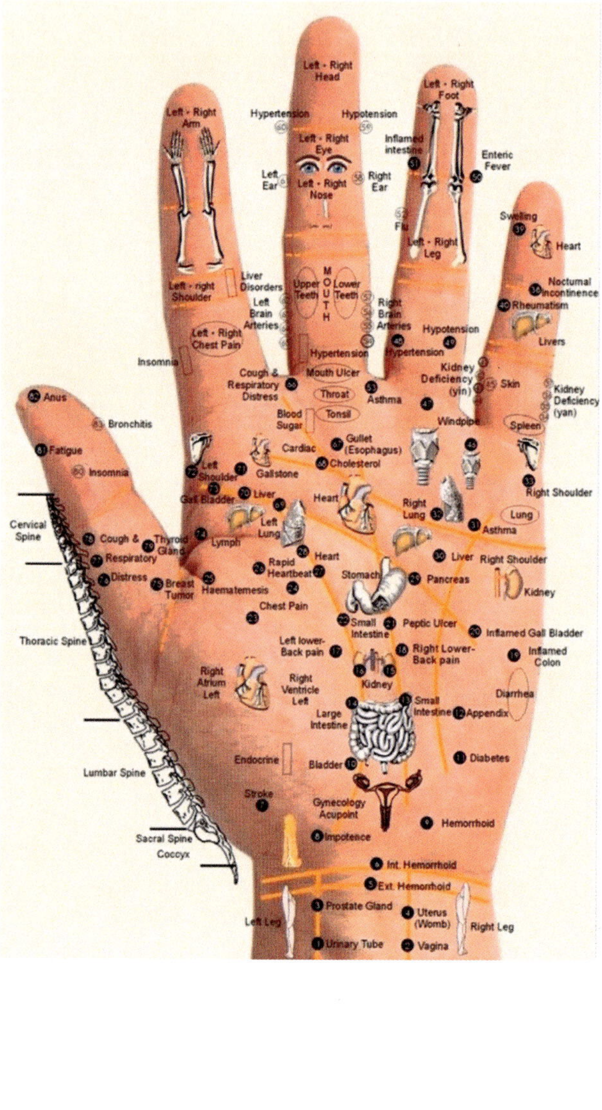

Left - Right Head
Left - Right Arm
Hypertension
Hypotension
Left - Right Eye
Left - Right Foot
Inflamed intestine
Enteric Fever
Left Ear
Left - Right Nose
Right Ear
Flu
Swelling
Heart
Left - Right Leg
Liver Disorders
Left - right Shoulder
Upper Teeth
MOUTH
Lower Teeth
Left Brain Arteries
Right Brain Arteries
Nocturnal Incontinence
Rheumatism
Left - Right Chest Pain
Hypotension
Livers
Insomnia
Hypertension
Hypertension
Cough & Respiratory Distress
Mouth Ulcer
Kidney Deficiency (yin)
Skin
Kidney Deficiency (yan)
Anus
Throat
Asthma
Blood Sugar
Tonsil
Windpipe
Spleen
Bronchitis
Cardiac
Gullet (Esophagus)
Cholesterol
Fatigue
Left Shoulder
Gallstone
Insomnia
Right Shoulder
Gall Bladder
Liver
Heart
Right Lung
Lung
Cervical Spine
Left Lung
Asthma
Cough &
Respiratory
Distress
Thyroid Gland
Lymph
Heart
Rapid Heartbeat
Liver
Right Shoulder
Stomach
Pancreas
Breast Tumor
Haematemesis
Kidney
Chest Pain
Small Intestine
Peptic Ulcer
Inflamed Gall Bladder
Thoracic Spine
Left lower-Back pain
Right Lower-Back pain
Inflamed Colon
Right Atrium Left
Right Ventricle Left
Kidney
Diarrhea
Large Intestine
Small Intestine
Appendix
Endocrine
Bladder
Diabetes
Lumbar Spine
Stroke
Gynecology Acupoint
Hemorrhoid
Sacral Spine
Coccyx
Impotence
Int. Hemorrhoid
Ext. Hemorrhoid
Prostate Gland
Left Leg
Uterus (Womb)
Right Leg
Urinary Tube
Vagina

Figure 2: Feet (Plantar Surface)

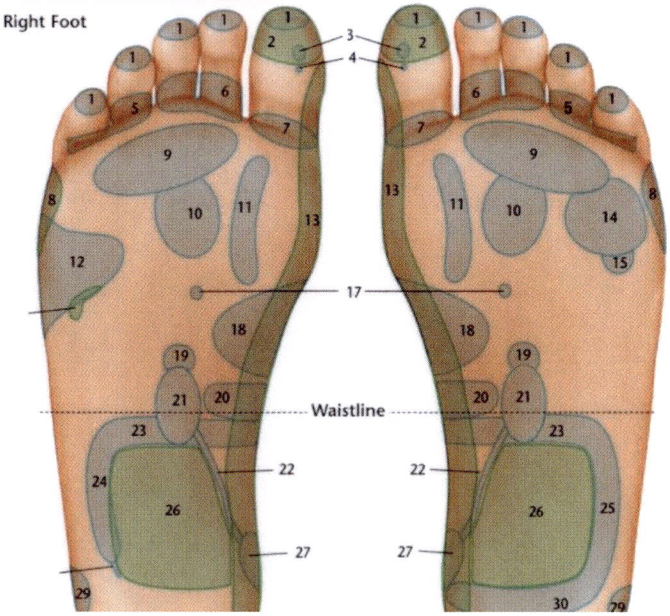
Right Foot
Waistline

1. Sinuses

2. Ovaries/testes

3. Uterus/prostate and rectum

4. Spine

2. Brain

3. Pituitary gland

4. Pineal gland

5. Ears

6. Eyes

7. Parathyroid gland/ neck and throat

8. Shoulders

9. Lungs and bronchi

10. Thymus

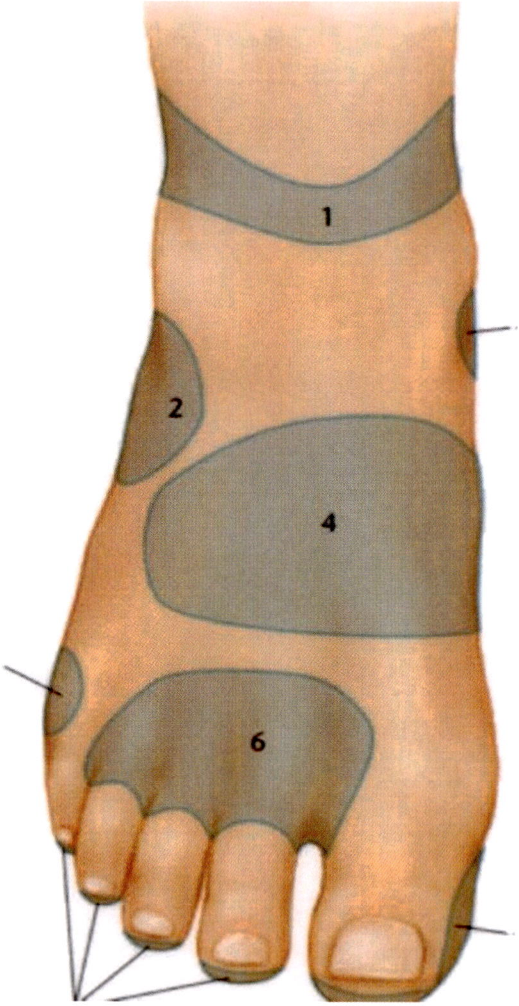
1
2
4
6

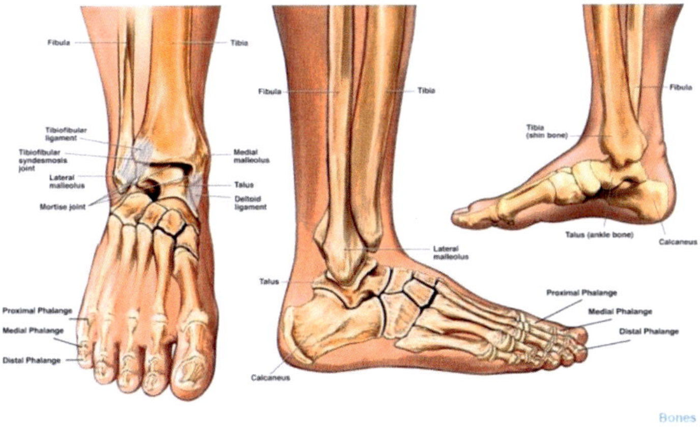
Fibula
Tibia
Tibiofibular ligament
Tibiofibular syndesmosis joint
Lateral malleolus
Mortise joint
Medial malleolus
Talus
Deltoid ligament
Proximal Phalange
Medial Phalange
Distal Phalange
Fibula
Tibia
Lateral malleolus
Talus
Calcaneus
Proximal Phalange
Medial Phalange
Distal Phalange
Fibula
Tibia (shin bone)
Talus (ankle bone)
Calcaneus
Bones

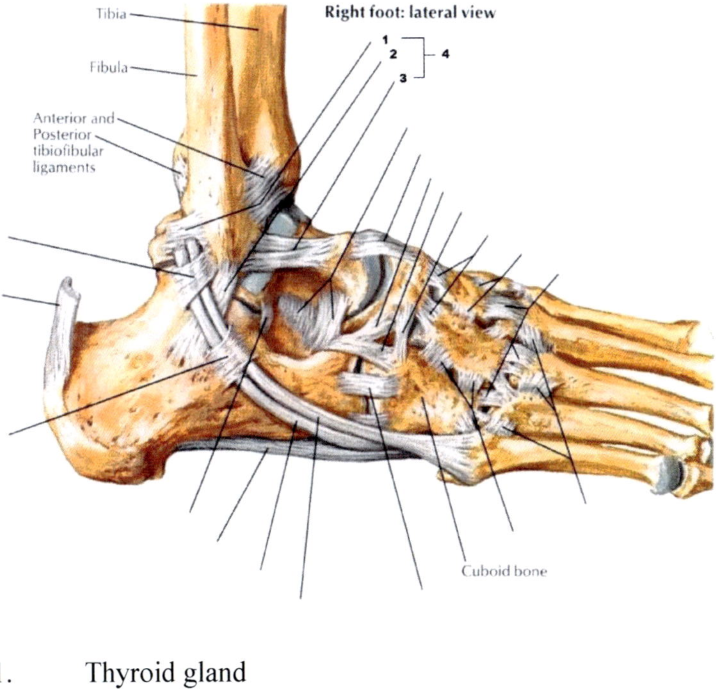
Right foot: lateral view
Tibia
Fibula
Anterior and Posterior tibiofibular ligaments
1
2
3
4
Cuboid bone

1. Thyroid gland
2. Liver
3. Spine

4. Heart, arteries, and veins

5. Spleen

6. Gall bladder

7. Solar plexus

8. Stomach

9. Adrenal glands

10. Pancreas

11. Kidneys

12. Ureter tubes

13. Transverse colon

14. Ascending colon

15. Descending colon

16. Small intestine

17. Bladder

18. Appendix

19. Hips

20. Sigmoid colon

21. Sciatic nerves

22. Hemorrhoids

Foot

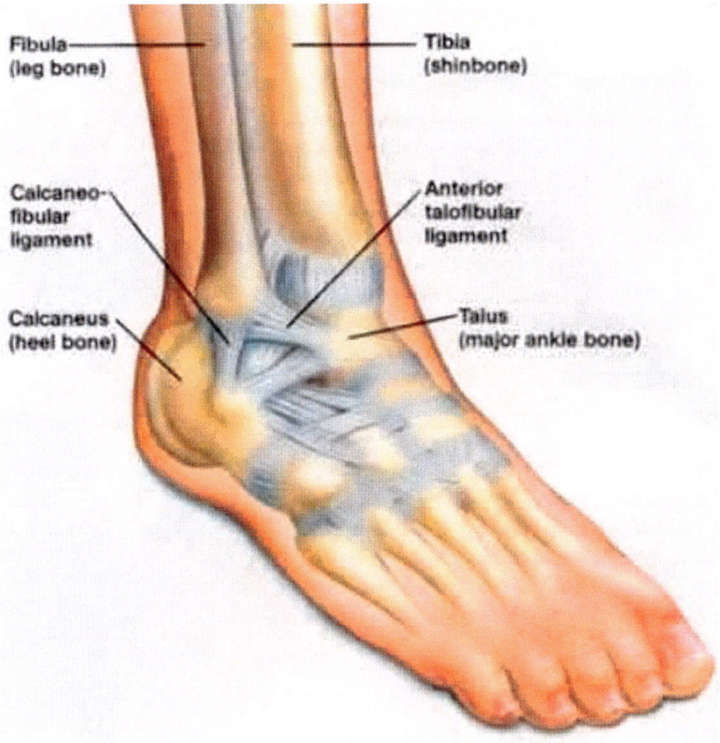
Fibula
(leg bone)
Tibia
(shinbone)
Calcaneo-
fibular
ligament
Anterior
talofibular
ligament
Calcaneus
(heel bone)
Talus
(major ankle bone)

1. Lymph glands and Fallopian tubes
2. Knee, hip, and lower back
3. Uterus/prostate gland
4. Breast
5. SLhuonuglsdaenrd bronchi
6. Sinuses
7. Top of head and brain

Hands

1. Eyes and ears

2. Shoulders

3. Spleen

4. Stomach and pancreas 5 Lymph drainage and back muscles

5. Neck

6. Hips

7. Lymph nodes

8. Liver

9. Gall bladder

10. Pancreas

11. Breast

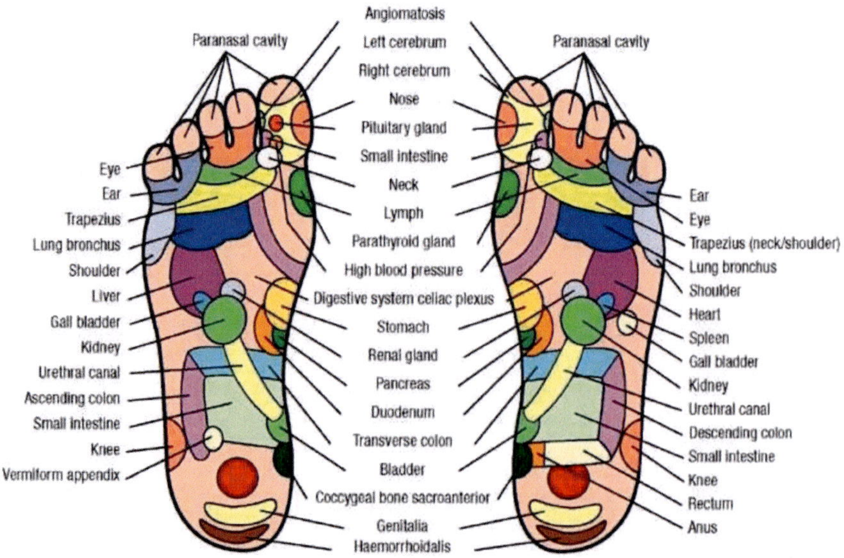
Paranasal cavity
Eye
Ear
Trapezius
Lung bronchus
Shoulder
Liver
Gall bladder
Kidney
Urethral canal
Ascending colon
Small intestine
Knee
Vermiform appendix
Angiomatosis
Left cerebrum
Right cerebrum
Nose
Pituitary gland
Small intestine
Neck
Lymph
Parathyroid gland
High blood pressure
Digestive system celiac plexus
Stomach
Renal gland
Pancreas
Duodenum
Transverse colon
Bladder
Coccygeal bone sacroanterior
Genitalia
Haemorrhoidalis
Paranasal cavity
Ear
Eye
Trapezius (neck/shoulder)
Lung bronchus
Shoulder
Heart
Spleen
Gall bladder
Kidney
Urethral canal
Descending colon
Small intestine
Knee
Rectum
Anus

Reflex Points of the Ear

1. Body warmer
2. Heel
3. Feet and toes
4. Ankle
5. Hand and fingers
6. Knees
7. Hips
8. Upper leg
9. Kidney
10. Back pain
11. Wrist
12. Lower back
13. Elbow
14. Liver
15. Upper arm
16. Spleen
17. Upper back
18. Shoulder
19. Forehead
20. Back of head

21. Neck

22. Face and body reflexes (under ear lobe)

Reflex Points of the Head and Face

1. Gonads

2. Internal organs

3. Stomach

4. Pituitary gland

Figure 4: Hands

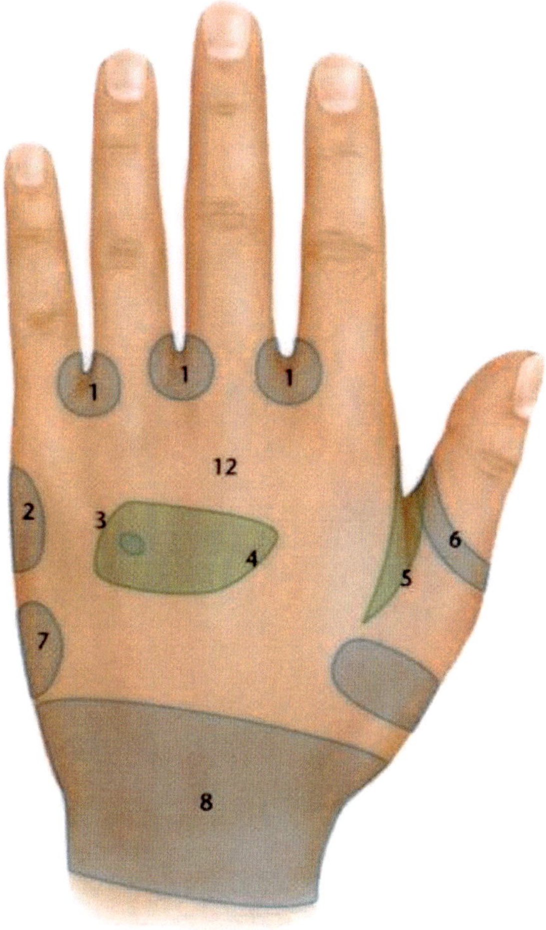
1
1
1
12
2
3
4
5
6
7
8

1. Blurred vision/mental conditions

2. Pineal gland

3. Headaches

4. Eye stress

Kidneys and adrenal glands

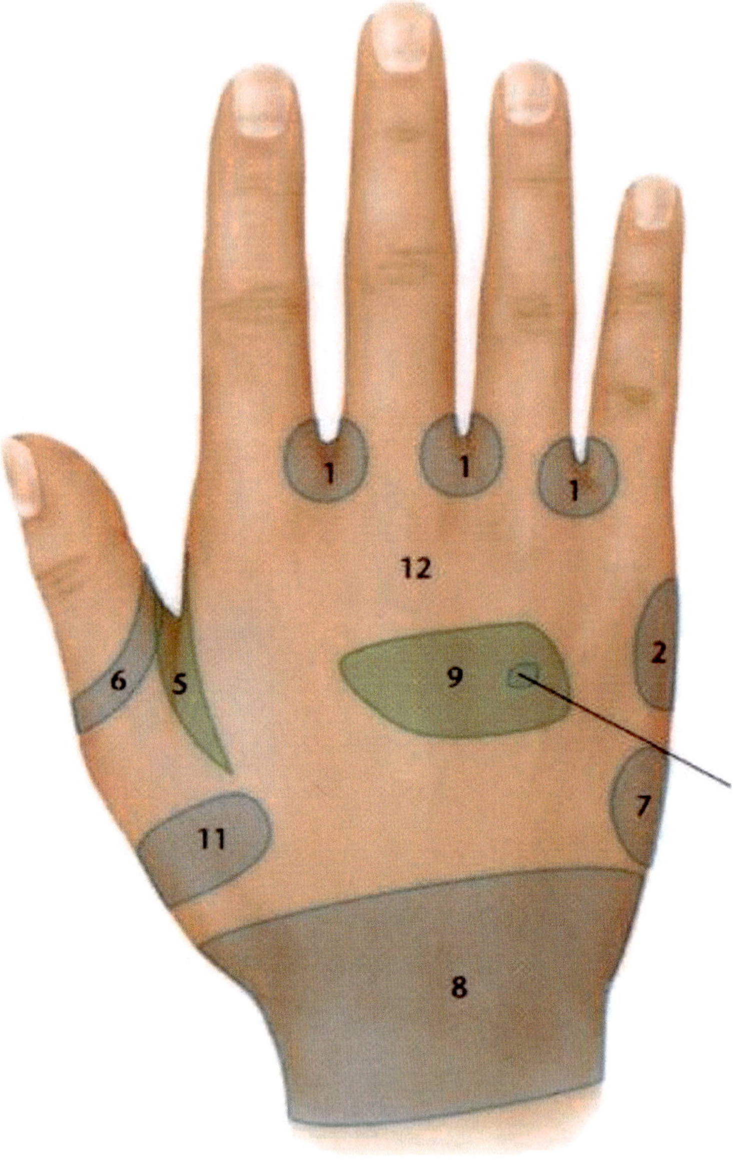

1
1
1
12
2
9
6
5
7
11
8

Flexors of Wrist

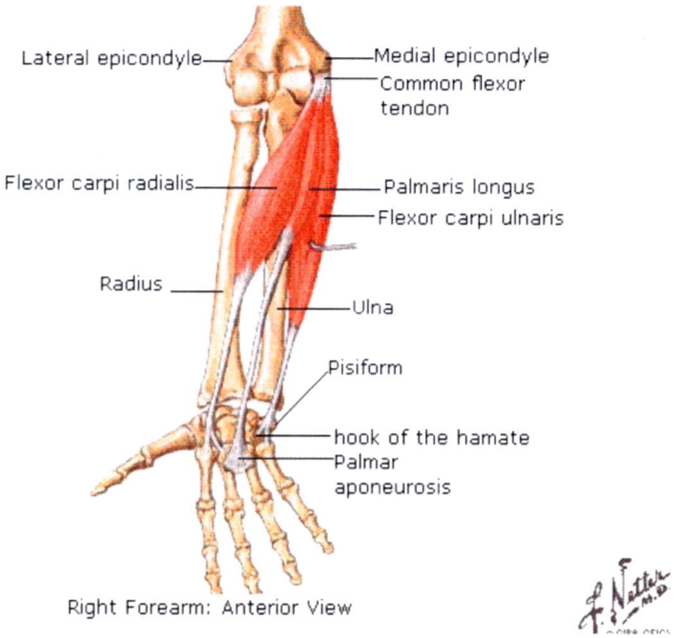
Lateral epicondyle
Medial epicondyle
Common flexor tendon
Flexor carpi radialis
Palmaris longus
Flexor carpi ulnaris
Radius
Ulna
Pisiform
hook of the hamate
Palmar aponeurosis
Right Forearm: Anterior View

Chase the pain until it goes

Look for secondary sign on the lower back closer to the spinal column often as vesicular rash. When reading Initial Reactions, as soon as the first two numbers appear on the screen, the device is removed from the skin. During this short time, the organism will not have time to react to the impulse so that an IR reading will be purely diagnostic and not therapeutic. When the SCENAR is left on the skin, the nervous system starts to respond. By comparing the final reactions (0's), the organism indicates an area of small asymmetry and treating with FmVar (maximum of dynamics from device) at this site will produce the best results. Maximum dynamics from the device will give maximum action from the organism. Before starting the procedure choose level of power of the impulse action.

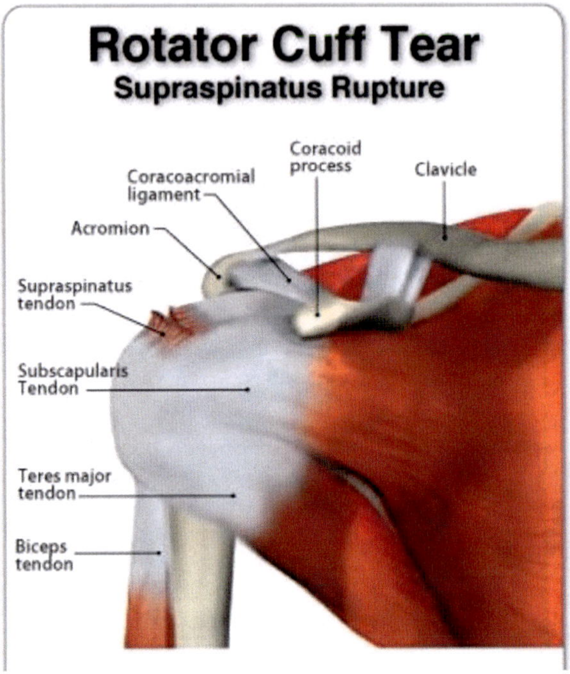

Rotator Cuff Tear
Supraspinatus Rupture
Coracoid process
Clavicle
Coracoacromial ligament
Acromion
Supraspinatus tendon
Subscapularis Tendon
Teres major tendon
Biceps tendon

Inflammation of a joint

Arthritis

Inflammation of a joint

Causes and Factors

Local or general infection, possibly specific (such as tuberculosis or chlamydiosis), trauma, allergy, autoimmune response, metabolic disorders etc.

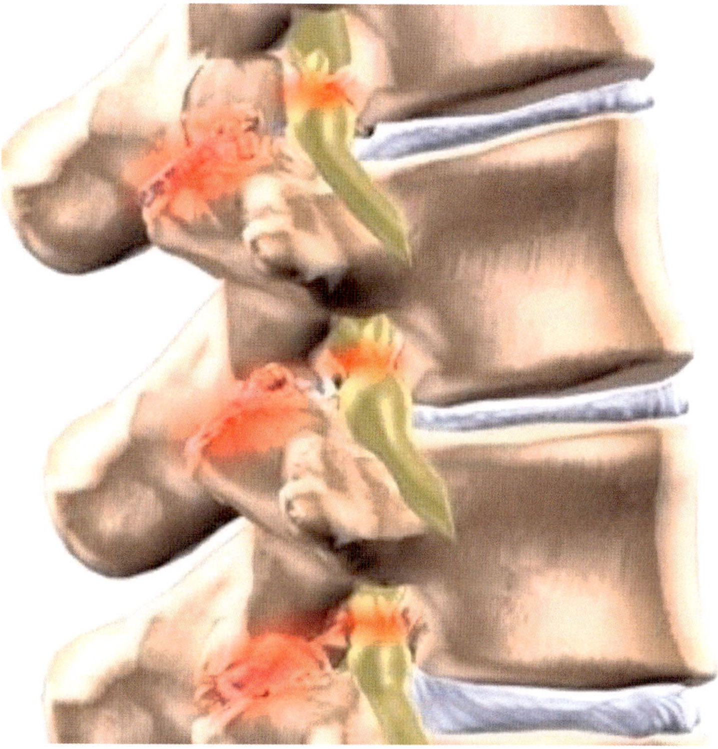

Arthritis can be caused by

- weakened immunity
- chronic focal infection (chronic tonsillitis etc.)
- overcooling
- large loads on a joint
- heredity

Clinical picture

General health condition: Poor health, high temperature, sometimes fevers. Pain is intensive, spontaneous, worse with movement and at night. There are more than 200 diseases with a clinical picture of mono- (1 joint is affected), or poly-(several joints are affected) arthritis (rheumatism, psoriasis, podagra, rheumatoid arthritis etc.). In arthritis, there are both general and specific symptoms of inflammations. Dermal integuments are hyperemic above the joint, their temperature is high. Except for neurodystrophic arthritis, where they are cyanotic, cold when palpated. Swelling and deformation of the joint involved are developed by inflammatory edema of soft tissues and cartilaginous coverings, and accumulation of exudate in joint. Functional changes are due to pain syndrome, from proliferative or fibrous process. Joint mobility: limited to complete absence of mobility. Laboratory data: changes in blood composition typical for inflammation.

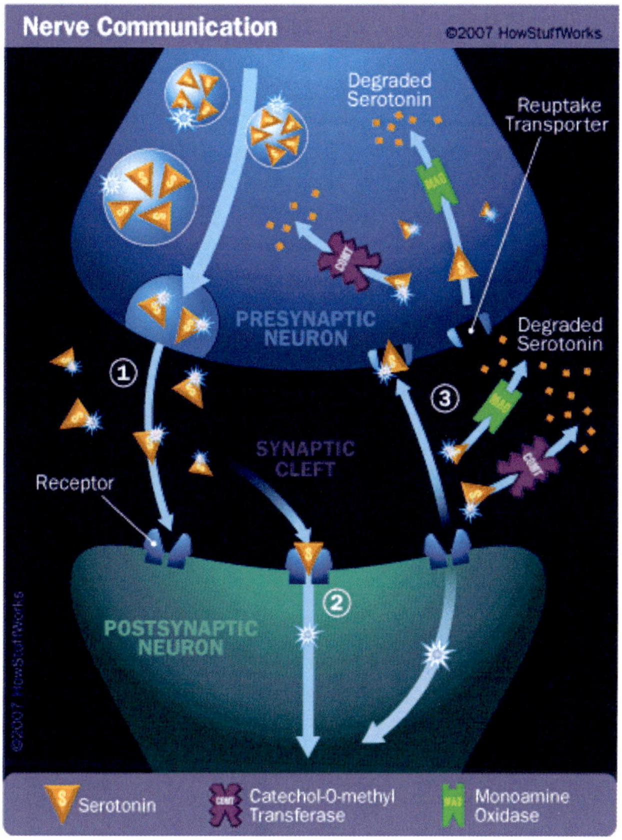
Nerve Communication
©2007 HowStuffWorks
Degraded Serotonin
Reuptake Transporter
PRESYNAPTIC NEURON
Degraded Serotonin
1
3
SYNAPTIC CLEFT
Receptor
2
POSTSYNAPTIC NEURON
Serotonin
Catechol-O-methyl Transferase
Monoamine Oxidase

Arthritis can be acute, sub-acute and chronic.

Acute arthritis is characterized with intensity of all above-mentioned symptoms, and mobility restriction is usually reversible.

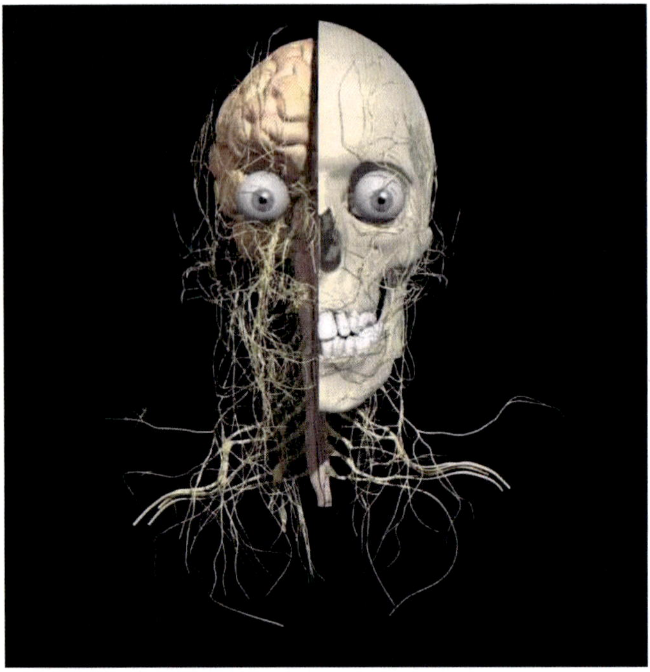

Sub-acute arthritis. General symptoms are the same but less intense, with longer periods of clinical symptoms, with tendency to more stable function disorder development is marked out.

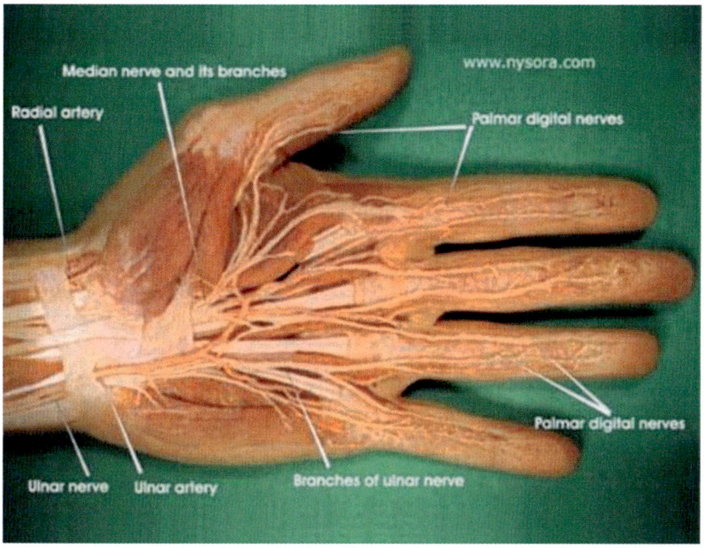
Median nerve and its branches
www.nysora.com
Radial artery
Palmar digital nerves
Palmar digital nerves
Ulnar nerve
Ulnar artery
Branches of ulnar nerve

Chronic arthritis. General symptomatology is less widespread; pain occurs at movements in a joint. Mobility is increasingly limited and proliferative, with fibrous changes, contractures, sub-dislocations, and ankylosis, which may result in the complete loss of joints function (such as bony or fibrous ankylosis from rheumatoid, septic arthritis).Chronic forms often result in disablement.

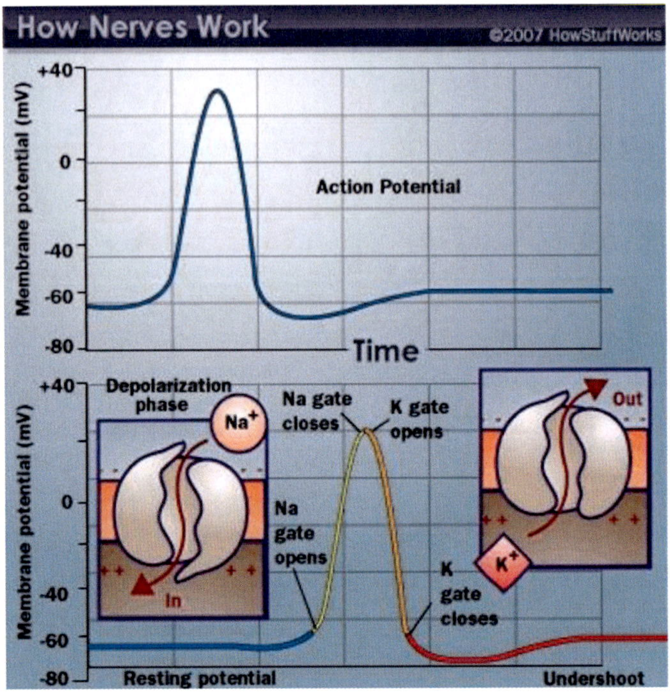

How Nerves Work
©2007 HowStuffWorks
Membrane potential (mV)
+40
0
-40
-60
-80
Action Potential
Time
Depolarization phase
Na+
Na gate closes
K gate opens
Out
Na gate opens
In
K+
K gate closes
Resting potential
Undershoot

The effectiveness of the SCENAR application depends on the location and stage of the condition.

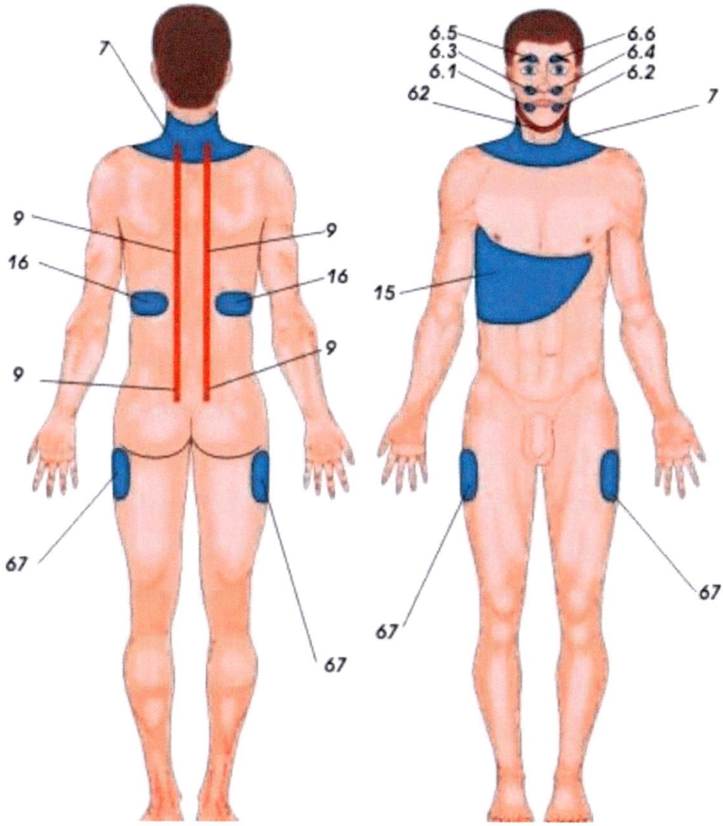
7
9
9
16
16
9
9
67
67
6.5
6.3
6.1
62
6.6
6.4
6.2
7
15
67
67

SCENAR treatment eliminates strain in the affected joint and ligaments and normalizes metabolic processes both locally and in the entire body. Treatment methods have been clinically proven for all types of arthritis.

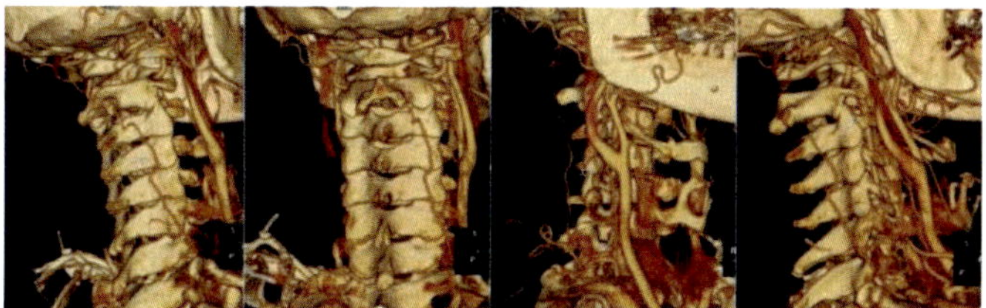

Treatment areas:

- Cervico-occipital area
- 6 facial exit points of trigeminal nerve
- paravertebral area
- liver-pancreas area
- adrenal area
- Pirogov's ring (tonsil projection)
- Points of the allergy

The device is applied to the projection of the affected and corresponding healthy joints and ligaments until pain disappears and the patient experiences a feeling of warmth. When several joints are affected, treatment should be started from the most painful joint followed by the corresponding healthy one. Treat any affected joints in the same way. If small joints are affected, treat all adjoining small joints. Treat healthy joints half the amount of time as the painful joint. Use high power level to treat arthritic conditions. Do one session daily for 15-20 days. Repeat treatment in 2 or 3 months.

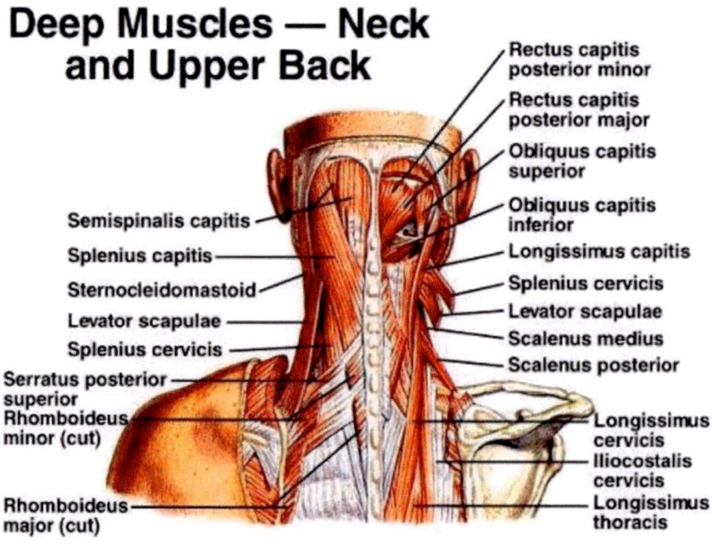
Deep Muscles — Neck and Upper Back
Rectus capitis posterior minor
Rectus capitis posterior major
Obliquus capitis superior
Obliquus capitis inferior
Longissimus capitis
Splenius cervicis
Levator scapulae
Scalenus medius
Scalenus posterior
Longissimus cervicis
Iliocostalis cervicis
Longissimus thoracis
Semispinalis capitis
Splenius capitis
Sternocleidomastoid
Levator scapulae
Splenius cervicis
Serratus posterior superior
Rhomboideus minor (cut)
Rhomboideus major (cut)

Chronic arthritis.

General symptomatology is less widespread; pain occurs at movements in a joint. Mobility is increasingly limited and proliferative, with fibrous changes, contractures, sub-dislocations, and ankylosis, which may result in the complete loss of joints function (such as bony or fibrous ankylosis from rheumatoid, septic arthritis).Chronic forms often result in disablement.

The effectiveness of the SCENAR application depends on the location and stage of the condition.

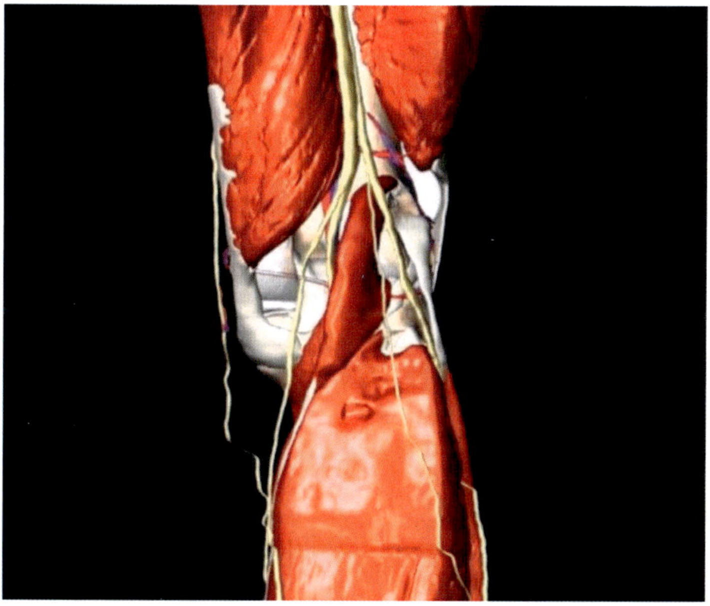

SCENAR treatment eliminates strain in the affected joint and ligaments and normalizes metabolic processes both locally and in the entire body. Treatment methods have been clinically proven for all types of arthritis.

Treatment areas:

Cervico-occipital area

6 facial exit points of trigeminal nerve

paravertebral area

liver-pancreas area

adrenal area

Pirogov's ring (tonsil projection)

Points of the allergy

The device is applied to the projection of the affected and corresponding healthy joints and ligaments until pain disappears and the patient experiences a feeling of warmth. When several joints are affected, treatment should be started from the most painful joint followed by the corresponding healthy one. Treat any affected joints in the same way. If small joints are affected, treat all adjoining small joints. Treat healthy joints half the amount of time as the painful joint. Use high power level to treat arthritic conditions. Do one session daily for 15-20 days. Repeat treatment in 2 or 3 months.

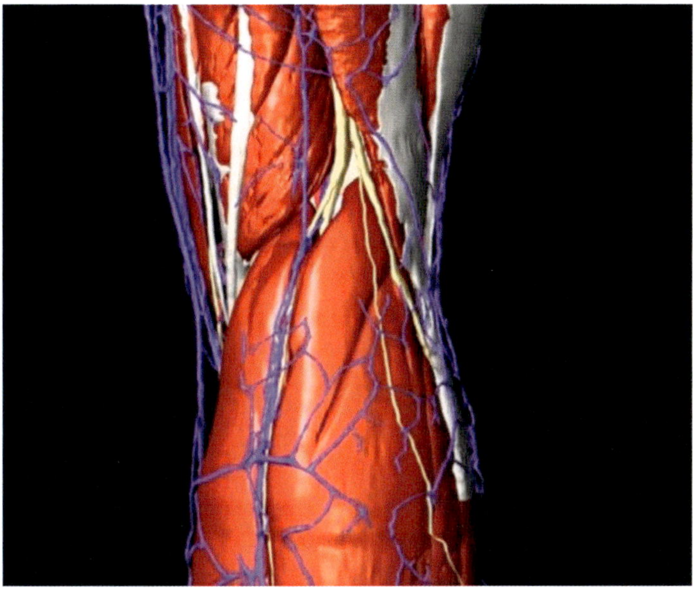

Causes and Factors

Local or general infection, possibly specific (such as tuberculosis or chlamydiosis), trauma, allergy, autoimmune response, metabolic disorders etc.

Arthritis can be caused by:

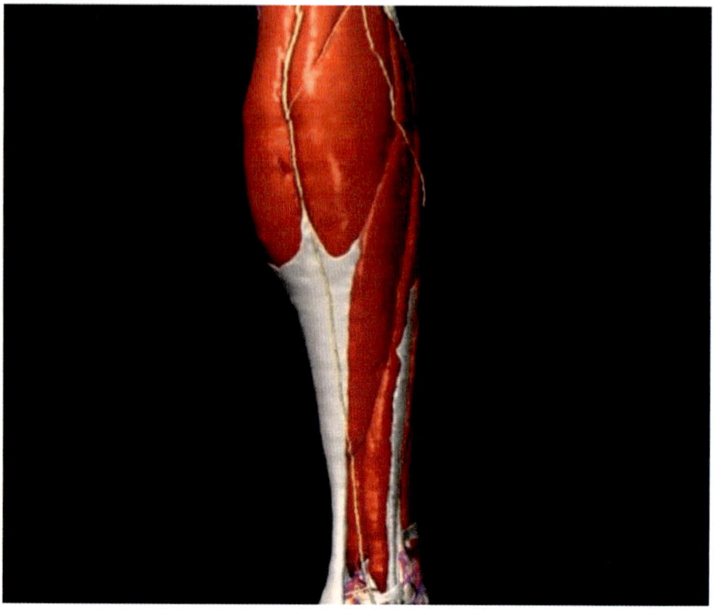

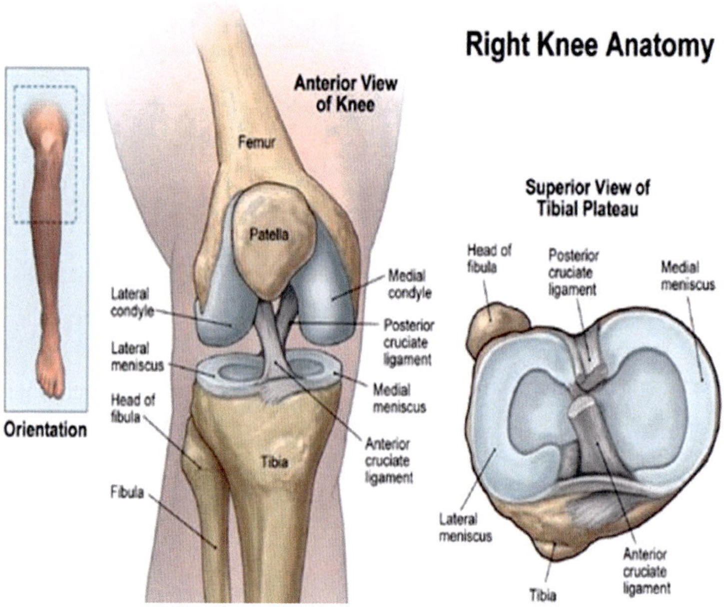

Right Knee Anatomy
Anterior View of Knee
Femur
Patella
Lateral condyle
Medial condyle
Posterior cruciate ligament
Lateral meniscus
Medial meniscus
Head of fibula
Anterior cruciate ligament
Tibia
Fibula
Orientation
Superior View of Tibial Plateau
Head of fibula
Posterior cruciate ligament
Medial meniscus
Lateral meniscus
Anterior cruciate ligament
Tibia

SCENAR treatment eliminates strain in the affected joint and normalizes metabolic process both locally and in the entire organism. Treatment methods have been clinically proven for all types of Arthrosis. The device is applied to the projection of the affected and corresponding healthy joints and ligaments until pain disappears and the patient experiences a feeling of warmth. Treat healthy joints half the amount of time as the painful joint. When several joints are affected, treatment should be started from the most painful joint followed by the corresponding healthy one. Treat any affected joints in the same way. If small joints are affected, treat all adjoining small joints.

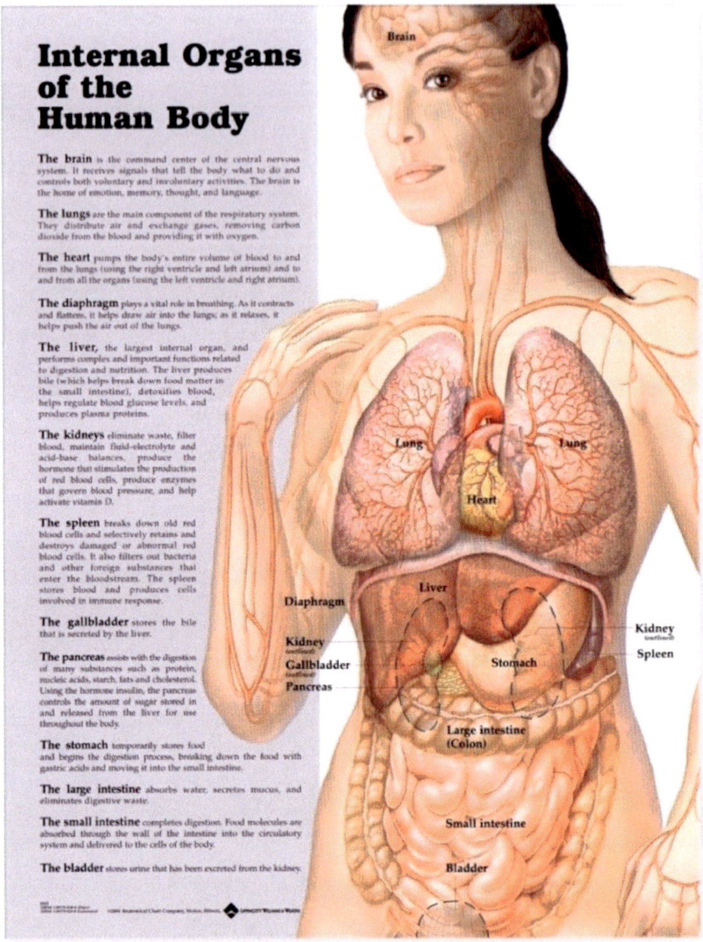
Internal Organs of the Human Body
The brain is the command center of the central nervous system. It receives signals that tell the body what to do and controls both voluntary and involuntary activities. The brain is the home of emotion, memory, thought, and language.
The lungs are the main component of the respiratory system. They distribute air and exchange gases, removing carbon dioxide from the blood and providing it with oxygen.
The heart pumps the body's entire volume of blood to and from the lungs (using the right ventricle and left atrium) and to and from all the organs (using the left ventricle and right atrium).
The diaphragm plays a vital role in breathing. As it contracts and flattens, it helps draw air into the lungs; as it relaxes, it helps push the air out of the lungs.
The liver, the largest internal organ, and performs complex and important functions related to digestion and nutrition. The liver produces bile (which helps break down food matter in the small intestine), detoxifies blood, helps regulate blood glucose levels, and produces plasma proteins.
The kidneys eliminate waste, filter blood, maintain fluid-electrolyte and acid-base balances, produce the hormone that stimulates the production of red blood cells, produce enzymes that govern blood pressure, and help activate vitamin D.
The spleen breaks down old red blood cells and selectively retains and destroys damaged or abnormal red blood cells. It also filters out bacteria and other foreign substances that enter the bloodstream. The spleen stores blood and produces cells involved in immune response.
The gallbladder stores the bile that is secreted by the liver.
The pancreas assists with the digestion of many substances such as protein, nucleic acids, starch, fats and cholesterol. Using the hormone insulin, the pancreas controls the amount of sugar stored in and released from the liver for use throughout the body.
The stomach temporarily stores food and begins the digestion process, breaking down the food with gastric acids and moving it into the small intestine.
The large intestine absorbs water, secretes mucus, and eliminates digestive waste.
The small intestine completes digestion. Food molecules are absorbed through the wall of the intestine into the circulatory system and delivered to the cells of the body.
The bladder stores urine that has been excreted from the kidney.
Brain
Lung
Lung
Heart
Liver
Diaphragm
Kidney
Gallbladder
Pancreas
Kidney
Spleen
Stomach
Large intestine
(Colon)
Small intestine
Bladder

Treatment areas:

- hip joints
- shoulder joints
- knee joints
- elbow joint
- ankle joint

Additional treatment zones:

- 6 facial exit points of trigeminal nerve
- Cervico-occipital area
- paravertebral area;
- Liver-pancreas area

Use high power level. Do one session daily for 15-20 days.

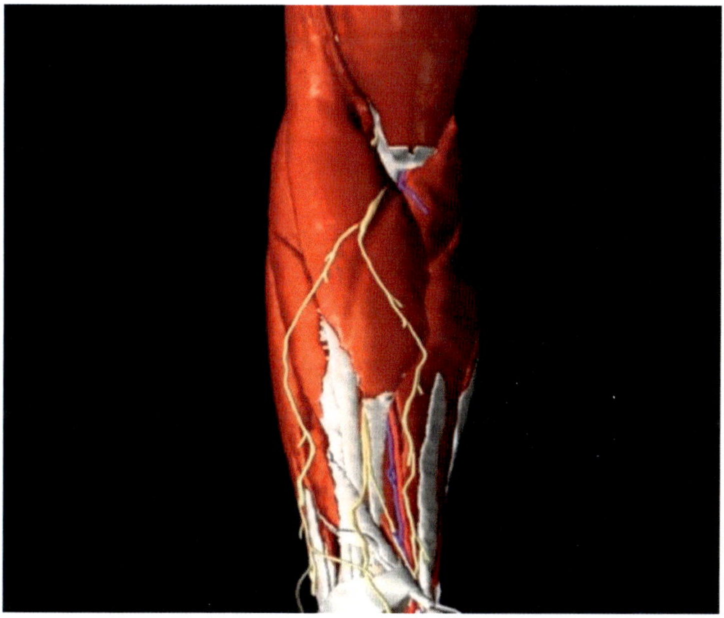

Treatment areas:

- lung fields - treat for one or two minutes, from the lung roots , in a circular (spiral) motion, upward to the left and downward - and to the area of departure;
- main bronchial area
- ribs and intercostal spaces;

- above the sternum from the jugular fossa (34) to the met sternum (79);
- infraclavicular area
- supraclavicular area from the bottom to the top;
- jugular fossa
- trachea

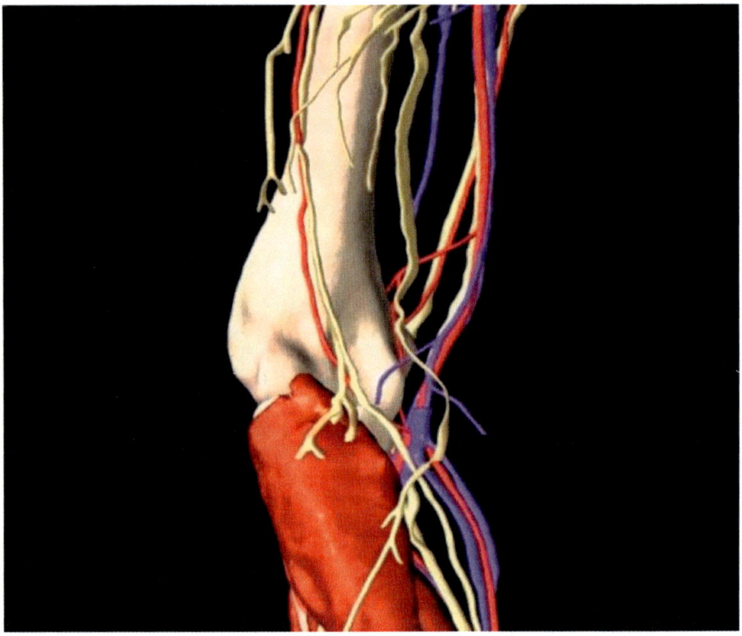

Additional treatment zones:

- nostrils and bridge of the nose
- maxillary sinus
- frontal sinus
- forehead between the eyebrows ("the third eye")
- Cervico-occipital area
- lumbosacral area

- sural muscle surface
- Pirogov's ring (tonsil projection)
- palms
- Plantar surface of the foot

It is recommended to change the beginning place of the procedure – one day you start from the left, next day – from the right. One should treat with medium intensity power (a patient feels moderate discomfort), changing intensity to the low one, then increasing it again until manifested hyperemia (reddening) comes up and sputum discharges.

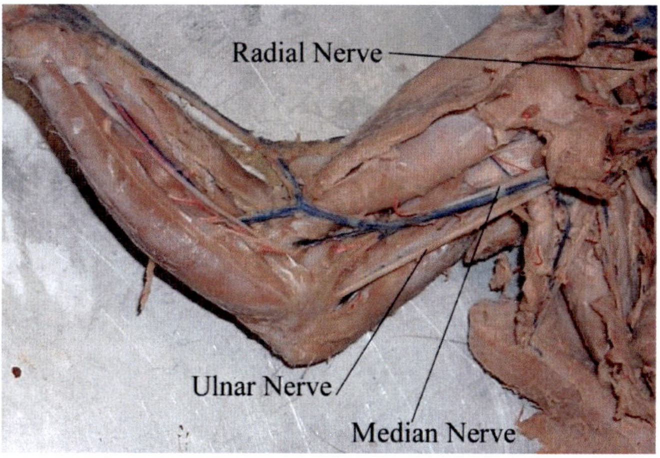
Radial Nerve
Ulnar Nerve
Median Nerve

Arthrosis

Arthrosis - degenerative and dystrophic disease of joints. Arthrosis is a wide-spread disease of joints, especially among elderly people. It affects both major (hip, knee, elbow, and ankle) and minor joints (wrist, interphalangeal, tars metatarsal and also vertebral joints – spondylarthrosis).

SCENAR treatment eliminates strain in the affected joint and normalizes metabolic process both locally and in the entire organism. Treatment methods have been clinically proven for all types of Arthrosis. The device is applied to the projection of the affected and corresponding healthy joints and ligaments until pain disappears and the patient experiences a feeling of warmth. Treat healthy joints half the amount of time as the painful joint. When several joints are affected, treatment should be started from the most painful joint followed by the corresponding healthy one. Treat any affected joints in the same way. If small joints are affected, treat all adjoining small joints.

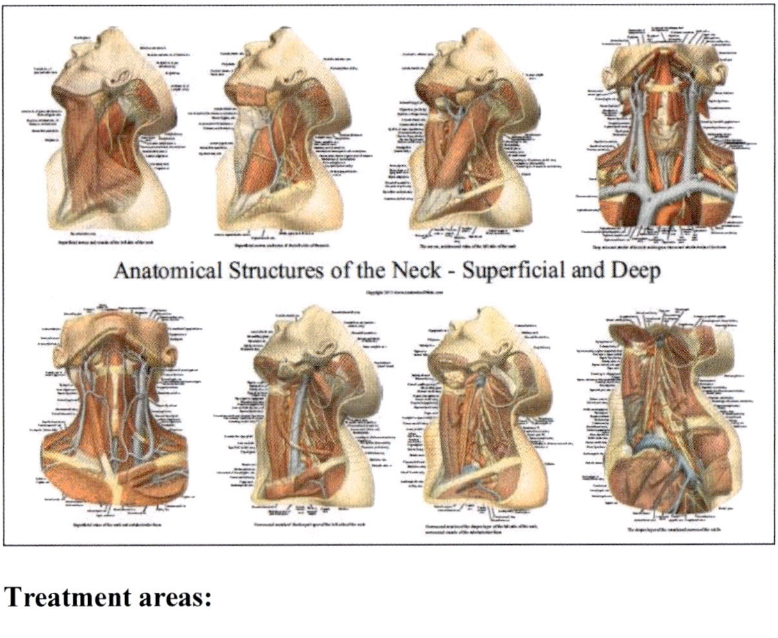
Anatomical Structures of the Neck - Superficial and Deep

Treatment areas:

- hip joints
- shoulder joints
- knee joints
- elbow joint

- Ankle joint .

Additional treatment zones:

- 6 facial exit points of trigeminal nerve
- Cervico-occipital area
- paravertebral area;
- Liver-pancreas area

Use high power level. Do one session daily for 15-20 days.

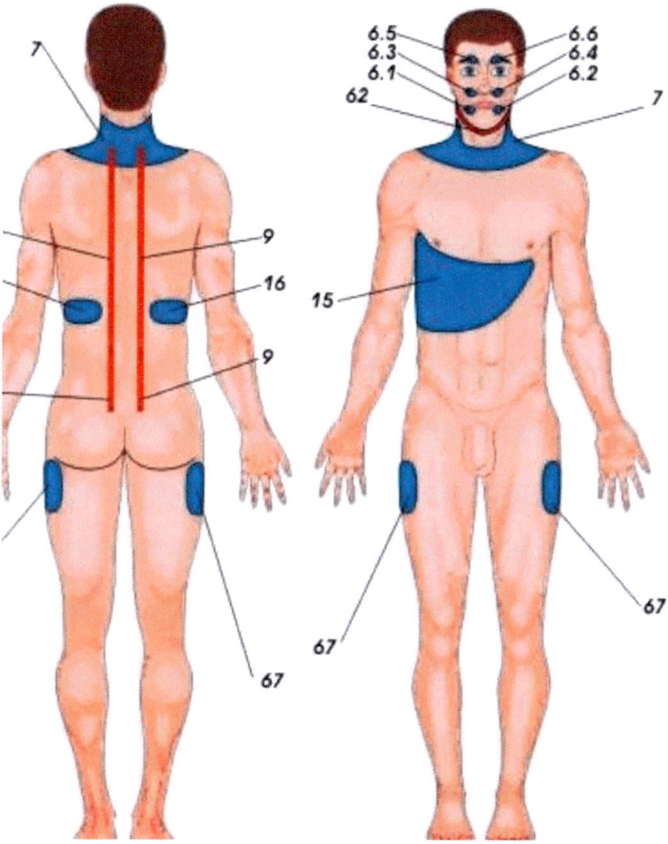
7
9
16
9
67
6.5
6.3
6.1
62
6.6
6.4
6.2
7
15
67
67

Bursitis

bursitis – inflammation of the periarthritic mucous bursa.

SCENAR treatment relieves pain symptom and eliminates inflammation.

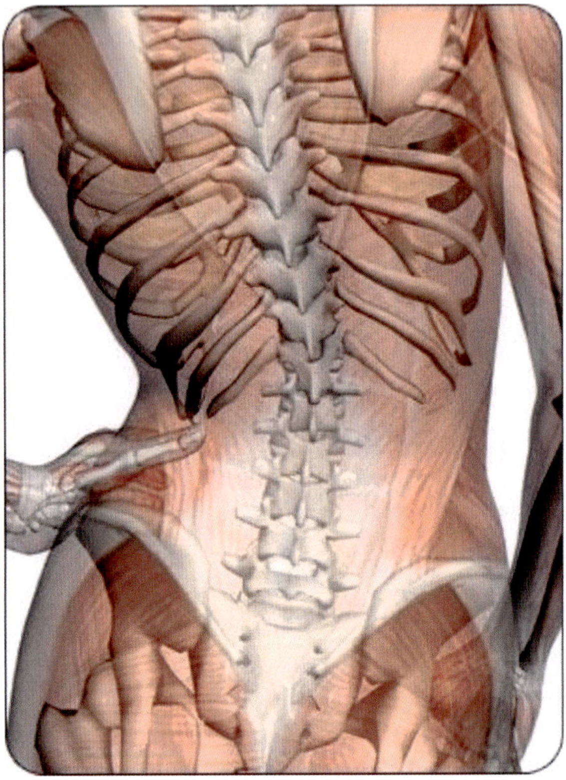

Treatment areas:

- pain location (affected joint, swelling);
- near-by muscles and tendons;
- Pirogov's ring (tonsil projection)
- axillary cavities
- inguinal area

- popliteal fossa
- Three tracks

Adrenal area

Additional treatment areas:

- plantar surface of the foot
- palm
- celiac plexus
- "100 diseases"
- Points of the allergy

Begin treatment on the healthy joint symmetric to the affected one. Use comfortable power level. Do 10-20 sessions for the treatment course. Repeat treatment in 2 or 3 months.

Contusion

Contusion – mechanical damage of soft tissues without damage of cutaneous (dermal) integuments.

Causes and Factors – trauma.

Clinical picture

Pain: is sharp at the moment of trauma, in some minutes it is reduced obviously without taking analgesics. As the swelling becomes larger the pain is increasing again. Swelling and edema on the place of damage come up either at once after trauma or sometime later. The hemorrhage is formed on the place of trauma at once or after some time. Hematoma can be formed later on in place of the bruise.

Lumbar Region of Back

Cross Section

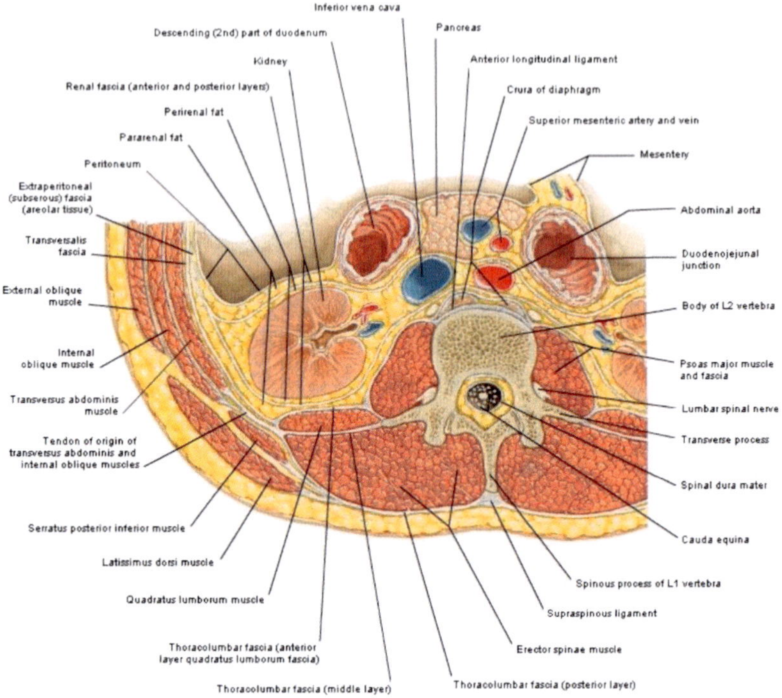

Inferior vena cava
Descending (2nd) part of duodenum
Pancreas
Kidney
Anterior longitudinal ligament
Renal fascia (anterior and posterior layers)
Crura of diaphragm
Perirenal fat
Superior mesenteric artery and vein
Pararenal fat
Mesentery
Peritoneum
Extraperitoneal (subserous) fascia (areolar tissue)
Abdominal aorta
Transversalis fascia
Duodenojejunal junction
External oblique muscle
Body of L2 vertebra
Internal oblique muscle
Psoas major muscle and fascia
Transversus abdominis muscle
Lumbar spinal nerve
Tendon of origin of transversus abdominis and internal oblique muscles
Transverse process
Spinal dura mater
Serratus posterior inferior muscle
Cauda equina
Latissimus dorsi muscle
Spinous process of L1 vertebra
Quadratus lumborum muscle
Supraspinous ligament
Thoracolumbar fascia (anterior layer quadratus lumborum fascia)
Erector spinae muscle
Thoracolumbar fascia (middle layer)
Thoracolumbar fascia (posterior layer)

Nerves of Heart

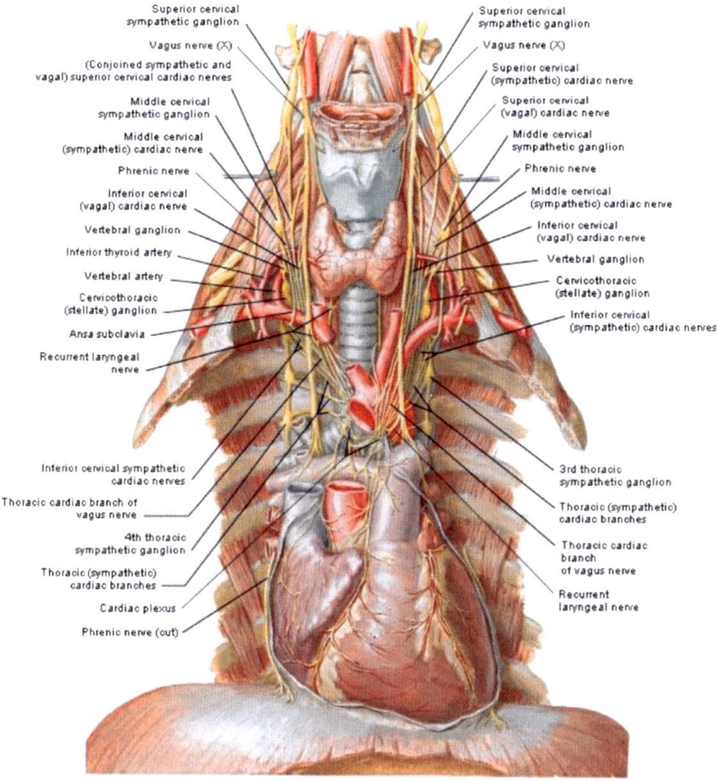

Superior cervical sympathetic ganglion
Vagus nerve (X)
(Conjoined sympathetic and vagal) superior cervical cardiac nerves
Middle cervical sympathetic ganglion
Middle cervical (sympathetic) cardiac nerve
Phrenic nerve
Inferior cervical (vagal) cardiac nerve
Vertebral ganglion
Inferior thyroid artery
Vertebral artery
Cervicothoracic (stellate) ganglion
Ansa subclavia
Recurrent laryngeal nerve
Inferior cervical sympathetic cardiac nerves
Thoracic cardiac branch of vagus nerve
4th thoracic sympathetic ganglion
Thoracic (sympathetic) cardiac branches
Cardiac plexus
Phrenic nerve (cut)
Superior cervical sympathetic ganglion
Vagus nerve (X)
Superior cervical (sympathetic) cardiac nerve
Superior cervical (vagal) cardiac nerve
Middle cervical sympathetic ganglion
Phrenic nerve
Middle cervical (sympathetic) cardiac nerve
Inferior cervical (vagal) cardiac nerve
Vertebral ganglion
Cervicothoracic (stellate) ganglion
Inferior cervical (sympathetic) cardiac nerves
3rd thoracic sympathetic ganglion
Thoracic (sympathetic) cardiac branches
Thoracic cardiac branch of vagus nerve
Recurrent laryngeal nerve

The aim of treatment is pain syndrome relieving, reducing of tension and normalization of metabolism in the trauma region.

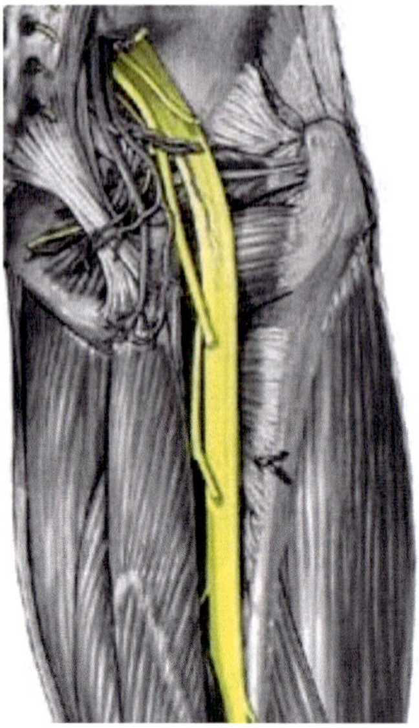

Motor nerves carry impulses from the brain to the skeletal muscles and somatic tissues, which creates voluntary movement

Treatment areas:

The device is applied directly in the area of trauma, the groups of neighboring muscles, involved joints and painful points occurring at minimal loading on the extremity (in joint's area contusion, strained muscles).

Additional treatment areas:

- 7-th & 8-th cervical vertebrae area
- area over thoracic vertebrae (thoracic spine area)
- scapula
- Lumbosacral area

Do 5-10 procedures daily.

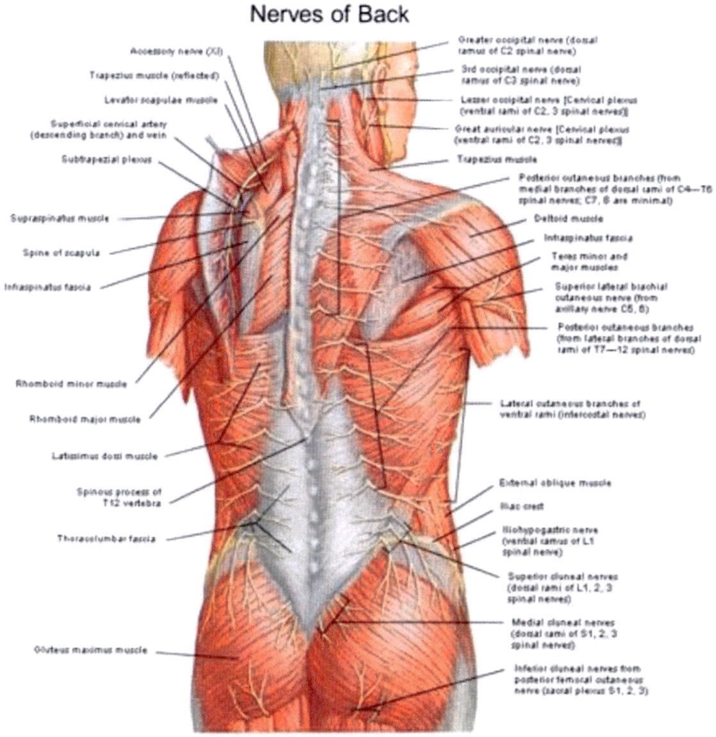
Nerves of Back
Accessory nerve (XI)
Trapezius muscle (reflected)
Levator scapulae muscle
Superficial cervical artery (descending branch) and vein
Subtrapezial plexus
Supraspinatus muscle
Spine of scapula
Infraspinatus fascia
Rhomboid minor muscle
Rhomboid major muscle
Latissimus dorsi muscle
Spinous process of T12 vertebra
Thoracolumbar fascia
Gluteus maximus muscle
Greater occipital nerve (dorsal ramus of C2 spinal nerve)
3rd occipital nerve (dorsal ramus of C3 spinal nerve)
Lesser occipital nerve [Cervical plexus (ventral rami of C2, 3 spinal nerves)]
Great auricular nerve [Cervical plexus (ventral rami of C2, 3 spinal nerves)]
Trapezius muscle
Posterior cutaneous branches (from medial branches of dorsal rami of C4—T6 spinal nerves; C7, 8 are minimal)
Deltoid muscle
Infraspinatus fascia
Teres minor and major muscles
Superior lateral brachial cutaneous nerve (from axillary nerve C5, 6)
Posterior cutaneous branches (from lateral branches of dorsal rami of T7—12 spinal nerves)
Lateral cutaneous branches of ventral rami (intercostal nerves)
External oblique muscle
Iliac crest
Iliohypogastric nerve (ventral ramus of L1 spinal nerve)
Superior cluneal nerves (dorsal rami of L1, 2, 3 spinal nerves)
Medial cluneal nerves (dorsal rami of S1, 2, 3 spinal nerves)
Inferior cluneal nerves from posterior femoral cutaneous nerve (sacral plexus S1, 2, 3)

Asthma

SCENAR treatment arrests attack, makes asphyxia less frequent, relieves strain in bronchi, and normalizes metabolic process both in the bronco-pulmonary system and in the entire organism.

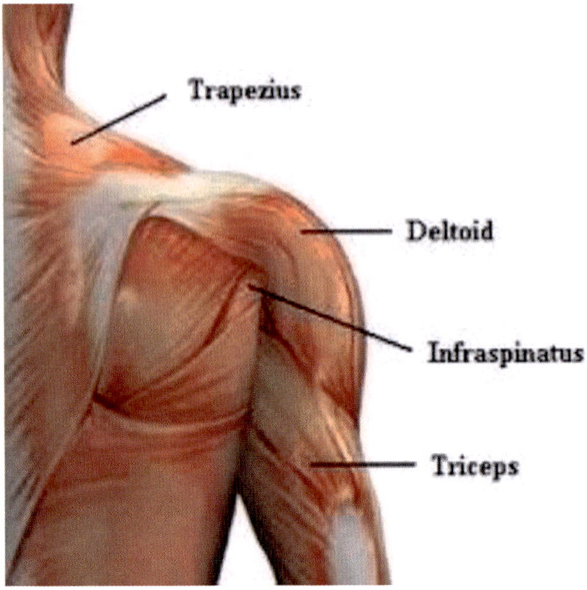
Trapezius
Deltoid
Infraspinatus
Triceps

SCENAR treatment eliminates inflammation and normalizes metabolic process in the broncho-pulmonary system.

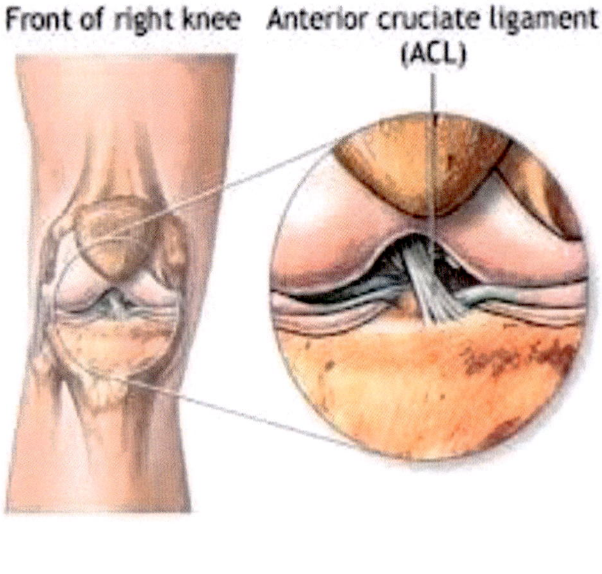
Front of right knee
Anterior cruciate ligament (ACL)

Treatment areas:

- lung fields - treat for one or two minutes, from the lung roots , in a circular (spiral) motion, upward to the left and downward - and to the area of departure;
- main bronchial area
- ribs and intercostal spaces;
- above the sternum from the jugular fossa (34) to the met sternum (79);
- infraclavicular area
- supraclavicular area from the bottom to the top;
- jugular fossa
- trachea

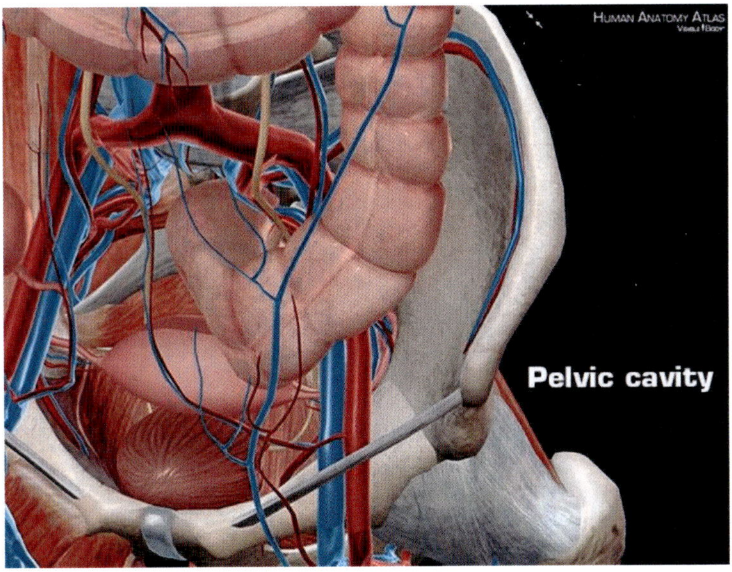
HUMAN ANATOMY ATLAS
Pelvic cavity

Additional treatment zones:

- nostrils and bridge of the nose
- maxillary sinus
- frontal sinus
- forchcad between the eyebrows ("the third eye")
- Cervico-occipital area
- lumbosacral area
- sural muscle surface
- Pirogov's ring (tonsil projection)
- palms
- Plantar surface of the foot

It is recommended to change the beginning place of the procedure – one day you start from the left, next day – from the right. One should treat with medium intensity power (a patient feels moderate discomfort), changing intensity to the low one, then increasing it again until manifested hyperemia (reddening) comes up and sputum discharges.

Ankylosing Spondelytis

Treatment areas

The affected and symmetric healthy joints and ligaments are influenced with the device in a projection until getting the feeling of "heat" or pains arresting. The time of influence on the healthy joint should be twice less. When several joints are affected the treatment is started from the most painful joint and its healthy symmetric one. When the process is located in large joints, the Hip joint anatomic hollow on a lateral surface of the joint projection should be treated.

Additional treatment zones:

- 6 facial exit points of the trigeminal nerve
- Cervico-occipital area
- paravertebral area
- liver-pancreas area

The procedures are carried out at the increased energy level. Use high power level to treat Ankylosing Spondylitis. Do 15-20 procedures daily.

Repeat treatment in 1.5 or 2 months

Attack Arresting

- jugular fossa 3-4 min;
- 7th – 8th cervical vertebrae area
- scapula
- area over the thoracic vertebrae (thoracic spine area)
- interscapular;
- along the lung fields go down paravertebrally and then go up with circular movements;
- after several cycles of movements we go to ribs & intercostal spaces (36), then we go back etc.;
- main bronchial area
- lung root
- Trachea

Additional treatment zones:

- most painful area;
- Cervico-occipital area
- liver-pancreas area

- adrenal area
- Sural muscle surface

You should work with slight pressure applied to the skin. It is recommended to revert to short treatment of the jugular fossa area at every spasm of bronchi coming up (whistling).The front surface of the chest is treated for 5-6 min. the projection of main bronchial area and trachea. Treatment is done at the high power level.

Bursitis

Bursitis – inflammation of the periarthric mucous bursa.

SCENAR treatment relieves pain symptom and eliminates inflammation.

Treatment areas:

- pain location (affected joint, swelling);
- near-by muscles and tendons;
- Pirogov's ring (tonsil projection)
- axillary cavities
- inguinal area
- popliteal fossa
- Three tracks
- Adrenal area

Additional treatment areas:

- plantar surface of the foot
- palm
- celiac plexus
- "100 diseases"
- Points of the allergy

Begin treatment on the healthy joint symmetric to the affected one. Use comfortable power level. Do 10-20 sessions for the treatment course. Repeat treatment in 2 or 3 months.

Brachial Plexis

Treatment areas:

- Cervico-occipital area
- scapular and humeral
- clavicle-scapula median

Additional treatment areas:

- 6 facial exit points of trigeminal nerve
- paravertebral area
- area over the thoracic vertebrae (thoracic spine area) (11);
- lumbosacral area
- external forearm surface
- elbow joint

Bronchitis

SCENAR treatment eliminates inflammation and normalizes metabolic process in the broncho-pulmonary system.

Treatment areas:

- lung fields treat for one or two minutes, from the lung roots in a circular (spiral) motion, upward - to the left and downward - and to the area of departure;
- main bronchial area

- ribs and intercostal spaces
- above the sternum from the jugular fossa to the met sternum
- infraclavicular area
- supraclavicular area from the bottom to the top;
- jugular fossa
- trachea.

Additional treatment zones:

- nostrils and bridge of the nose
- maxillary sinus
- frontal sinus
- forehead between the eyebrows ("the third eye")
- Cervico-occipital area
- sacral area
- sural muscle surface
- Pirogov's ring (tonsil projection)
- palms
- Plantar surface of the foot

It is recommended to change the beginning place of the procedure – one day you start from the left, next day – from the right. One should treat with medium intensity power (a patient feels moderate discomfort), changing intensity to the low one, then increasing it again until manifested hyperemia (reddening) comes up and sputum discharges.

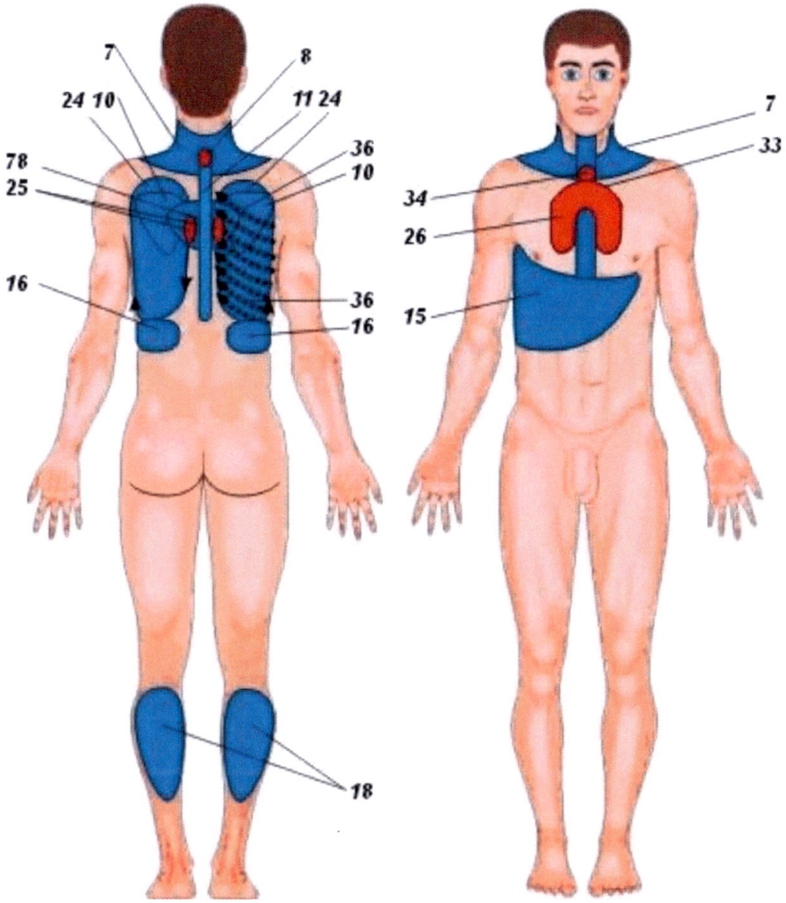

7
8
24 10
11 24
78
25
36
10
16
36
16
18
7
33
34
26
15

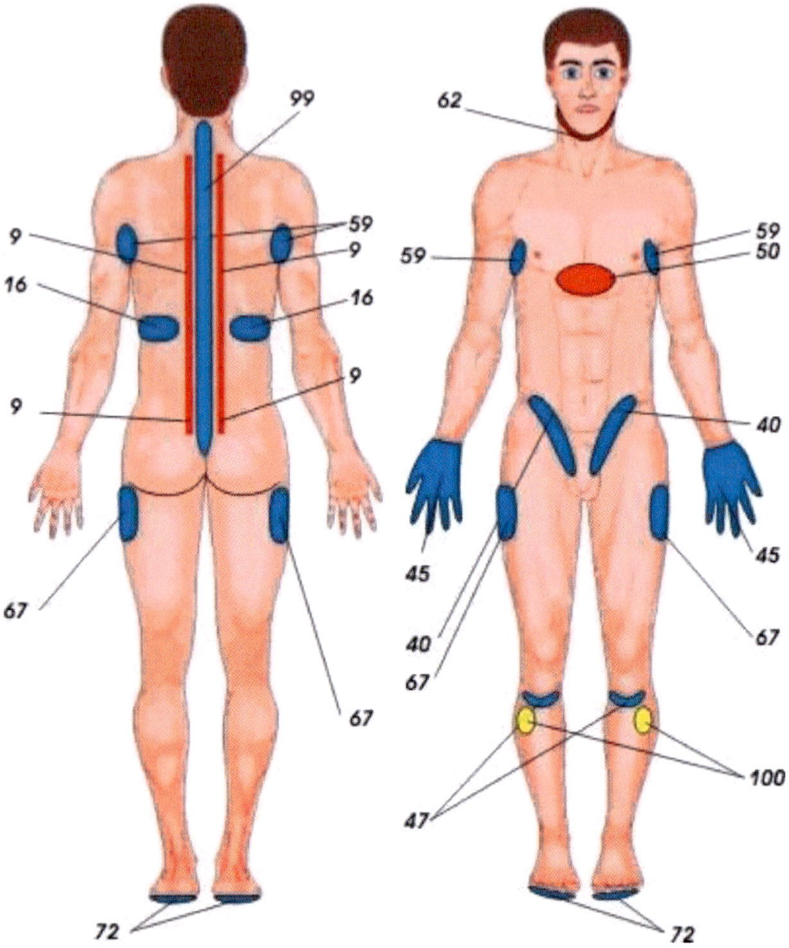
99
62
9
59
9
16
16
59
59
50
9
9
40
45
45
67
67
40
67
67
100
47
72
72

Contusion

Contusion – mechanical damage of soft tissues without damage of cutaneous (dermal) integuments.

Causes and Factors – trauma.

Clinical picture

Pain: is sharp at the moment of trauma, in some minutes it is reduced obviously without taking analgetic. As the swelling becomes larger the pain is increasing again. Swelling and edema on the place of damage come up either at once after trauma or sometime later. The hemorrhage is formed on the place of trauma at once or after some time. Hematoma can be formed later on in place of the bruise.

The aim of treatment: pain syndrome relieving, reducing of tension and normalization of metabolism in the trauma region.

The device is applied directly in the area of trauma, the groups of neighboring muscles, involved joints and painful points occurring at minimal loading on the extremity (in joint's area contusion, strained muscles).

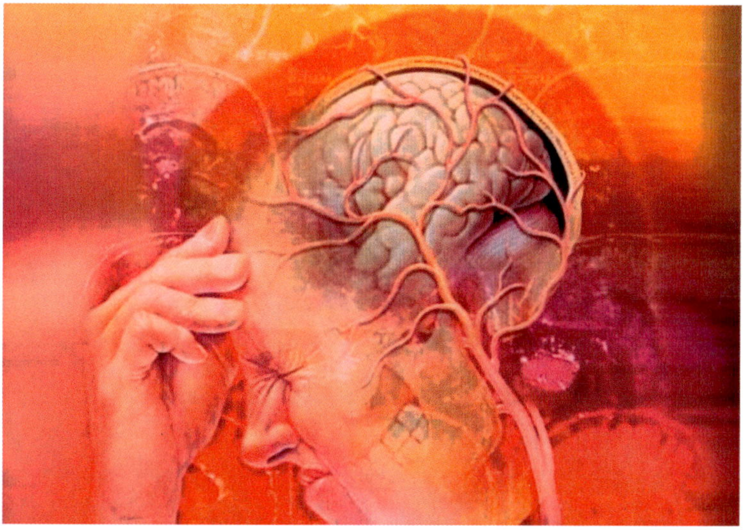

Additional treatment areas:

- 7-th & 8-th cervical vertebrae area
- area over thoracic vertebrae (thoracic spine area)
- scapula
- Lumbosacral area

Do 5-10 procedures daily.

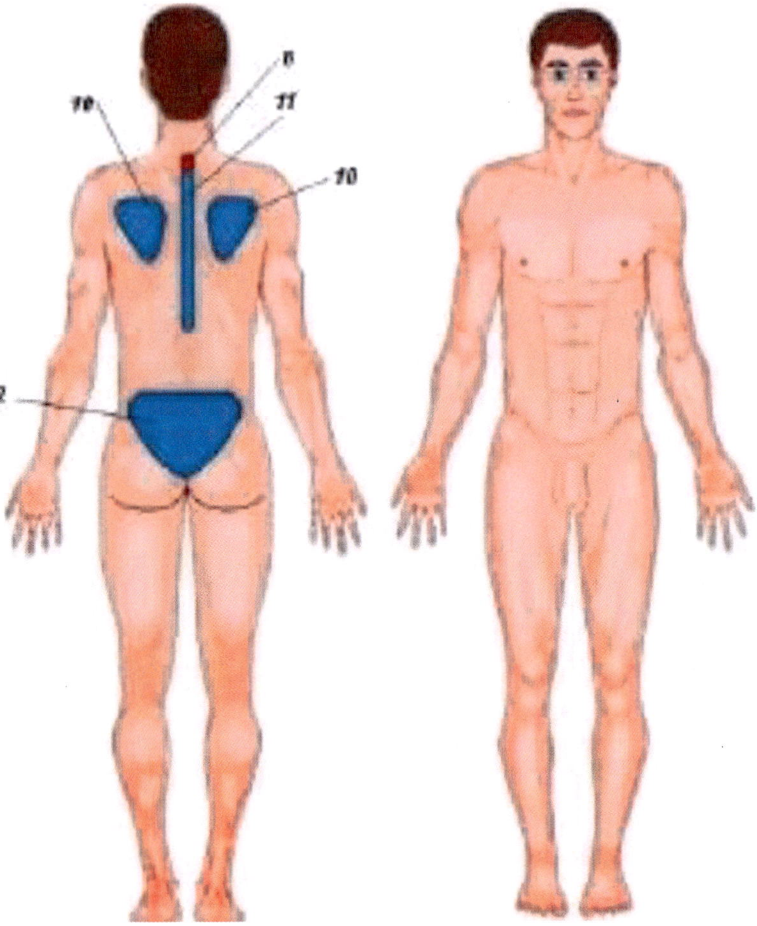

8
10
11
10
12

Craniocerebral Injury

Craniocerebral injury is the injury resulted from a blow and accompanied with damage of the brain. Open injury (fracture of the vault or other departments of the skull) and closed injury (concussion, contusion of the brain, hematoma) are distinguished.

Clinical picture

Seriousness of patient's state is determined by the degree of damage. The level of consciousness can be expressed as a light form of stun and the hardest coma. Peripheral neurological symptomatology depends on the location and character of the damage. Craniocerebral injury is a frequent cause of death.

The aim of medical treatment is relieving of brain edema, decompression (intracranial pressure reducing), and stopping of bleeding.

Treated areas:

- the site of injury;
- the occipital region
- the 1st cervical vertebra
- 6 facial exit points of trig minus
- area of the carotic artery
- Cervico-occipital area
- The abdomen region, additionally treated areas:
- eliac plexus area ,
- all joints;
- regions of the liver and pancreas
- Area of the spleen

Treat at high power level for 10-15 min, repeating the influence several times per day.

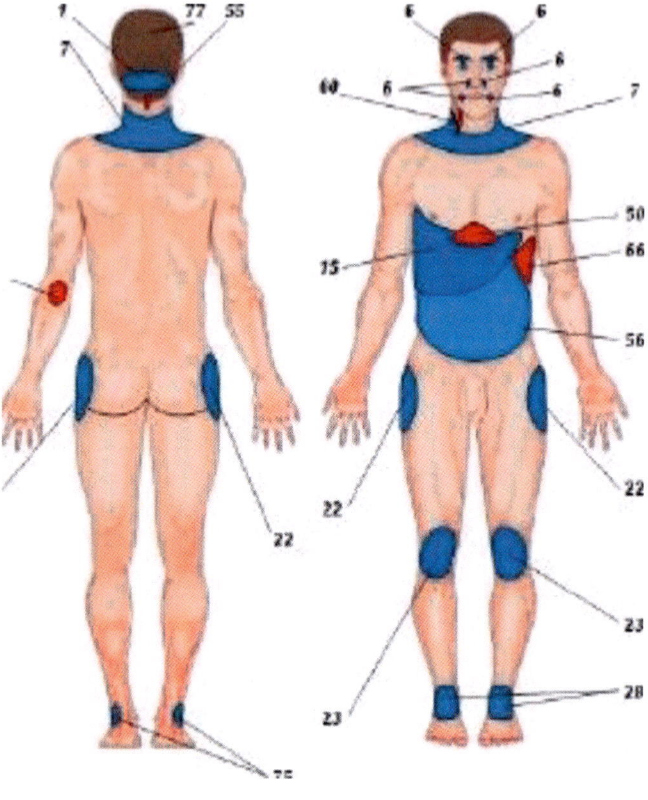

7
77
55
7
22
6
6
6
6
6
7
50
66
15
56
22
22
23
23
28

Chronic Fatigue Syndrome

SCENAR treatment provides general relaxation of the organism (“relaxation phase”), tones up its essential functions (“phase of sufficient tonus”), and stabilizes energy at a proper level.

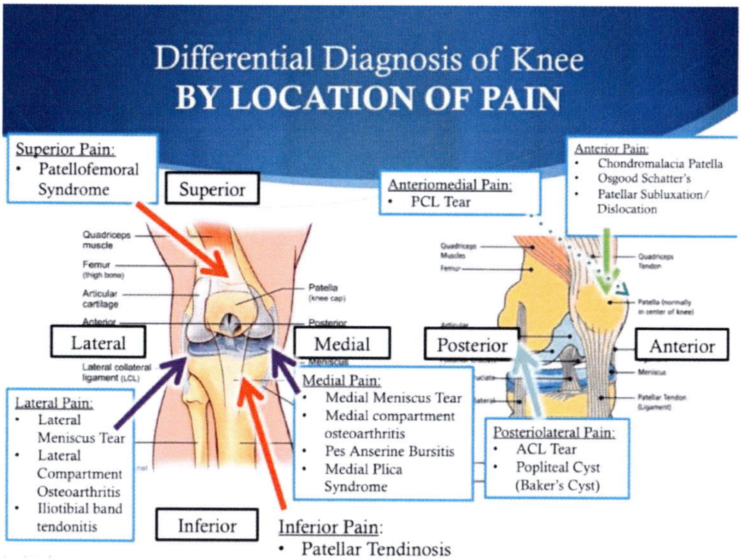
Differential Diagnosis of Knee
BY LOCATION OF PAIN
Superior Pain:
• Patellofemoral Syndrome
Superior
Anteriomedial Pain:
• PCL Tear
Anterior Pain:
• Chondromalacia Patella
• Osgood Schatter's
• Patellar Subluxation/ Dislocation
Quadriceps muscle
Femur (thigh bone)
Articular cartilage
Patella (knee cap)
Lateral
Medial
Posterior
Anterior
Lateral collateral ligament (LCL)
Medial Pain:
• Medial Meniscus Tear
• Medial compartment osteoarthritis
• Pes Anserine Bursitis
• Medial Plica Syndrome
Lateral Pain:
• Lateral Meniscus Tear
• Lateral Compartment Osteoarthritis
• Iliotibial band tendonitis
Posteriolateral Pain:
• ACL Tear
• Popliteal Cyst (Baker's Cyst)
Inferior
Inferior Pain:
• Patellar Tendinosis

Treatment areas:

- occipital
- forehead between the eyebrows ("the third eye ")
- nostrils and bridge of the nose
- 6 facial exit points of trigeminal nerve
- Cervico-occipital area
- 7-th & 8-th cervical vertebrae area
- Paravertebral area

Additional treatment areas:

- scapula
- lumbosacral area
- elbow joint
- liver-pancreas area
- adrenal area (treated if patient is calm and not in excited state)

- front thigh, lower third
- sural muscle surface ;
- front and outer surfaces of the feet
- palm
- scrotum
- Umbilical

Do one session daily for10-15 days. Each session lasts for 20-30 min.

Repeat treatment in one - three months.

Dermatitis

Find the area of the skin which is affected. Choose the power level outside the area of lesion. Start working on the symmetrical area first, and then gently move to work over the affected area, until you achieve the relief from the symptoms (itchiness, pain, soreness, etc.). Stop the procedure when you achieved significant improvement. Repeat the procedure as soon as symptoms reoccur.

Facial Nerve Palsy

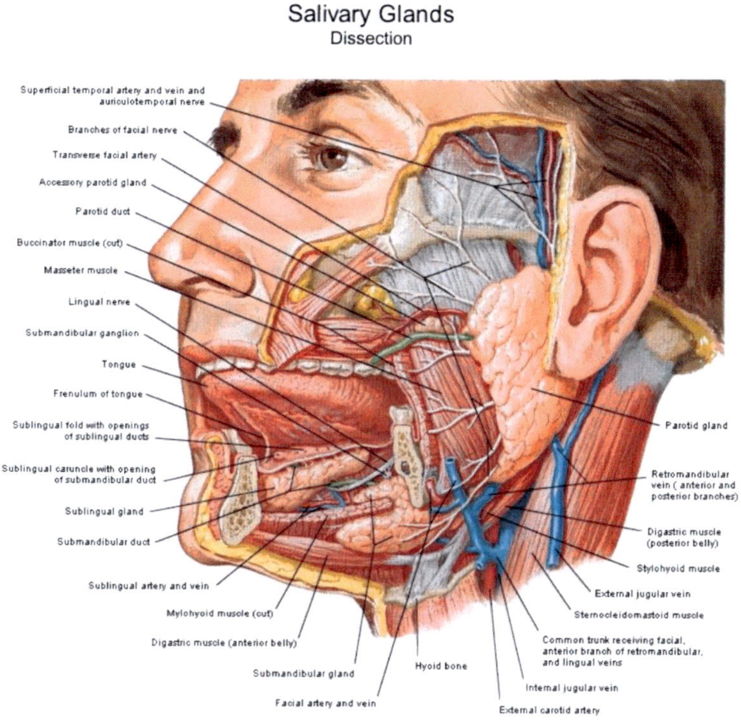

Salivary Glands
Dissection
Superficial temporal artery and vein and auriculotemporal nerve
Branches of facial nerve
Transverse facial artery
Accessory parotid gland
Parotid duct
Buccinator muscle (cut)
Masseter muscle
Lingual nerve
Submandibular ganglion
Tongue
Frenulum of tongue
Sublingual fold with openings of sublingual ducts
Sublingual caruncle with opening of submandibular duct
Sublingual gland
Submandibular duct
Sublingual artery and vein
Mylohyoid muscle (cut)
Digastric muscle (anterior belly)
Submandibular gland
Facial artery and vein
Hyoid bone
Parotid gland
Retromandibular vein (anterior and posterior branches)
Digastric muscle (posterior belly)
Stylohyoid muscle
External jugular vein
Sternocleidomastoid muscle
Common trunk receiving facial, anterior branch of retromandibular, and lingual veins
Internal jugular vein
External carotid artery

Specific areas:

- Six points
- Beneath and behind the ear
- Collar zone

Start from the healthy side.

Frequency of Treatment:

- Acute - Treat daily or more often.
- Refer to Emergency if necessary.

Not Acute - Treat once a day, three times a week.

A complete treatment usually consists of one to ten sessions.

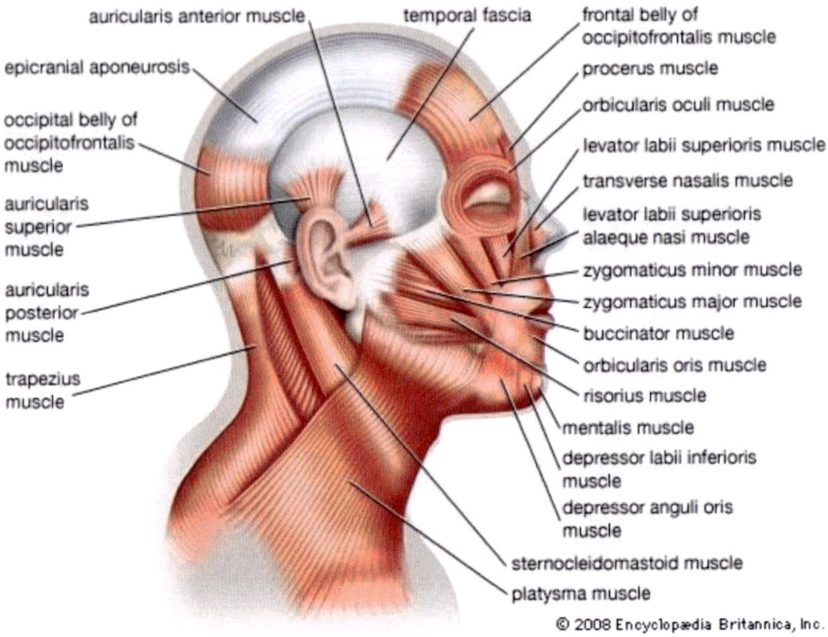
auricularis anterior muscle
temporal fascia
frontal belly of occipitofrontalis muscle
epicranial aponeurosis
procerus muscle
occipital belly of occipitofrontalis muscle
orbicularis oculi muscle
levator labii superioris muscle
transverse nasalis muscle
auricularis superior muscle
levator labii superioris alaeque nasi muscle
zygomaticus minor muscle
auricularis posterior muscle
zygomaticus major muscle
buccinator muscle
orbicularis oris muscle
trapezius muscle
risorius muscle
mentalis muscle
depressor labii inferioris muscle
depressor anguli oris muscle
sternocleidomastoid muscle
platysma muscle
© 2008 Encyclopædia Britannica, Inc.

Facial Paresis

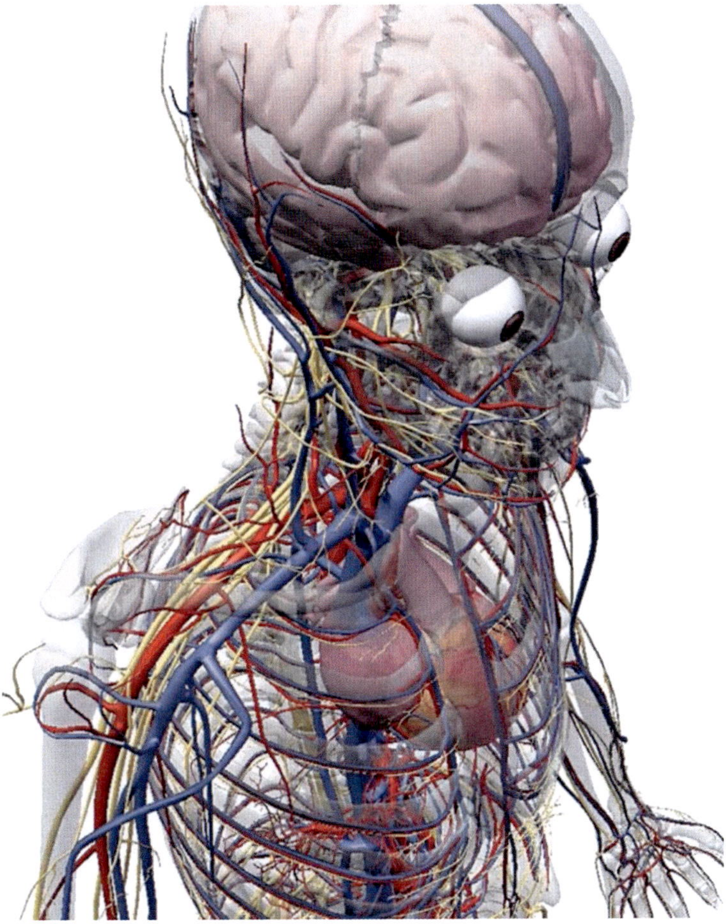

SCENAR treatment eliminates paresis of the mimic muscles.

Treatment areas:

- behind-the-ear
- ear lobule-temple (mastoid projection)
- “Three tracks”

- 6 facial exit points of trigeminal nerve
- upper forehead edge, the beginning of the hair part
- mid-chin
- mouth angle-chin
- Cervico-occipital area

Additional treatment areas:

- maxillary sinus
- nostrils and bridge of the nose
- nasal active points
- nostril-eye
- over-and-under-the-eyebrow
- lower jaw angle
- nosalabial fold
- periocular
- sub maxillary
- gum
- "100 diseases"

Initiate treatment on the healthy side and continue according to the treatment areas. Use high power level for the paresis area and comfortable one for the rest areas.

Do 15-40 sessions for the treatment course..

Gastritis

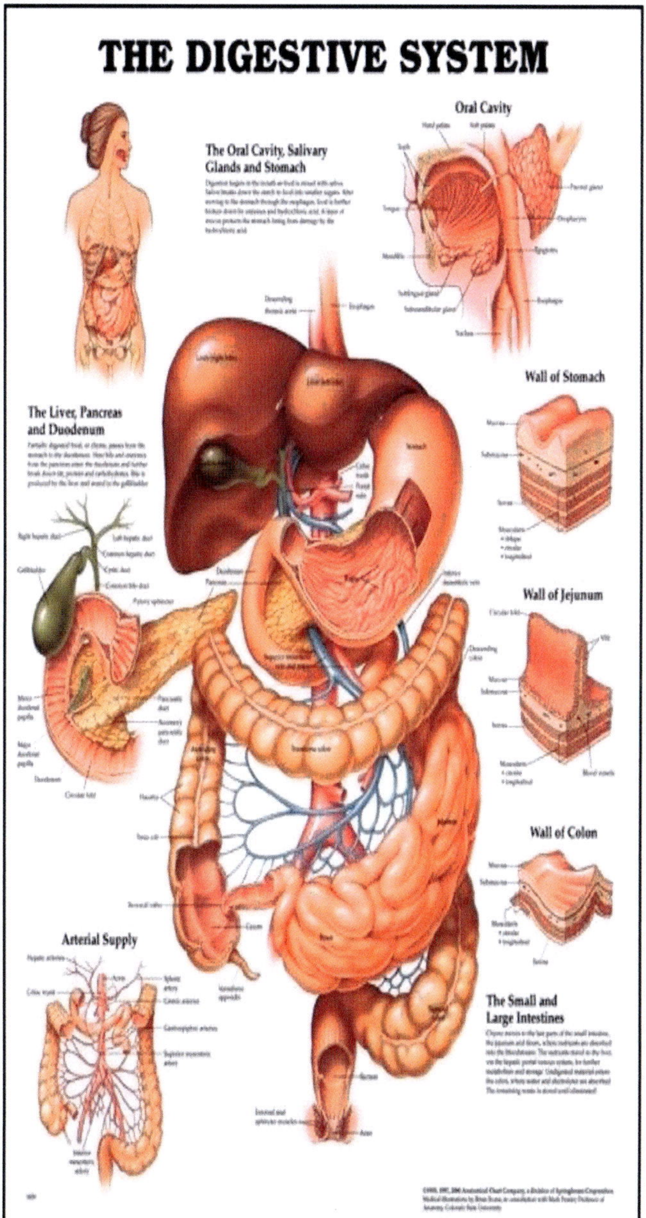
THE DIGESTIVE SYSTEM
Oral Cavity
The Oral Cavity, Salivary Glands and Stomach
The Liver, Pancreas and Duodenum
Wall of Stomach
Wall of Jejunum
Wall of Colon
Arterial Supply
The Small and Large Intestines

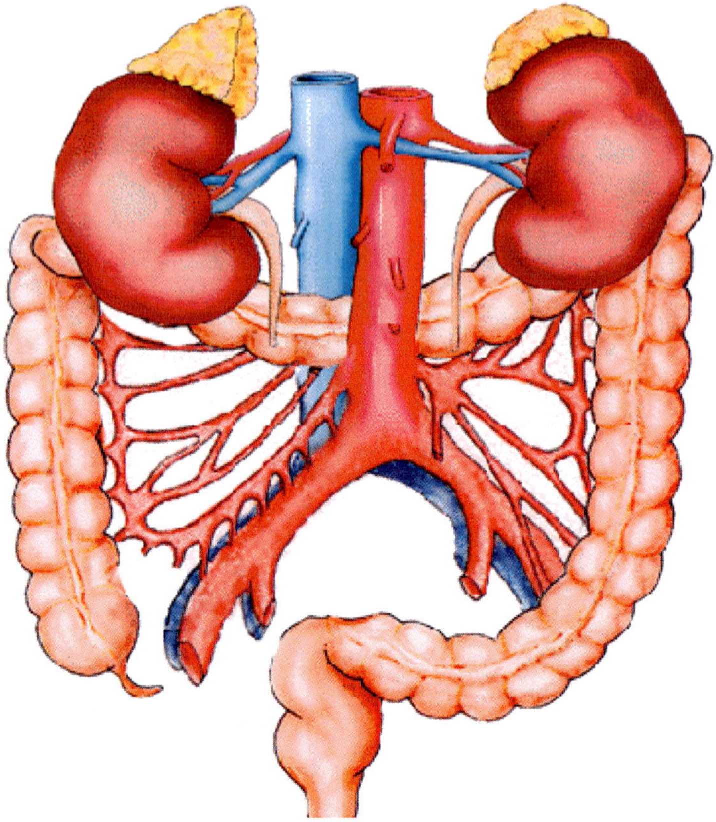

Treatment areas:

- Cervico-occipital area
- paravertebral area
- 6 facial exit points of trigeminal nerve
- adrenal area
- tip of the tongue
- abdomen (projection of the intestine)
- umbilical
- liver-pancreas area
- gall-bladder
- female perineal and genital scrotum.

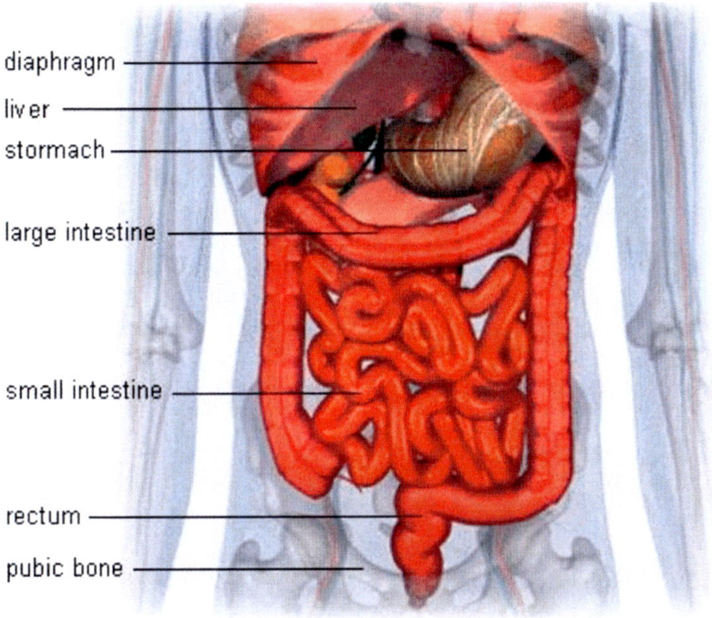
diaphragm
liver
stormach
large intestine
small intestine
rectum
pubic bone

The treatment course - from 2 weeks to 25 days

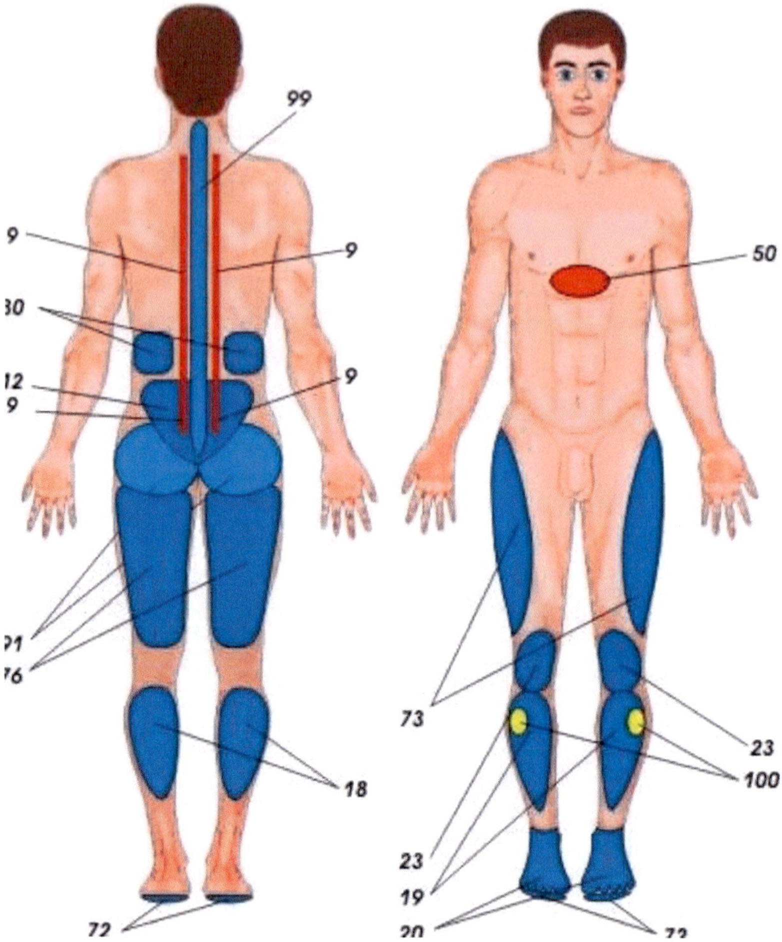
99
9
9
12
9
9
18
72
50
73
23
100
23
19

Headache

Specific areas:

- Collar zone
- Venous sinuses
- Pirogovring
- Point PC3

- Opposite side of head to sensation of origin of headache
- Craniotherapy from eye sockets up and over the head

Chase the pain until it goes

Look for secondary sign on the lower back closer to the spinal column often as vesicular rash.

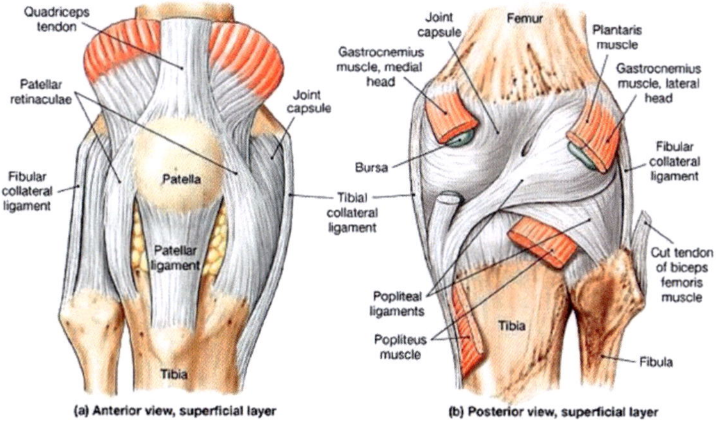

Quadriceps tendon
Patellar retinaculae
Joint capsule
Fibular collateral ligament
Patella
Patellar ligament
Tibia
Joint capsule
Femur
Plantaris muscle
Gastrocnemius muscle, medial head
Gastrocnemius muscle, lateral head
Bursa
Fibular collateral ligament
Tibial collateral ligament
Cut tendon of biceps femoris muscle
Popliteal ligaments
Popliteus muscle
Tibia
Fibula

(a) Anterior view, superficial layer (b) Posterior view, superficial layer

When reading Initial Reactions, as soon as the first two numbers appear on the screen, the device is removed from the skin. During this short time, the organism will not have time to react to the impulse so that an IR reading will be purely diagnostic and not therapeutic. When the SCENAR is left on the skin, the nervous system starts to respond. By comparing the final reactions (0's), the organism indicates an area of small asymmetry and treating with FmVar (maximum of dynamics from device) at this site will produce the best results. Maximum dynamics from the device will give maximum action from the organism. Before starting the procedure choose level of power of the impulse action.

- Below-threshold level of energy does not give subjective sensation;
- Threshold level is sensed as slight vibration;
- Above-threshold level is sensed as comfortable electro-action;
- Supra-threshold level is sensed as painful electro-action (as shooting pain).

Specific areas:

- Collar zone
- Venous sinuses
- Pirogov's ring
- Point PC3
- Opposite side of head to sensation of origin of headache
- Craniotherapy from eye sockets up and over the head

Facial Paresis

SCENAR treatment eliminates paresis of the mimic muscles.

Treatment areas:

- behind-the-ear
- ear lobule-temple (mastoid projection)
- "Three tracks 6 facial exit points of trigeminal nerve
- upper forehead edge, the beginning of the hair part
- mid-chin
- mouth angle-chin

- Cervico-occipital area

Additional treatment areas:

- maxillary sinus
- nostrils and bridge of the nose
- nasal active points
- nostril-eye
- over-and-under-the-eyebrow
- lower jaw angle
- nosalabial fold
- periocular
- sub maxillary
- gum
- "100 diseases"

Initiate treatment on the healthy side and continue according to the treatment areas. Use high power level for the paresis area and comfortable one for the rest areas.

Do 15-40 sessions for the treatment course.

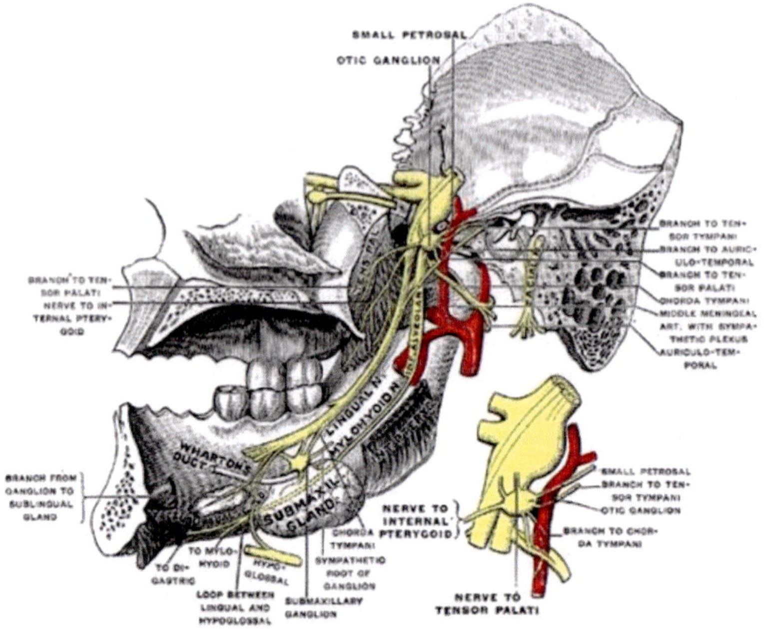
SMALL PETROSAL
OTIC GANGLION
BRANCH TO TENSOR PALATI
NERVE TO INTERNAL PTERYGOID
BRANCH TO TENSOR TYMPANI
BRANCH TO AURICULO-TEMPORAL
BRANCH TO TENSOR PALATI
CHORDA TYMPANI
MIDDLE MENINGEAL ART. WITH SYMPATHETIC PLEXUS
AURICULO-TEMPORAL
LINGUAL N.
MYLOHYOID N.
WHARTON'S DUCT
SUBMAXIL. GLAND
BRANCH FROM GANGLION TO SUBLINGUAL GLAND
TO MYLO-HYOID
TO DI-GASTRIC
HYPO-GLOSSAL
LOOP BETWEEN LINGUAL AND HYPOGLOSSAL
SUBMAXILLARY GANGLION
CHORDA TYMPANI
SYMPATHETIC ROOT OF GANGLION
NERVE TO INTERNAL PTERYGOID
SMALL PETROSAL
BRANCH TO TENSOR TYMPANI
OTIC GANGLION
BRANCH TO CHORDA TYMPANI
NERVE TO TENSOR PALATI

Ischalgia

Ischialgia (sciatica, sciatic neuralgia): a pain caused by injury or inflammation of the sciatic nerve.

SCENAR treatment relieves painful sensations and prevents recurrent pains. Do the procedure while patient lies on his side. Use comfortable power level.

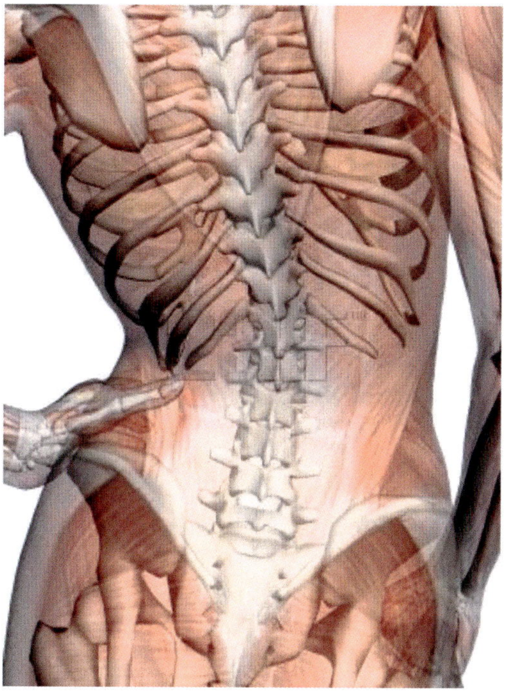

Treatment areas:

- pain location;
- Three Pathways
- lumbosacral area
- gluteal
- back surface of the femurs
- sural muscle surface
- anterior and lateral surface of the femur
- front and outer surface of the calves

Additional treatment areas:

- knee joints
- kidneys
- plantar surface of the foot

- front and outer surface of the feet
- "100 diseases"
- celiac plexus

Do 7-15 sessions for the treatment course. Repeat treatment in 3 or 4 months

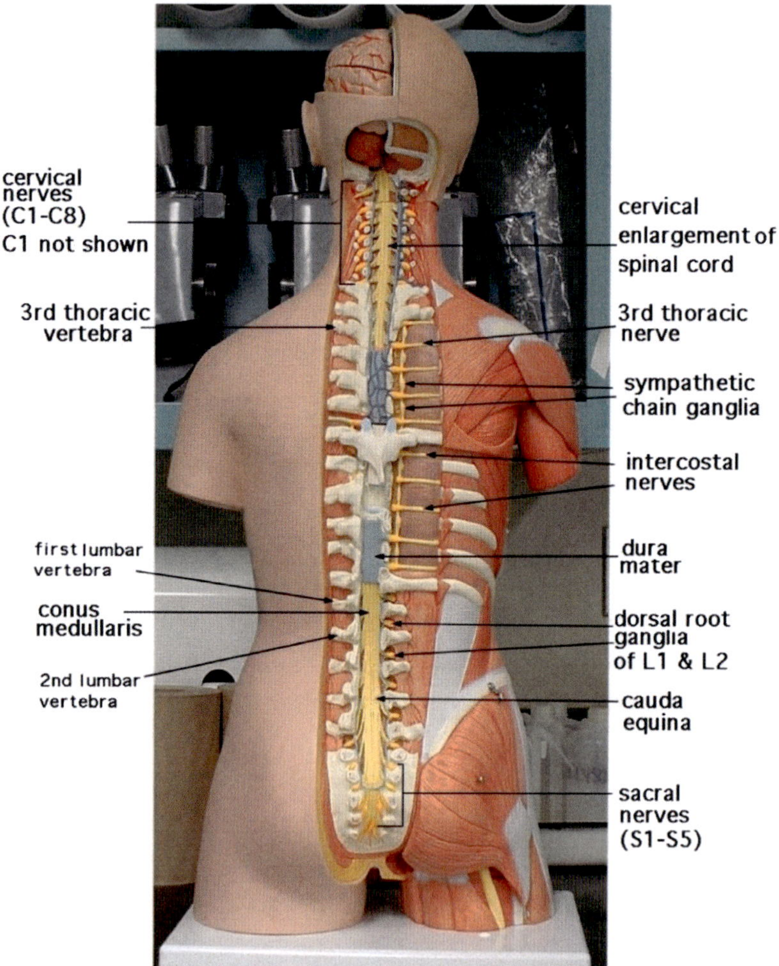
cervical nerves (C1-C8)
C1 not shown
3rd thoracic vertebra
first lumbar vertebra
conus medullaris
2nd lumbar vertebra
cervical enlargement of spinal cord
3rd thoracic nerve
sympathetic chain ganglia
intercostal nerves
dura mater
dorsal root ganglia of L1 & L2
cauda equina
sacral nerves (S1-S5)

Faster wound healing

Faster wound healing: This is due to faster regeneration of tissues as a result of the above processes.

General effect:

- Normal sleep patterns
- Better appetite
- Improved sense of well-being due to higher levels of energy

Priority Areas for Treatment

- Direct projection of the pain.
- Primary signs as described in the "Treatment Reaction Indicators" above;
- Asymmetry
- Small Asymmetry
- Horizontals
- General Zones
- Symmetrical Areas
- Reciprocal areas

Levator Scapula

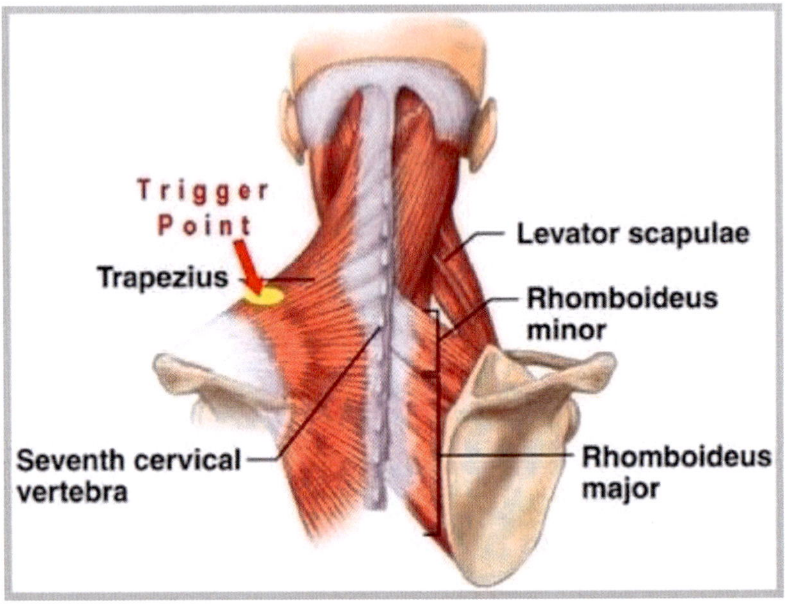
Trigger
Point
Trapezius
Levator scapulae
Rhomboideus
minor
Seventh cervical
vertebra
Rhomboideus
major

The **levator scapulae** help raise the shoulder blade and thereby raise the shoulder. Trigger points in levator scapulae muscles cause pain and stiffness in the angle of the neck. Also to a lesser degree send pain along the inner edge of the shoulder blade and to the back of the shoulder. This trigger point is what keeps you from turning your head to look behind you when you are backing up your car. You may not be able to turn your head at all towards the side that has the trigger point.

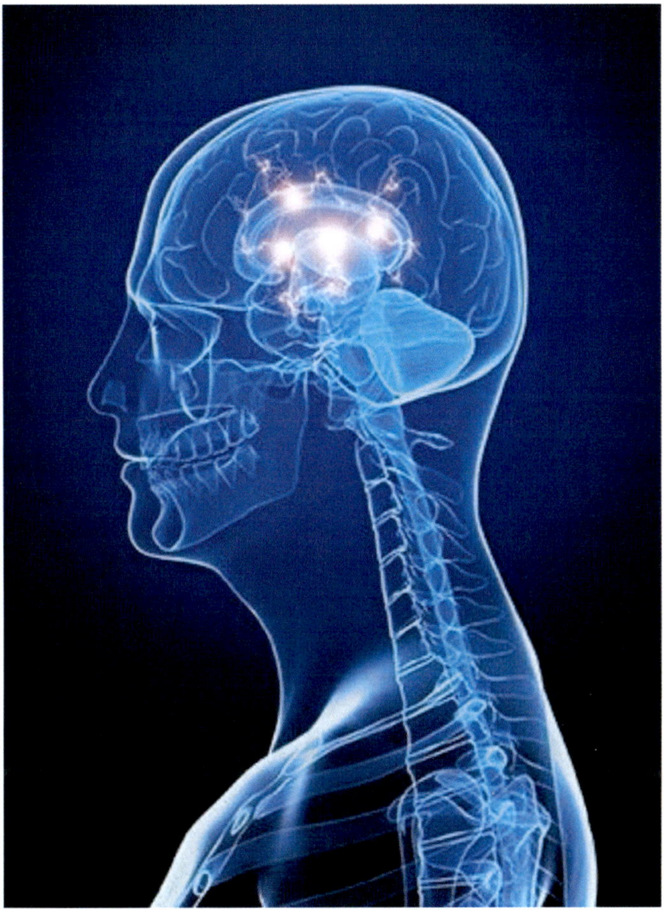

Lumbosacral Plexitis

Treatment areas:

- Cervico-occipital area
- paravertebral area
- Lumbosacral area

Additional treatment areas:

- 6 facial exit points of trigeminal nerve

- 7-th & 8-th cervical vertebrae area
- elbow joint
- Front thigh, lower third

The treatment is carried out at the comfortable and a little bit higher power level.

Do 5-15 procedures daily. Repeat treatment in 1-1, 5 months

Muscular spasm

Treat the full length of the muscle first

Then treat both sides of the muscular attachments to bones sequentially.

When comparing IRs, we need a difference of +4 or higher.

When comparing Doses and '0's, we work on a difference of + 1 or higher.

For the first Dose, the IR should be +4 or greater than the following (preceding) IR.

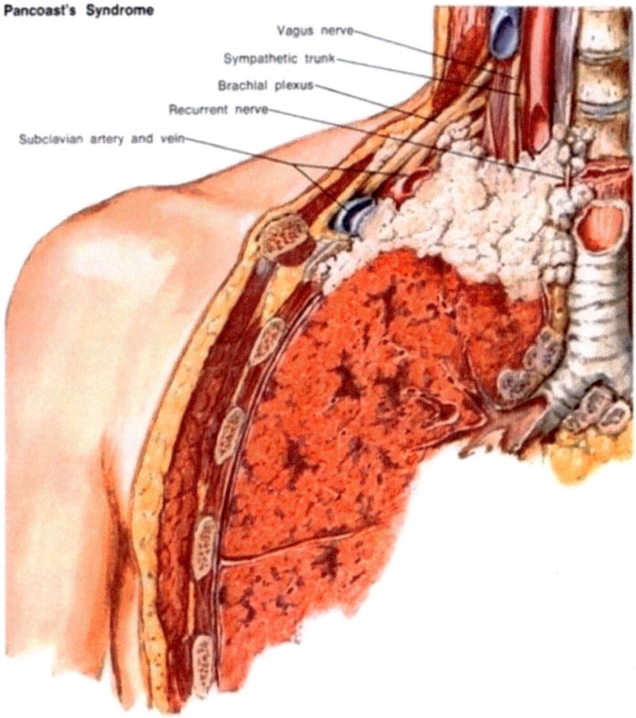
Pancoast's Syndrome
Vagus nerve
Sympathetic trunk
Brachial plexus
Recurrent nerve
Subclavian artery and vein

After you give the first Dose on higher reading, any subsequent IR which is greater than the IR you have just dosed by +4 should be also dosed when working on the vertical line and greater by +1 when working on the horizontal line.

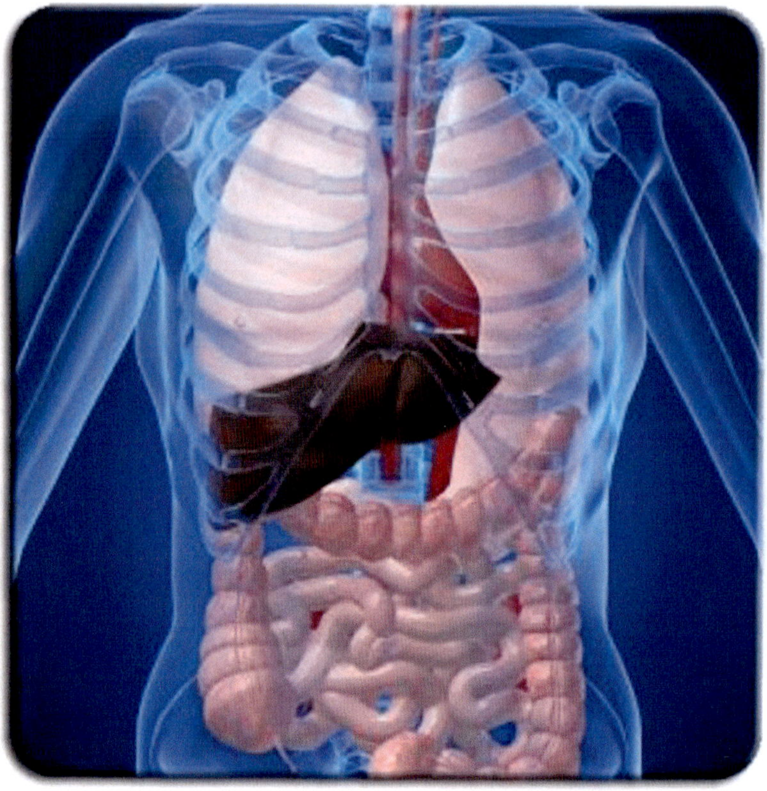

Choose the highest Dose within the route and bring the speed of reaction down to '0' (give 0 / Dose 2).

Get several different '0's completing treatment on the back and then on the highest 0 reading set FmVar / Altemat for 2 minutes.

Complete the procedure on the face using the principles above.

Treat any one zone applying the same principles.

If you did not get any "0"s, move onto the next zone.

For acute pain or in an emergency:

- Use high level of power

For chronic pain or on children and elderly:

- Use comfortable level of power

Myositis

The aim of treatment: to relieve muscle tension, to arrest pain syndrome, to normalize metabolism in affected area and in the whole organism. The device should be applied along the affected muscles and their tendons within the limits of pains localization. It is expedient to apply power massage treatment with the device of the affected muscle and tendon sheath at the comfortable level of power intensity with low speed of moving.

Additional treatment zones:

- paravertebral area
- elbow joint
- lumbosacral area
- Cervico-occipital area
- Occipital

Muscle Tears

For edema and acute pain treatment during first 5 days after trauma happens, it's optimal to work with:

Subjective-dosed mode (Diag=0).

Frequency 180-350 Hz and Intensity mode - in alternation (by the comfort feelings).

For the maximal pain area - Swing mode (Mod=Sw1) for 2-3 minutes.

In addition periodically treat the symmetric area, also backbone and next-to-backbone area (paravertebral) on the same horizontal level as the muscle tear is.

It's desirable to provide SCENAR procedures 3-5 time per day.

On the 6th day and later you can use lower frequencies 45-60-90 Hz and Fm Var Mode in alternation. Not less than 2-3 procedures per day.

The main task during each procedure is the searching of the small-asymmetry signs in the treatment area (see Instructions) and then treating them untill dynamical (contrary) changes. Wish you quick and full recovery!

Neurological Disorders

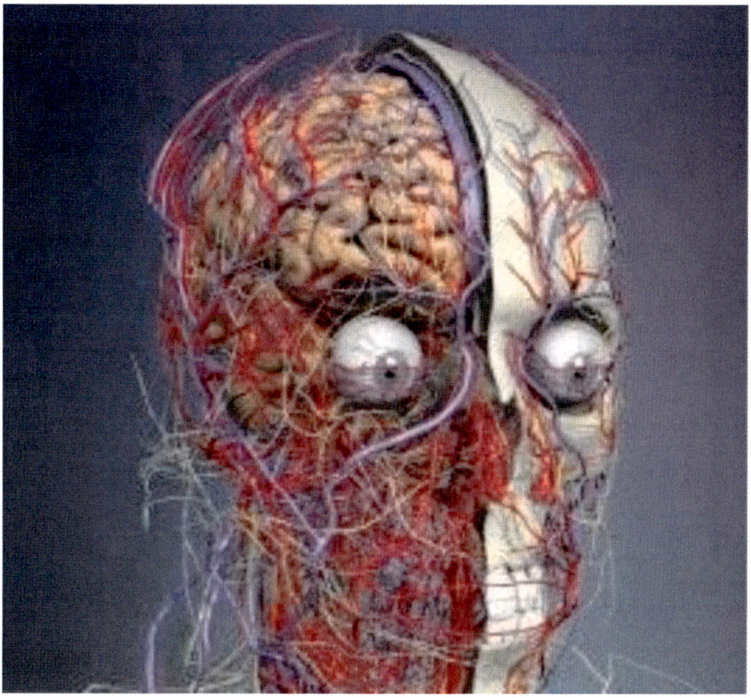

It is necessary to work on General zones as well as on Specific zones.

Better to start with the limbs rather than the head.

Start from the healthy side (symmetrical area) before treating the affected area.

When treating a stroke victim, treat all limbs.

Use reciprocal principles in chronic cases.

Treat only two joints if they are affected (pair of symmetrical normally) at any one time, no more.

Preferably treat the horizontals rather than segments.

If there is pain in the spinal column, treat general zones and a pair of adjacent joints involved in the process.

Frequently change the settings. Once the smallest asymmetry has been found, change the settings.

Results are often delayed. Be patient and warn the patient to keep a positive attitude.

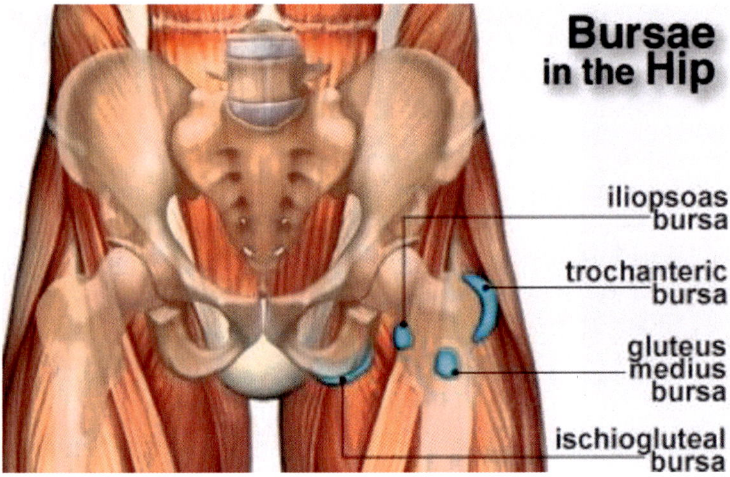
Bursae
in the Hip
iliopsoas
bursa
trochanteric
bursa
gluteus
medius
bursa
ischiogluteal
bursa

Skin Functions

One square inch (6.5 sq. cm) of skin contains up to 4.5 m (15 ft.) of blood vessels, which have as one of their functions the regulation of body temperature. It contains over 4 million various receptors.

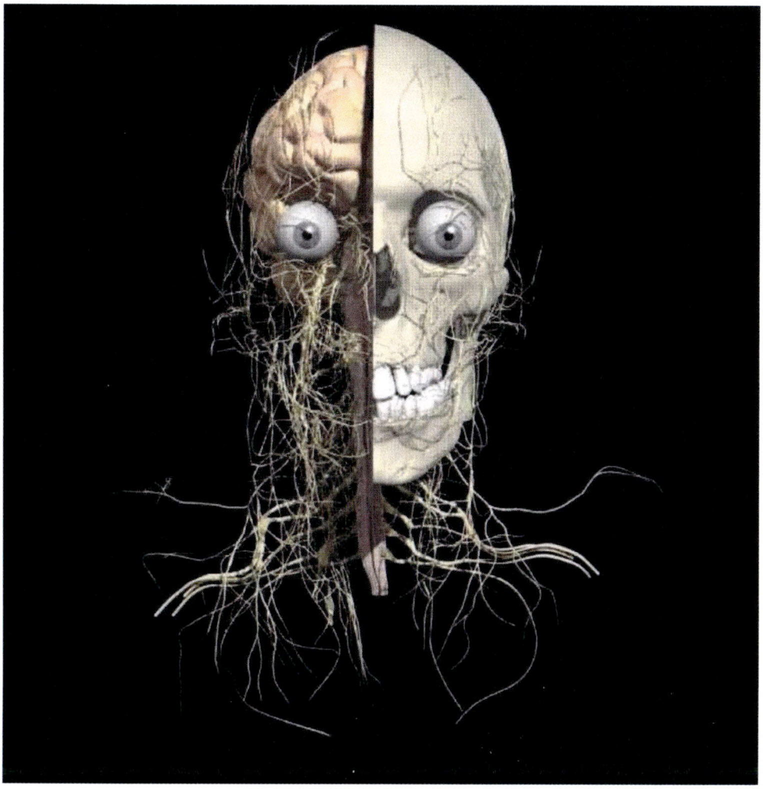

The skin comes into direct contact with the environment and plays a great role in vital functions of the human organism. Covering our whole body, it is the first organ to react to environmental factors.

The skin is of great significance in maintaining the organism's internal balance (homeostasis).

The brain controls all the organs and tissues by means of electric pulses. We can act on the body's nervous system through the skin, using electric pulses similar to the body.

The Scenar influences and is influenced by, the reaction of the skin.

The SCENAR activates nearly all organism systems through the specialized sensory nerves in the skin.

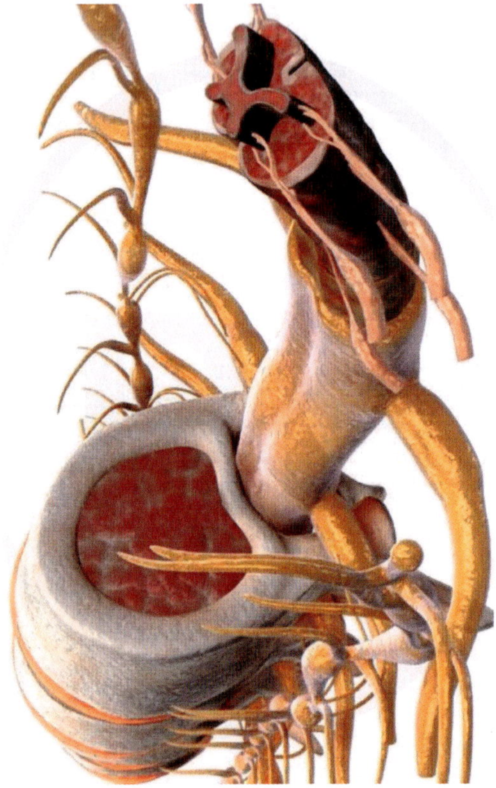

By using SCENAR-signals, it is possible to achieve significant therapeutic effects due to the activation of the somatic or autonomic nervous system neurons in the tissues. These effects are considerable when compared to other methods of electro-therapy. The therapeutic mechanisms involved reflect those as known in physiotherapy. So why and by which physiologic mechanisms, are these therapeutic effects achieved? To answer this question, we would like to look into the modern view regarding the structure, function and chemical physiology of nerve excitation. First of all, let us examine aspects of the SCENAR signal.

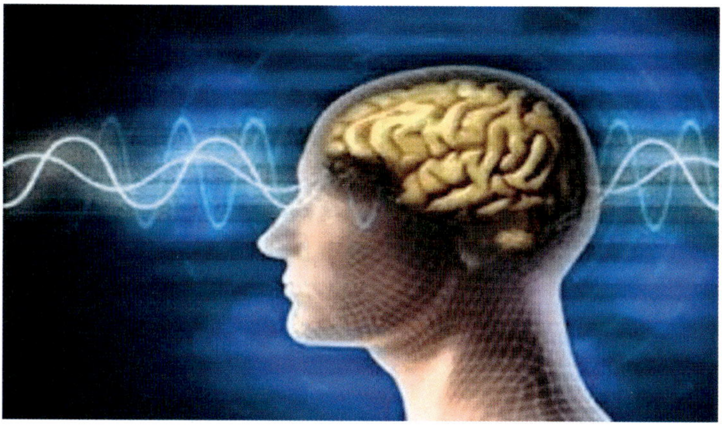

A high amplitude and at the same time, a short, non-damaging action.

An absence or essential diminishing of the process of adaptation resulting from them biofeedback process, in which each impulse differs from the previous one. The neutralization of the possible effect of accommodation because of the high curve of the front of the action signal.

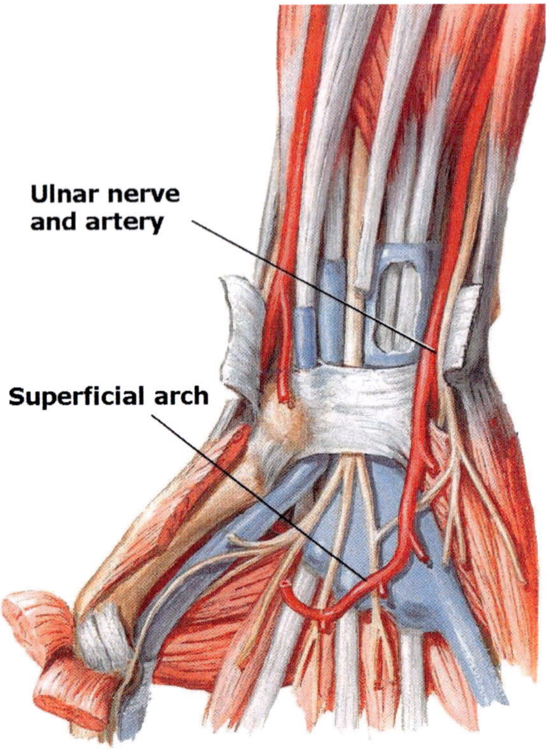
Ulnar nerve
and artery
Superficial arch

So every impulse is actually different from the preceding input. The organism is unable to accommodate to the stimuli and there action to the impulses does not diminish, i.e., there is no process of accommodation.

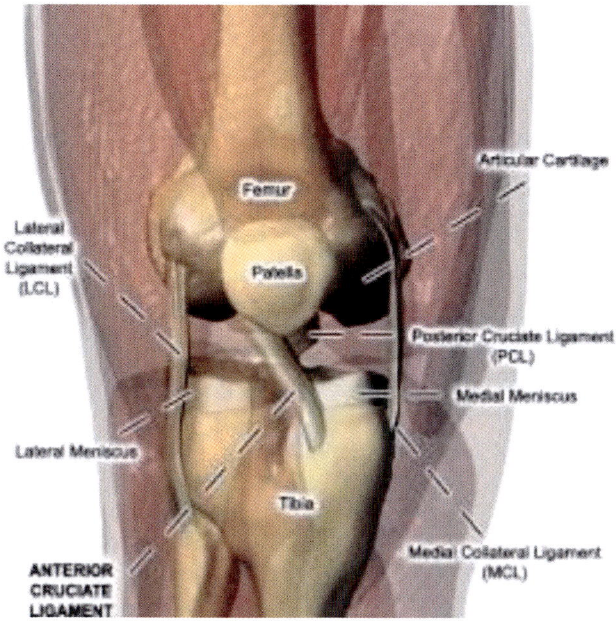
Articular Cartilage
Femur
Lateral
Collateral
Ligament
(LCL)
Patella
Posterior Cruciate Ligament
(PCL)
Medial Meniscus
Lateral Meniscus
Tibia
Medial Collateral Ligament
(MCL)
ANTERIOR
CRUCIATE
LIGAMENT

The moving of the device over the skin's surface while treating creates a dynamic response from the body.

The treatment of the special zones (the choice of small asymmetry, etc.) is aimed to activate numerous nervous endings.

Spinal Column Disorders

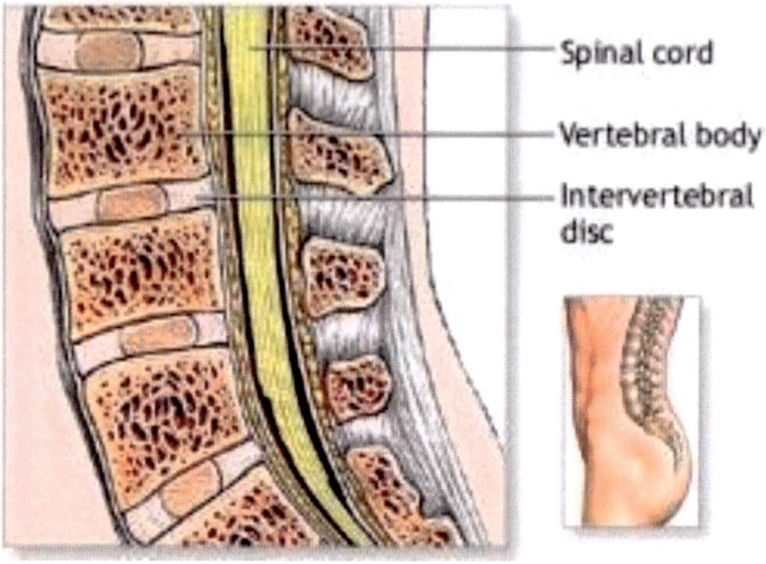
Spinal cord
Vertebral body
Intervertebral disc

Specific areas and Tips:

Observe and examine the back and limbs

Assess the muscles: tension/relaxation

Test muscles with physical load to pinpoint the pain

Test strength of the muscles. With a complaint of pain, work on high power.

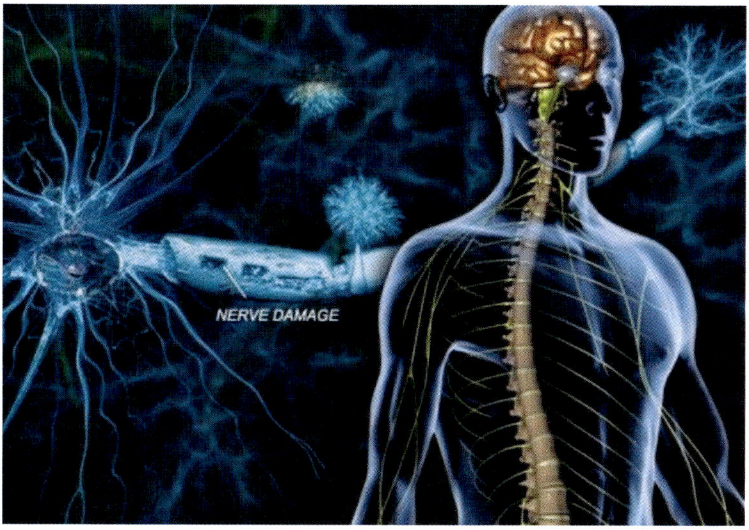
NERVE DAMAGE

When working in Constant (Subjectively dosed) mode (Diag 0 / Diag=OFF / CONSTANT) on paravertebral route, assess according to three positions of the electrode, looking for and treating asymmetries.

Treat muscles in spasm, starting from the healthy side.

In case of a complaint of pain without muscular spasm, treat the point of pain.

Find a small asymmetry on the opposite reciprocal limb; work out that small asymmetry and only then work on the painful limb.

Use Reciprocal principle: arm/leg; external/internal; flexor/extensor.

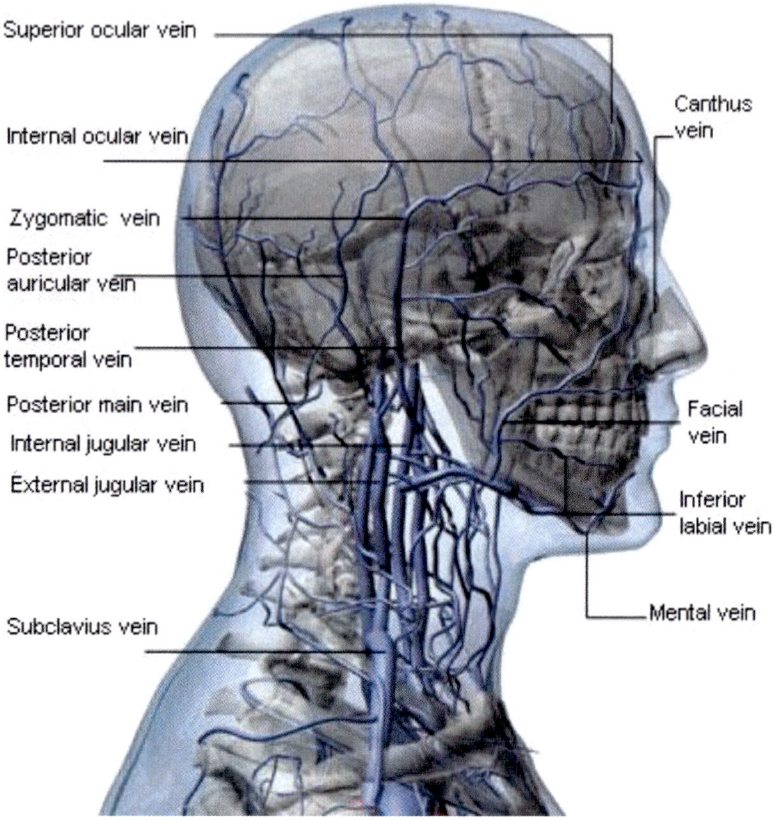
Superior ocular vein
Internal ocular vein
Zygomatic vein
Posterior
auricular vein
Posterior
temporal vein
Posterior main vein
Internal jugular vein
External jugular vein
Subclavius vein
Canthus
vein
Facial
vein
Inferior
labial vein
Mental vein

Joint Disorders, Strains & Sprains

Work on any of the painful sites which appear at the moment of movement on high power, with the settings for pain.

Move the electrode around the area trying to find the most painful spot or any other small asymmetry. Work it out.

Once you have completed the treatment, try for any signs of pain, reinforcing the joint.

If you have found the spot of pain, work on it (you may use Fm Var (Altemat) mode for 2min).

Test the joint for pain and mobility in the end of the procedure. Finish the session with a significant improvement.

If only one joint is involved in the process, work on the symmetrical joint, spending halftime less on the healthy joint. Treat the damaged joint as well as adjacent muscles.

If there are many joints involved, choose the most painful, and work on that pair of joints until complete recovery, then move on to treat another pair of joints.

When working on small joints treat all areas adjacent to the affected area.

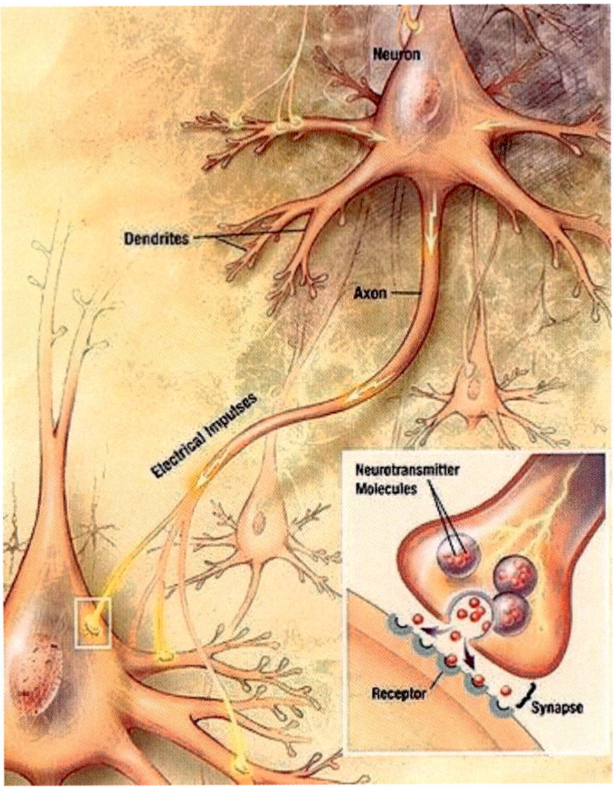
Neuron
Dendrites
Axon
Electrical Impulses
Neurotransmitter Molecules
Receptor
Synapse

Trapezius

Trapezius trigger point number 2 is deeper in the upper trapezius and sends pain to the base of the skull. This referred pain predictably induces secondary trigger points in the muscles of the back of the neck. When neck massage feels good but doesn't get rid of the pain, the problem may be in the trapezius muscles, not the neck. No. 3 also refers pain to the base of the skull and to a small place on top of the shoulder. It is responsible for the burning pain between shoulder blades that comes after a long spell at the computer without elbow support. This is one of the many causes of a stiff neck. Trapezius trigger point number 4 occurs next to the inner border of the shoulder blade in the broad middle part of the trapezius. This causes a burning kind of pain nearby, alongside the spine. Superficial trigger points in this area can cause goose bumps on the back of the upper arm and sometimes on the thighs. Medical diagnosis includes spinal disk compression, spinal stenosis, and bursitis of the shoulder or neuralgia.

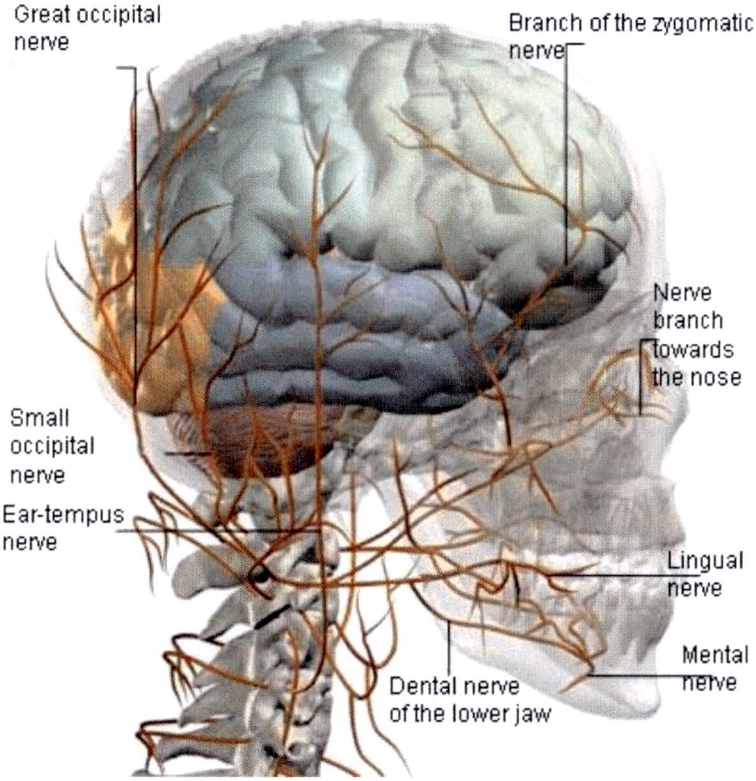

Great occipital nerve
Branch of the zygomatic nerve
Nerve branch towards the nose
Small occipital nerve
Ear-tempus nerve
Lingual nerve
Mental nerve
Dental nerve of the lower jaw

Toothache

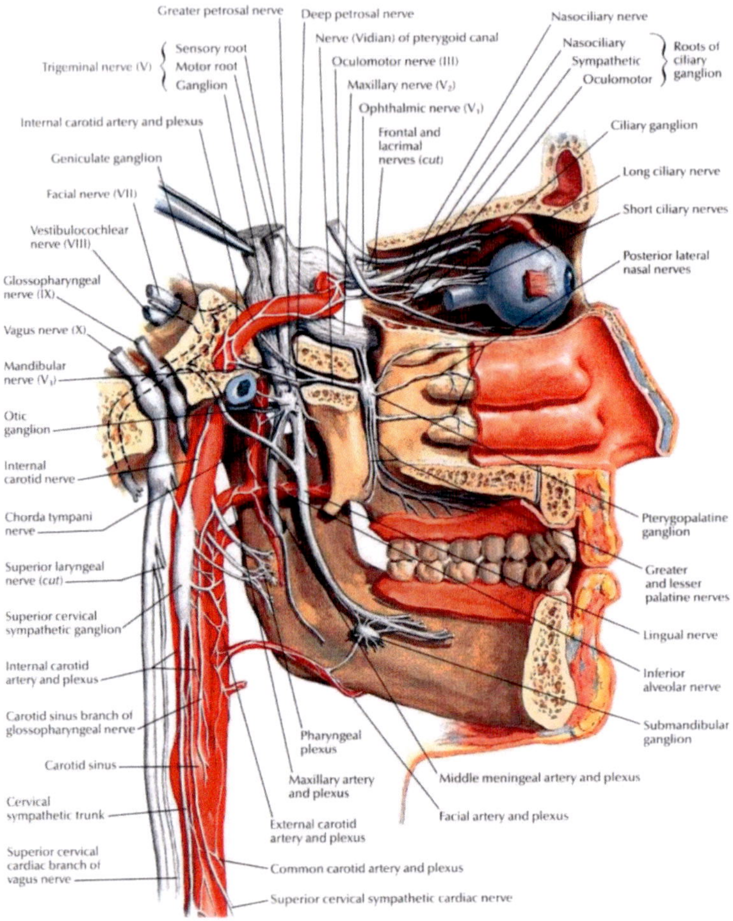

Greater petrosal nerve
Deep petrosal nerve
Nasociliary nerve
Trigeminal nerve (V)
Sensory root
Motor root
Ganglion
Nerve (Vidian) of pterygoid canal
Oculomotor nerve (III)
Maxillary nerve (V2)
Ophthalmic nerve (V1)
Nasociliary
Sympathetic
Oculomotor
Roots of ciliary ganglion
Internal carotid artery and plexus
Geniculate ganglion
Frontal and lacrimal nerves (cut)
Ciliary ganglion
Long ciliary nerve
Facial nerve (VII)
Short ciliary nerves
Vestibulocochlear nerve (VIII)
Posterior lateral nasal nerves
Glossopharyngeal nerve (IX)
Vagus nerve (X)
Mandibular nerve (V3)
Otic ganglion
Internal carotid nerve
Chorda tympani nerve
Pterygopalatine ganglion
Superior laryngeal nerve (cut)
Greater and lesser palatine nerves
Superior cervical sympathetic ganglion
Lingual nerve
Internal carotid artery and plexus
Inferior alveolar nerve
Carotid sinus branch of glossopharyngeal nerve
Submandibular ganglion
Pharyngeal plexus
Carotid sinus
Maxillary artery and plexus
Middle meningeal artery and plexus
Cervical sympathetic trunk
External carotid artery and plexus
Facial artery and plexus
Superior cervical cardiac branch of vagus nerve
Common carotid artery and plexus
Superior cervical sympathetic cardiac nerve

Acute toothache: spontaneous paroxysm of the toothache, which is very often felt in the ear or temple.

Treatment areas:

- most painful area
- 6 facial exit points of trigeminal nerve
- Pirogov's ring (tonsil projection)

- ear lobule-temple (mastoid projection)
- Sub maxillary
- frontal sinus
- maxillary sinus
- Cervico-occipital area
- nasal active points
- lower jaw angle
- "100 diseases"
- Tip of the tongue

Do 7-10 sessions for the treatment course. Repeat treatment in 3 months

Trigeminal Neuralgia

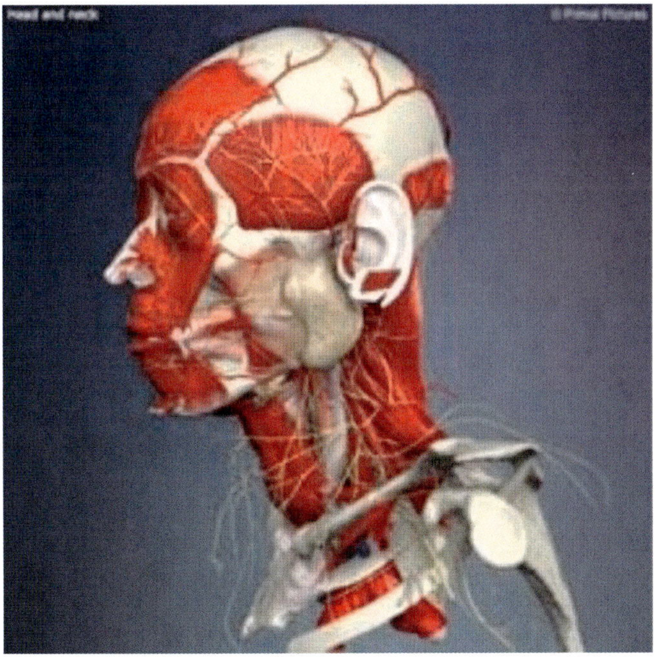

The aim of the treatment is to arrest pain syndrome, to relieve edema and inflammation.

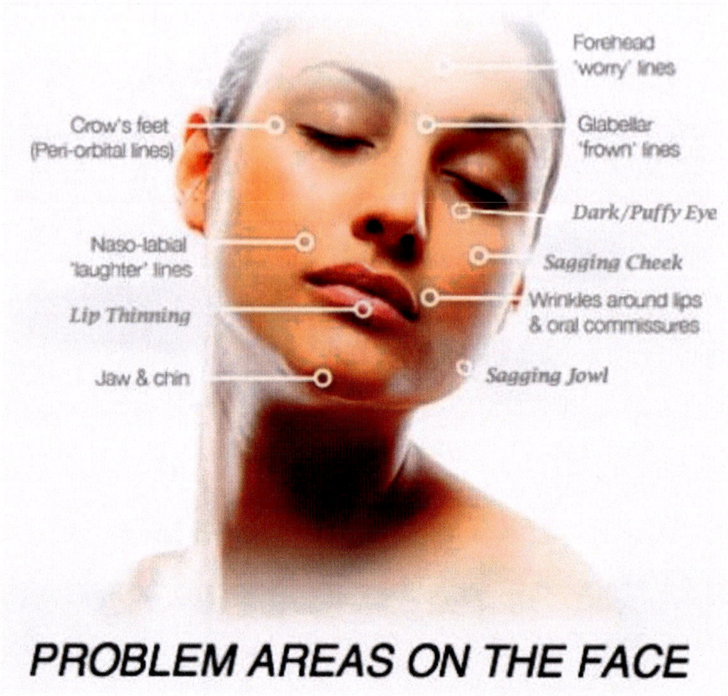
Forehead
'worry' lines
Crow's feet
(Peri-orbital lines)
Glabellar
'frown' lines
Dark/Puffy Eye
Naso-labial
'laughter' lines
Sagging Cheek
Lip Thinning
Wrinkles around lips
& oral commissures
Jaw & chin
Sagging Jowl
PROBLEM AREAS ON THE FACE

Treatment areas:

- mouth angle-chin
- nostril-eye
- over-and-under-the-eyebrow
- lower jaw angle
- ear lobule-temple (mastoid projection)
- behind-the-ear
- Frontal

Additional treatment areas:

- occipital
- forehead between the eyebrows ("the third eye")

- Cervico-occipital area
- 7-th & 8-th cervical vertebrae area
- Paravertebral area

Start working on the healthy side and don't treat the sore side on the first day. The next day carry out the procedure on the sore side. Carry out 2-3 procedures per day until the pain is reduced or stopped. Do 5-15 procedures daily.

Set the device to DIAGN 1 and prepare to look for the highest of the initial reactions (IPs). To make it simple, use your arm as the area in which to search for the IP's. 15)

Practicing using DIAGN 1:

Place the device on the skin outside of the intended area to treat. Press the button t to increase the level of power until the patient feels a comfortable pricking sensation.

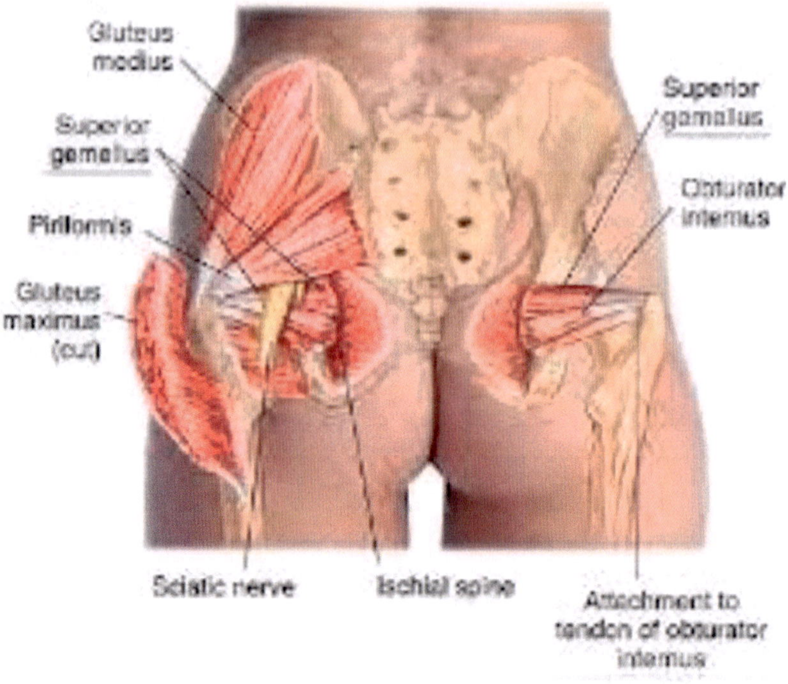
Gluteus medius
Superior gemellus
Piriformis
Gluteus maximus (cut)
Superior gemellus
Obturator internus
Sciatic nerve
Ischial spine
Attachment to tendon of obturator internus

Visual Disturbances

The inner ear functions as guidance system for the focusing of the eyes. They can make things appear to be jumping around in front of your eyes. Though not related to the inner ear, a droopy eyelid, excessive tearing or reddening of the eyes can also often is traced to SCM trigger points.

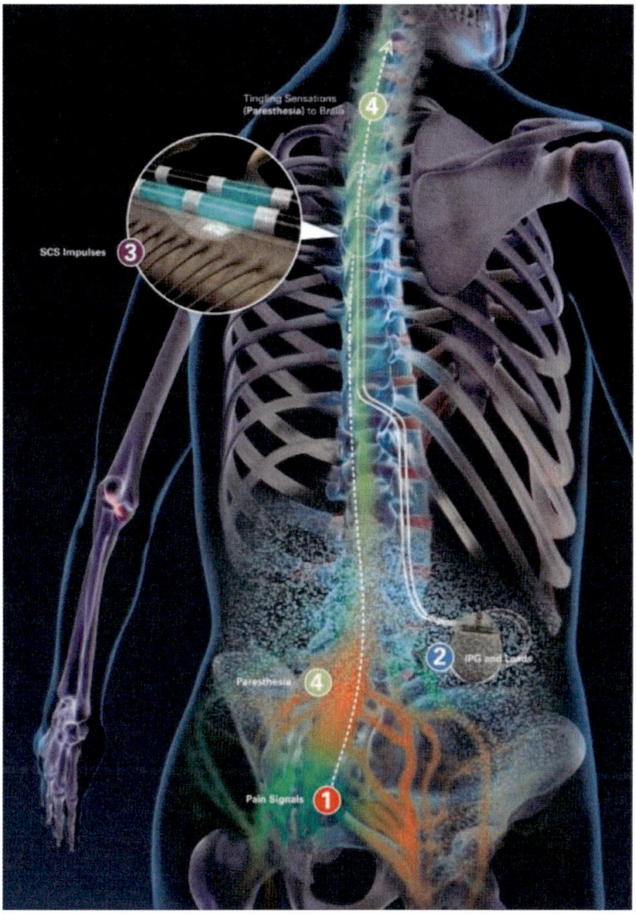
4
Tingling Sensations (Paresthesia) to Brain
3
SCS Impulses
2
IPG and Leads
4
Paresthesia
1
Pain Signals

Systemic Symptoms:

These symptoms involve the generation of excess mucus in the sinuses, nasal cavities, and throat. They can be the simple explanation for your sinus congestion, sinus drainage, glop in the throat, chronic cough, rhinitis, and persistent hay fever or cold symptoms. A persistent dry cough can often be stopped with SCENAR work applied to the sternal branch near its attachment to the breastbone. Trapezius number 1 trigger point causes pain in the temple, at the back corner of the jaw, down the side of the neck behind the ear, and even behind the eye. Occasionally, pain occurs in the back of the head. Their effects are most often identified as a tension headache. This trigger point is also a frequent cause of dizziness that is indistinguishable from that caused by the trigger point in the SCM. Moreover, it's capable of inducing secondary trigger points in muscles in the temple and jaw, making it an indirect cause of jaw pain and toothache.

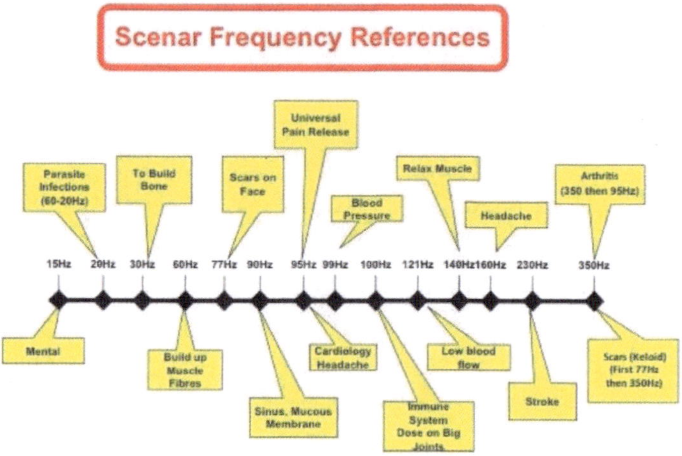
Scenar Frequency References
Parasite Infections (60-20Hz)
To Build Bone
Scars on Face
Universal Pain Release
Blood Pressure
Relax Muscle
Headache
Arthritis (350 then 95Hz)
15Hz
20Hz
30Hz
60Hz
77Hz
90Hz
95Hz
99Hz
100Hz
121Hz
140Hz
160Hz
230Hz
350Hz
Mental
Build up Muscle Fibres
Sinus, Mucous Membrane
Cardiology Headache
Immune System Dose on Big Joints
Low blood flow
Stroke
Scars (Keloid) (First 77Hz then 350Hz)

Chapter 17.
Nerve Regeneration

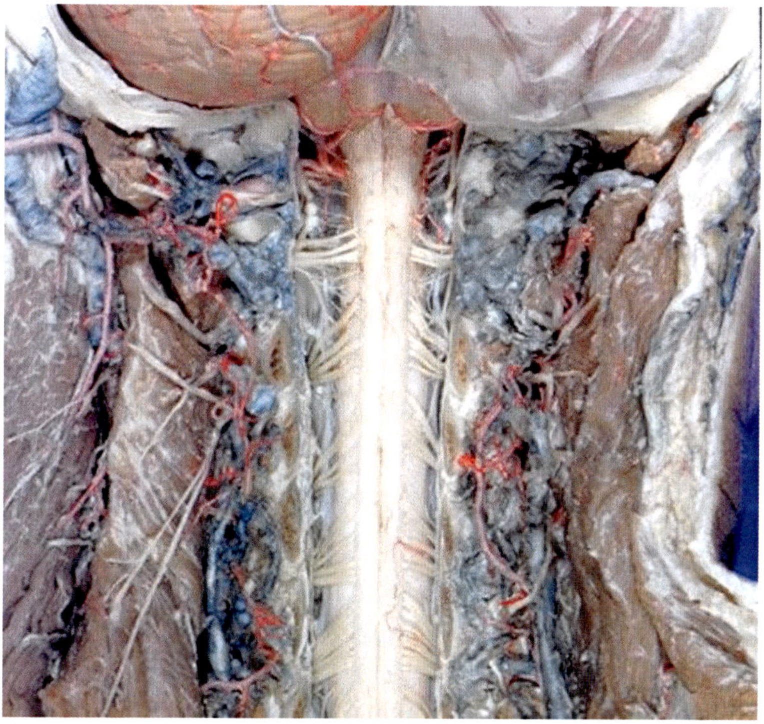

Tissue regeneration

Tissue regeneration is a series of endothermic and electrochemical reactions. This means that minute amounts of electricity are needed by the cells to provide energy to fuel the regenerative process. The body normally contains more than enough energy to produce this desired effect. When we have an injury this produces what is called "**the current of injury**" or a reversal of the normal process.

Electronic stimulation of mitochondrial function (again, the powerhouse of the cell) causes the **replenishment of ATP** and then the **conversion of ATP** (Adenosine Triphosphate) **to ADP** (Adenosine Diphosphate) at the cellular level resulting in stimulation of the sodium potassium pump. Thus, the membrane active transport is increased, thus allowing the intracellular flow of nutrients and extracelluar flow of waste materials. This leads to increased protein synthesis (as **ATP provides the energy source that tissues need to build proteins), cell regeneration and acceleration of tissue healing.**

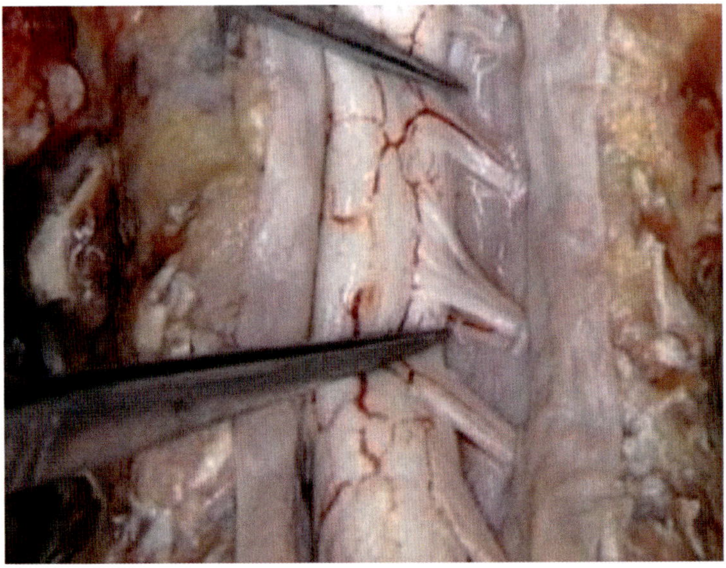

Electronic stimulation produces electrochemical changes in the body that set the stage for healing. Electro-Therapy initiates the healing process by replenishing ATP, increasing the membrane transport of ions, and facilitating protein synthesis. With recharged cellular batteries, the body can take over and perform the healing of which it is capable.

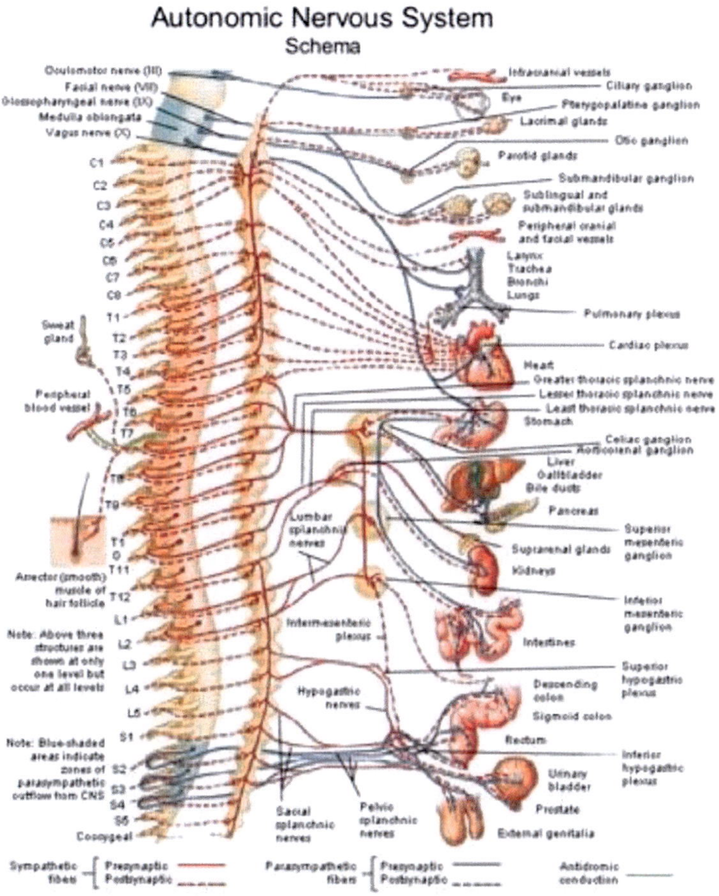
Autonomic Nervous System
Schema
Oculomotor nerve (III)
Facial nerve (VII)
Glossopharyngeal nerve (IX)
Medulla oblongata
Vagus nerve (X)
C1
C2
C3
C4
C5
C6
C7
C8
T1
T2
T3
T4
T5
T6
T7
T8
T9
T10
T11
T12
L1
L2
L3
L4
L5
S1
S2
S3
S4
S5
Coccygeal
Sweat gland
Peripheral blood vessel
Arrector (smooth) muscle of hair follicle
Note: Above three structures are shown at only one level but occur at all levels
Note: Blue-shaded areas indicate zones of parasympathetic outflow from CNS
Intracranial vessels
Ciliary ganglion
Eye
Pterygopalatine ganglion
Lacrimal glands
Otic ganglion
Parotid glands
Submandibular ganglion
Sublingual and submandibular glands
Peripheral cranial and facial vessels
Larynx
Trachea
Bronchi
Lungs
Pulmonary plexus
Cardiac plexus
Heart
Greater thoracic splanchnic nerve
Lesser thoracic splanchnic nerve
Least thoracic splanchnic nerve
Stomach
Celiac ganglion
Aorticorenal ganglion
Liver
Gallbladder
Bile ducts
Pancreas
Superior mesenteric ganglion
Suprarenal glands
Kidneys
Lumbar splanchnic nerves
Inferior mesenteric ganglion
Intermesenteric plexus
Intestines
Superior hypogastric plexus
Descending colon
Sigmoid colon
Hypogastric nerves
Rectum
Inferior hypogastric plexus
Urinary bladder
Prostate
Sacral splanchnic nerves
Pelvic splanchnic nerves
External genitalia
Sympathetic fibers
Presynaptic
Postsynaptic
Parasympathetic fibers
Presynaptic
Postsynaptic
Antidromic conduction

Medical science has established that there are extensive electrical fields at work in the body. The nervous system, for example, has long been known to work through both electrochemical and purely electrical signals. In fact, electrical bonding at the atomic level holds all molecules together. A cell, like all units comprised of atomic and molecular assemblies, thus has an electronic moment which results from the interaction of all its electrochemical constituents.

We now know that the body is composed of an interconnected semiconductor fibrous matrix that extends into its every nook and cranny. Macroscopically, this system consists of the connective tissues that form bones, tendons, fascia, cartilage, and ligaments and that also form the matrix of all organs and glands. All of the systems of the body, the musculature, vasculature, nervous system, digestive tract, integument, and lymphatics are composed of connective tissue that gives them their characteristic form and physical properties.

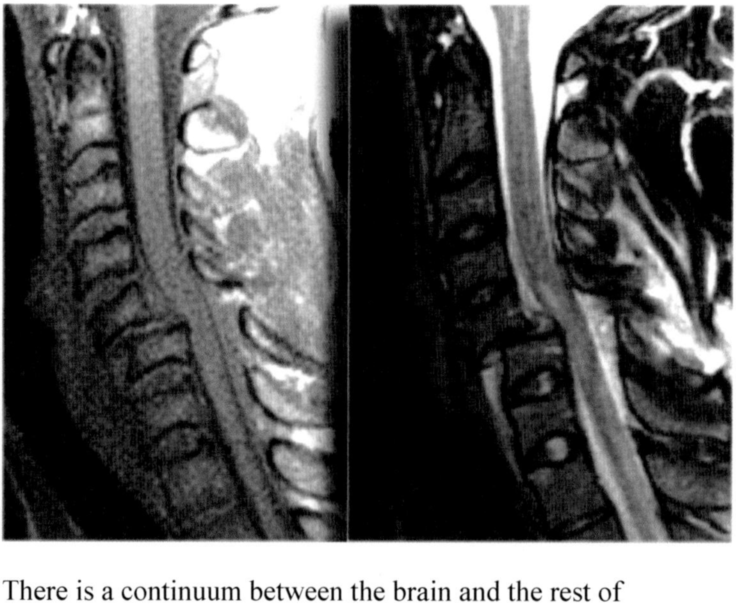

There is a continuum between the brain and the rest of the body through the perineurium (tissue of mesodermal origin consisting of collagen fibroblasts and fatty cells; supports organs and fills spaces between them and forms tendons and ligaments) and an electromagnetic field deep within.

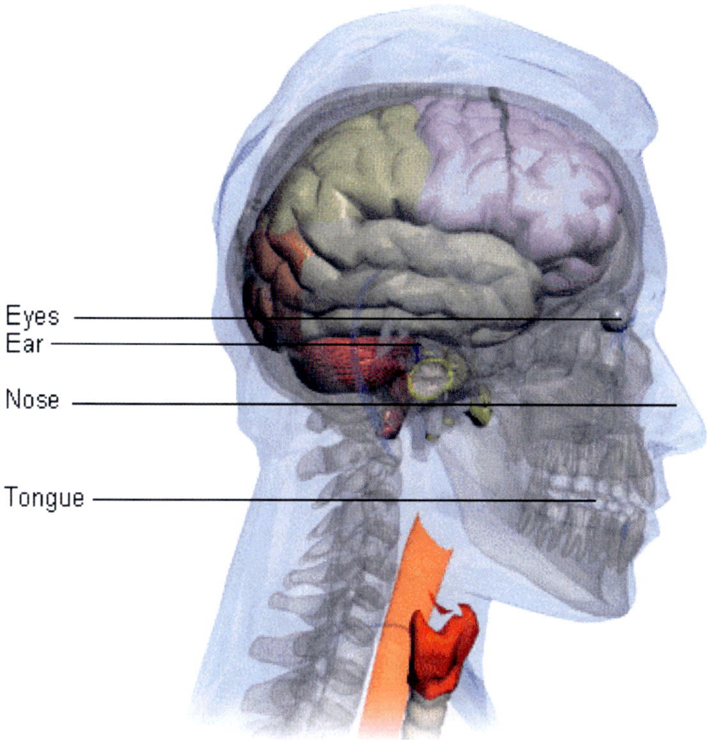
Eyes
Ear
Nose
Tongue

The electromagnetic field holds energetic vibrational or frequency patterns that are characteristic of specific events that had occurred which have been either traumatically physical or emotional. This explains how the effects of physical injury remain in the tissue long after the tissue should have healed. This also explains how emotional trauma and memory is "stored" in physical tissue and then affects physical function.

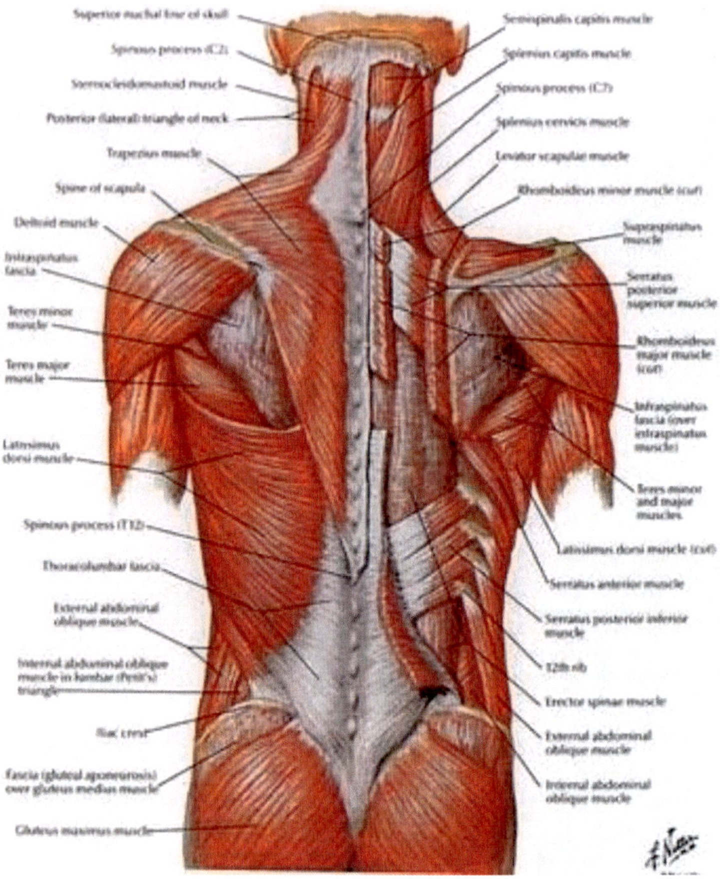
Trapezius muscle
Spine of scapula
Deltoid muscle
Teres minor muscle
Teres major muscle
Latissimus dorsi muscle
Spinous process (T12)

Trauma and internal disease manifest themselves as a dysfunction of the autonomic homeostasis. Areas affected by a disease are shown to be detectable as more electro-conductive than the surrounding skin. Therefore, any physical disorder which increases autonomic activity can be measured at specific points using a point-specific probe. If the biochemical system is in a state of imbalance or non-homeostasis, it is probably due to the fact that the **capacitive elements of the cells are not relaying the energy distribution system properly.** Either there is not enough energy or there is too much energy stored in the capacitors in the cell. This state of misalignment resulting from imbalance in the capacitor system in the cell is thus an imbalance in energy flow, resulting in a state of systemic trauma caused by the body's attempt to compensate for the imbalance. This trauma results in pain-producing signals being transmitted throughout the involved areas of the central nervous system. As these tissue areas receive the correct flow of electrical energies, circulation is improved and the normal healing process is quickened. This is characterized by an immediate reduction in pain. Case in point, **after the body receives a bioelectric therapy, there is electronic input into various points regulating the functioning of cells and neuro-muscular systems of the body.** Glycogen utilization of the muscle tissue increases and the amino acid content of the brain tissue also increase. At the same time, activities of some enzymes in the tissue are stronger. These changes indicate that treatment can promote the metabolic process of tissues in their apparent movement to help invigorate the body's power of resistance to unfavorable factors, thereby promoting the recovery of damaged tissues.

Regeneration is a series of endothermic electrochemical reactions. This means that electricity is used in miniscule quantities by cells to provide the energy to fuel the regenerative process. The tissue in the area of involvement needs energy in the form of electricity. The patient's body contains more that an adequate quantity of energy to produce the desired effect. Unfortunately, the electrical resistance in the area of involvement is so elevated that the body's energy flow cannot enter the area because the laws of physics require that energy travel only via the path of least resistance.

The result, energy traveling in the body will circumvent the area of pathology because it always takes the path of least resistance, which is around, rather than through, the area of pathology.

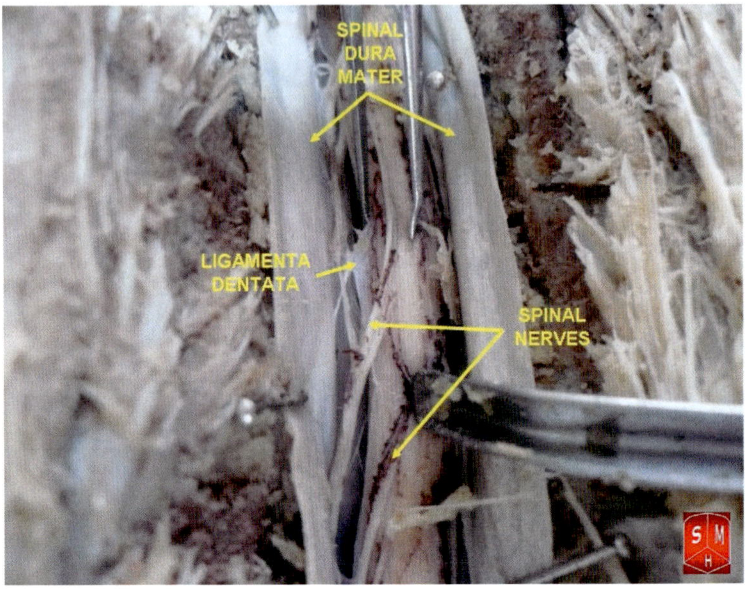
SPINAL
DURA
MATER
LIGAMENTA
DENTATA
SPINAL
NERVES

We must enable the energy to pass into the pathology. In addition, **we can aid the process by increasing the body's ability to actually produce and store energy in the area of involvement**. As we have discussed, this is done by charging the tissue in a manner similar to charging a battery. The greater the charge on the cell, the less resistant it is to the flow of electrical energy.

Additionally, as the cell charge increases, the molecular kinetic energy in the cell increases. Physics provides the equation which reveals that at this point the **electro-vibratory rate (EVR)** of the cell's molecular structure must increase with the increased kinetic energy (energy of movement). An increased EVR will be coupled in direct proportion with an increased electroconductivity (decreased electrical resistance). Finally, while functioning as a battery, the charged cell provides some of the energy which is involved in the energy flow equation. Now, the entire skin layer of the body and obviously at the site of injury is composed of epidermis and dermis and ranges in depth from less than 0.5 to 3 to 4 mm. **It can be represented by an electrical circuit consisting of resistors and capacitors.** One way to increase current density beneath the skin is to increase carrier frequency. An increase in frequency decreases the capacitive resistance and the general health of the cells improve. As a result, a greater amount of current density should be available beneath tissue layers.

The first phase of a typical electrotherapy treatment is typically designed to stimulate the tissue and affect the electrical resistance of the skin. The increased activity of the mitochondria enhances the production of ATP in the cytoplasm. **The ATP provides the fuel for the transmigration of metabolite and metabolic waste across the cell membranes as well as the re-establishment of cellular bioelectronic ionic concentration gradient.** What this means is that cell membrane potential is re-established levels of intra-cellular metabolic waste (i.e., lactic acid) are reduced and fresh concentrations of usable cellular metabolites are introduced into the exhausted cell. At this point the cell can enter its regenerative phase.

The SCENAR facilitates the healing process:

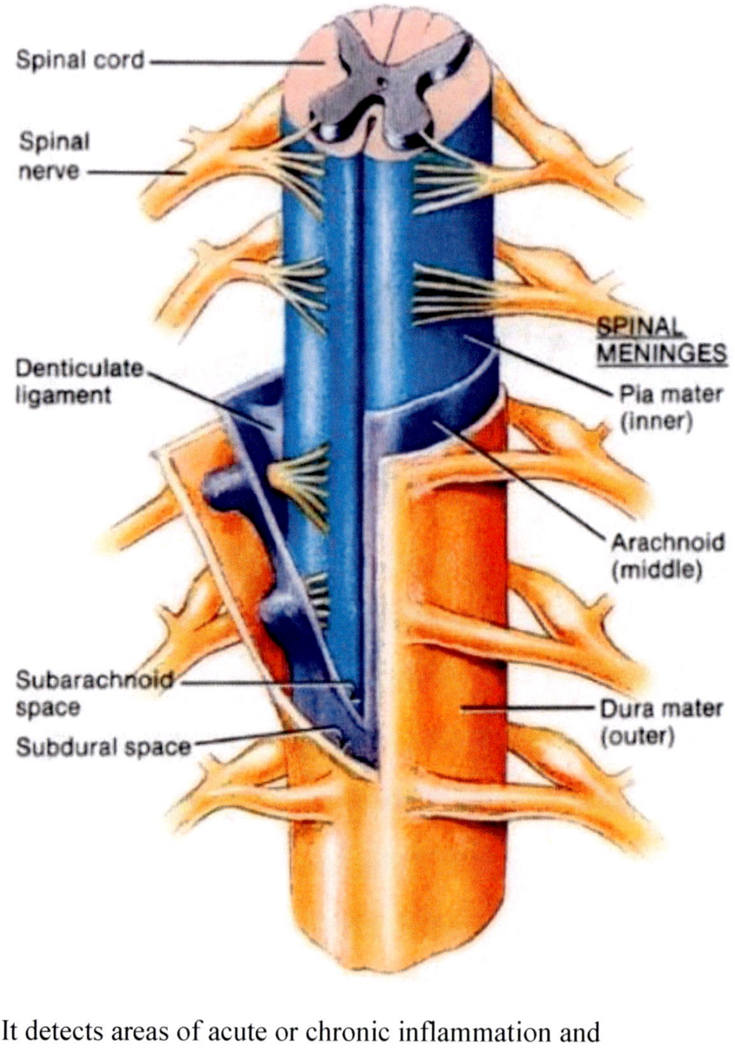
Spinal cord
Spinal nerve
SPINAL MENINGES
Denticulate ligament
Pia mater (inner)
Arachnoid (middle)
Subarachnoid space
Subdural space
Dura mater (outer)

It detects areas of acute or chronic inflammation and areas of adaptation or degeneration

It pumps in biocompatible energy to provide the energetic resources needed in order to initiate repair

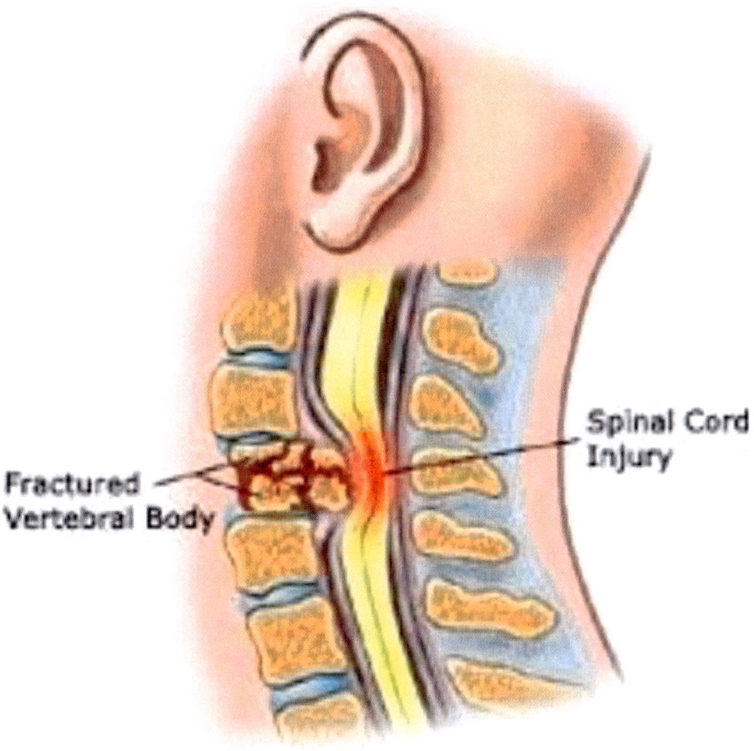
Spinal Cord
Injury
Fractured
Vertebral Body

It reconnects the brain to the injury so nutrients and healing can be directed to the area

It reverses the polarity of adapted injured tissue from negative to positive so resources for repair are attracted and the electropositive current of injury is restored, thereby notifying the brain of the situation.

It provides a signal that stimulates the release of neuropeptides from the pharmacy of chemicals in the skin to augment the ingredients needed for repair. It tones down the sympathetic nervous system and tunes up the parasympathetic nervous system. It provides a sequenced series of nerve-like impulses alternating with pauses to prevent adaptation/habituation to the signals. It dynamically changes the signal characteristics in accordance with the bio-feedback from the body. Using biofeedback, the **Scenar continuously monitors the body's response to its signals and modifies each successive signal to affect a normalization of pathological signals.** The Scenar reads the skin impedance, which changes according to the varying and constantly changing capacitance and inductance of the tissues being tested. These properties vary from moment to moment and place to place throughout the body. This is the reason the Scenar was designed with the unique capability of dynamic measurement of tissue imbalance. In other words, the Scenar measures the time dynamics of the underlying tissue.

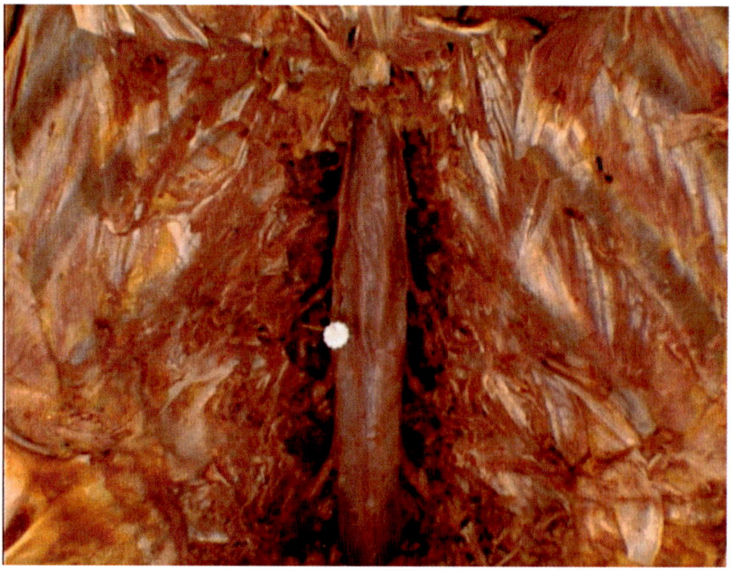

When the Scenar is activated, an electrical pulse is sent into the tissue. The time reaction of the tissue to

the pulse is measured. The pulse is then modified and sent back in to nudge the tissue towards a more normal response pattern.

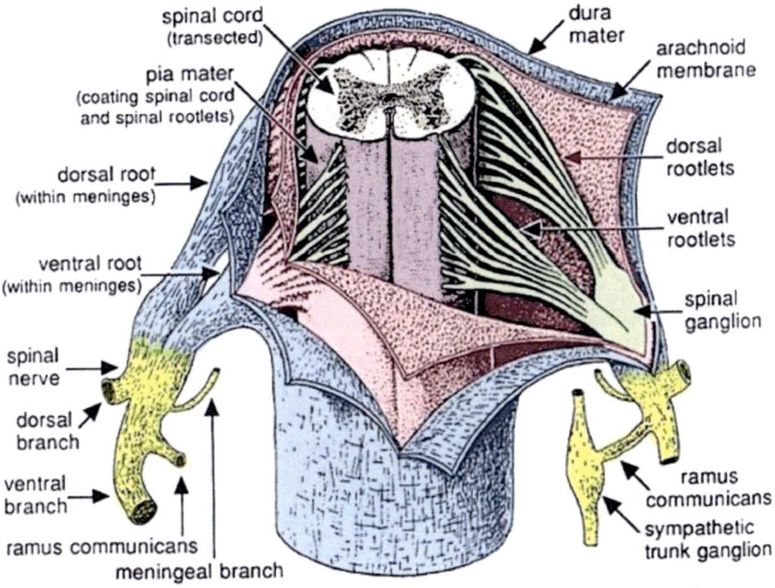
spinal cord
(transected)
dura
mater
arachnoid
membrane
pia mater
(coating spinal cord
and spinal rootlets)
dorsal
rootlets
dorsal root
(within meninges)
ventral
rootlets
ventral root
(within meninges)
spinal
ganglion
spinal
nerve
dorsal
branch
ventral
branch
ramus
communicans
sympathetic
trunk ganglion
ramus communicans
meningeal branch

It is applied on the skin surface, stimulating all structures of the skin. The skin develops from the same embryological layer as the nervous system. This allows for treatment of internal organs as the Scenar stimulates reflexive zones on the surface of the skin.

It works along acupuncture meridians and neurological zones.

It releases a regulative healing-peptide cascade.

It helps to restore homeostasis.

It eliminates repetitive central nervous system patterns.

It works along ascending pathways in the spinal cord to affect the cortex of the brain. This causes efferent pathways from the cortex to convey impulses, which affect a response in the organs associated with the reflex area on the skin.

It works directly on local spinal reflexes.

It re-establishes normal membranous resonance.

Through molecular polarization it normalizes adapted tissue polarities.

By microphoresis it stimulates selective reabsorption of trace elements and minerals from the skin.

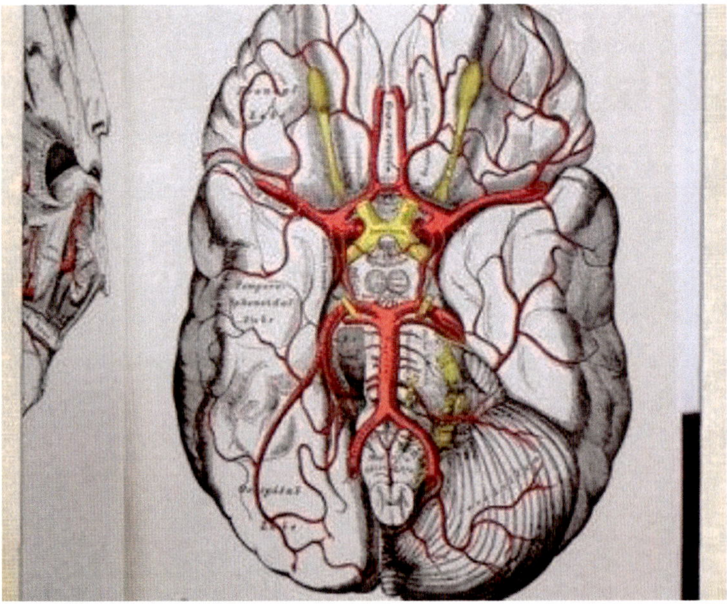

The RITM SCENAR is marketed for the following indications:

- **Symptomatic relief and management of chronic intractable pain.**
- **Acute and chronic pain relief and the resulting increase in range of motion.**
- **Adjunctive treatment in the management of post-surgical and post traumatic pain.**
- **Muscle relaxation, reducing muscle cramps and spasms.**

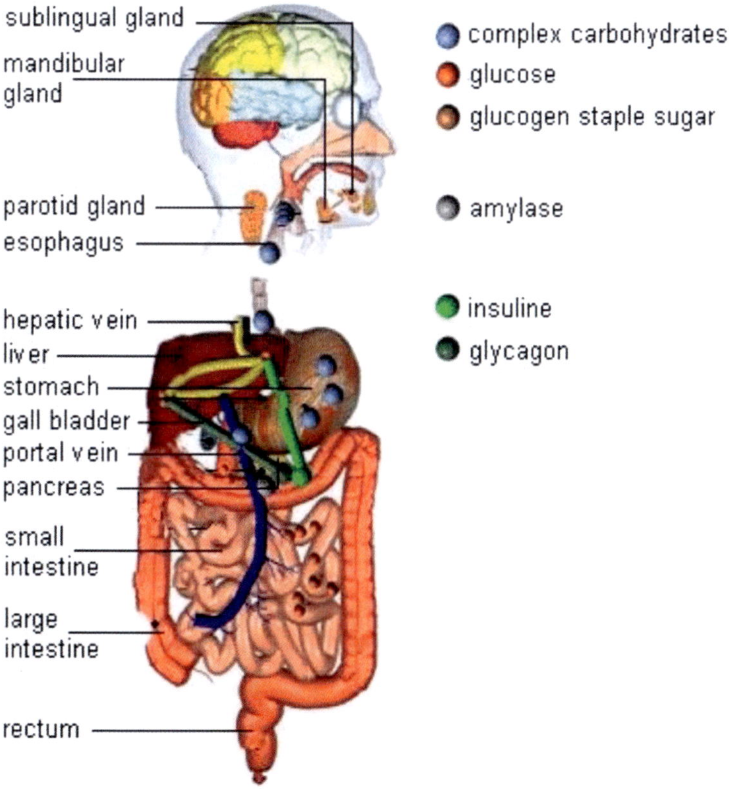
sublingual gland
mandibular gland
parotid gland
esophagus
hepatic vein
liver
stomach
gall bladder
portal vein
pancreas
small intestine
large intestine
rectum
complex carbohydrates
glucose
glucogen staple sugar
amylase
insuline
glycagon

It is applied on the skin surface, stimulating all structures of the skin. The skin develops from the same embryological layer as the nervous system. This allows for treatment of internal organs as the SCENAR stimulates reflexive zones on the surface of the skin.

It works along acupuncture meridians and neurological zones.

It releases a regulative healing-peptide cascade.

It helps to restore homeostasis.

It eliminates repetitive central nervous system patterns.

It works along ascending pathways in the spinal cord to affect the cortex of the brain. This causes efferent pathways from the cortex to convey impulses, which affect a response in the organs associated with the reflex area on the skin.

It works directly on local spinal reflexes.

It re-establishes normal membranous resonance.

I offer a new healthcare technology that can directly influence the human body with individually dosed pulse current and activate the brain to respond to an injury so healing can be directed to the area.

SCENAR Therapy is non-drug medical technology, which is directed at **activating the self-healing resources of the human organism**. These devices are non-invasive energy regulators of the body's systems.

The Nervous System

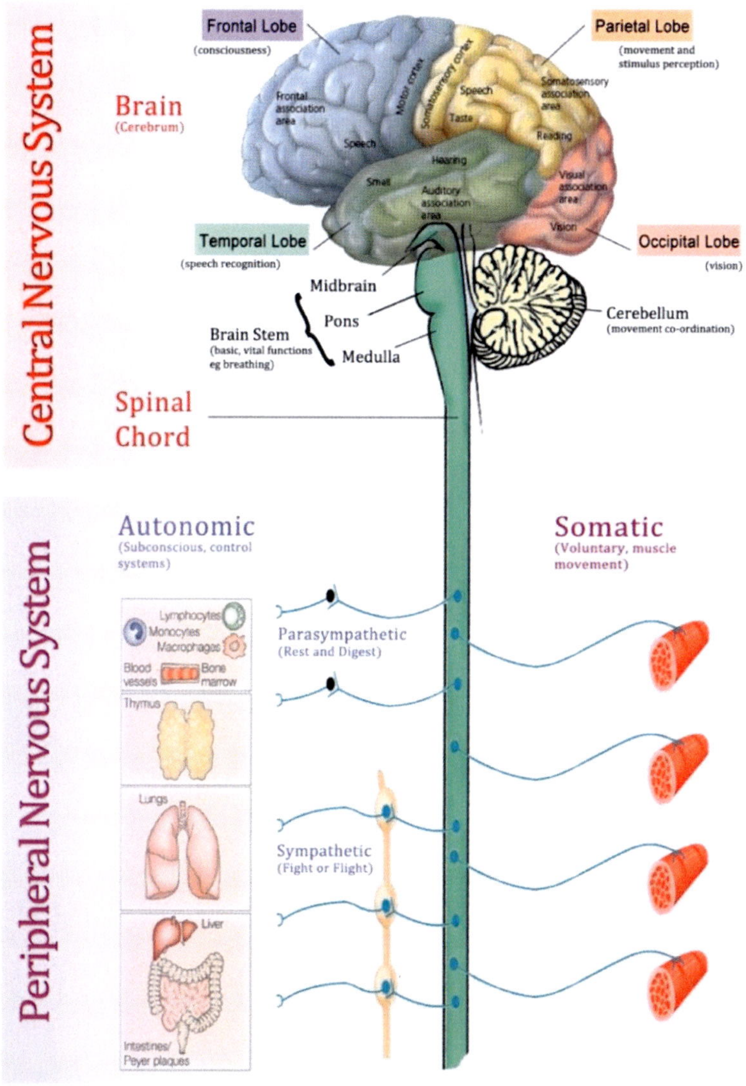
Central Nervous System
Brain
(Cerebrum)
Frontal Lobe
(consciousness)
Parietal Lobe
(movement and stimulus perception)
Temporal Lobe
(speech recognition)
Occipital Lobe
(vision)
Midbrain
Pons
Medulla
Brain Stem
(basic, vital functions eg breathing)
Cerebellum
(movement co-ordination)
Spinal
Chord
Peripheral Nervous System
Autonomic
(Subconscious, control systems)
Somatic
(Voluntary, muscle movement)
Parasympathetic
(Rest and Digest)
Sympathetic
(Fight or Flight)
Lymphocytes
Monocytes
Macrophages
Blood vessels
Bone marrow
Thymus
Lungs
Liver
Intestines/
Peyer plaques

Scenar devices were invented in Russia nearly 20 years ago in order to keep cosmonauts in good health while in space. In 1986 the first SCENAR device, having passed clinical trials, was given permission by USSR Medical Council to be used in hospitals and homes.

These devices are intended to **stimulate the body's self-recovery program** by using its own "internal pharmacy" of neuropeptides. This enables the body to choose the most appropriate chemical combination for each particular case.

Lately, great popularity has been associated with the medicine-free methods of treatment that would help our organism to fight diseases in the most natural way and considerably reduce or even exclude drug taking at all.

The Scenar stimulates cellular reactions to help restore respiratory capacity in tissues and organs, lower concentration of hydrogen ions in tissues, restore or improve utilization of free oxygen by the cell and restore metabolic processes in the body.

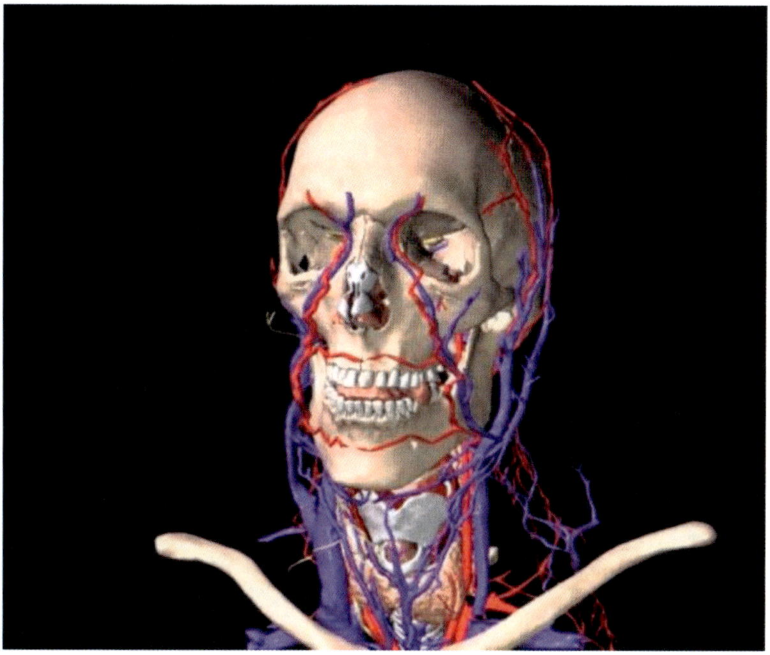

This is called homeostasis, which is the state in which all the processes responsible for energy transformations in the organism are dynamically balanced and stable despite environmental changes.

Since the brain controls the tissues and organs with electric pulses, it is natural that Scenar generated pulses can influence the internal organs and systems through feedback from the body.

The Scenar is effective in managing pain associated with soft tissue dysfunction and in controlling chronic, severe pain.

The outcome of the neurostimulation is that it affects the area of pathological activity locally through increased blood circulation, neuropeptide release, stimulation of the lymph flow, reduction of acute or chronic inflammation and muscle relaxation.

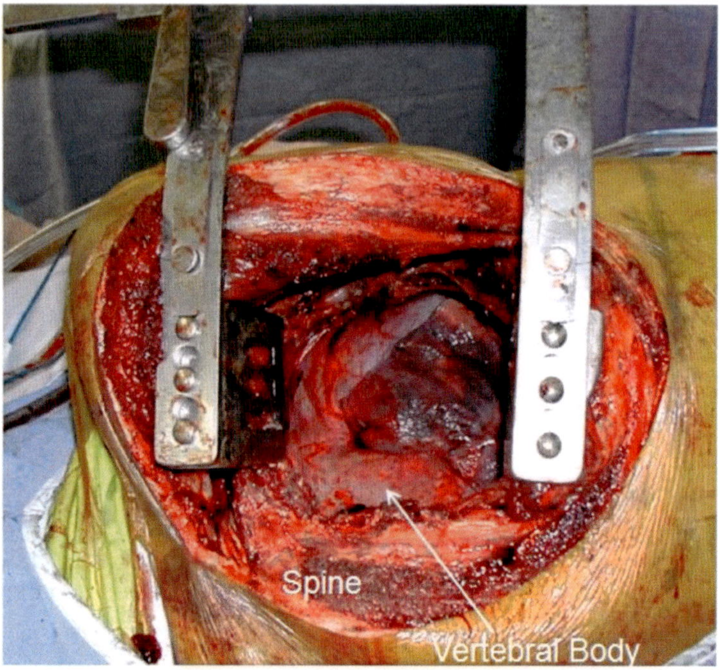
Spine
Vertebral Body

As the pathological systems are eliminated, there is disappearance of complaints and restoration of function.

It detects areas of degeneration. Then it pumps in biocompatible energy to provide the energetic resources needed to initiate repair.

It reverses the polarity of adapted injured tissue from negative to positive so resources for repair are attracted and the electropositive current of injury is restored, thereby notifying the brain of the situation.

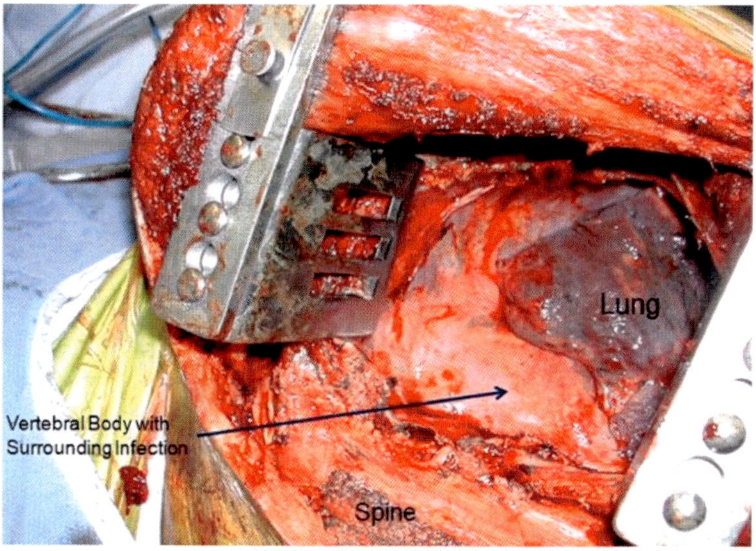
Lung
Vertebral Body with
Surrounding Infection
Spine

It provides a signal that stimulates the release of neuropeptides from the pharmacy of chemicals in the skin to augment the ingredients needed for repair.

The Scenar is applicable in a wide variety of clinical situations from acute injury to post-operative recovery, and the treatment of chronic pain.

It is portable, small and easy to use as the Scenar is hand held, lightweight and battery operated.

SCENAR stands for Self-Controlled-Energo-Neuro-Adaptive-Regulator Therapy. It may be defined as a new healthcare technology that can directly influence the human (animal) body with individually dosed pulse current and activate reflex and biochemical processes in skin receptors.

SCENAR Therapy is non-drug medical technology, which is directed at activating the self-healing resources of the human organism.

SCENAR devices are non-invasive energy-neuro-adaptive regulators of the body's systems. These devices are intended to stimulate the body's self-recovery program by using its own "internal pharmacy" of neuropeptides. This enables the body to choose the most appropriate chemical combination for each particular case.

Lately, great popularity has been associated with the medicine-free methods of treatment that would help our organism to fight diseases in the most natural way and considerably reduce or even exclude drug taking at all.

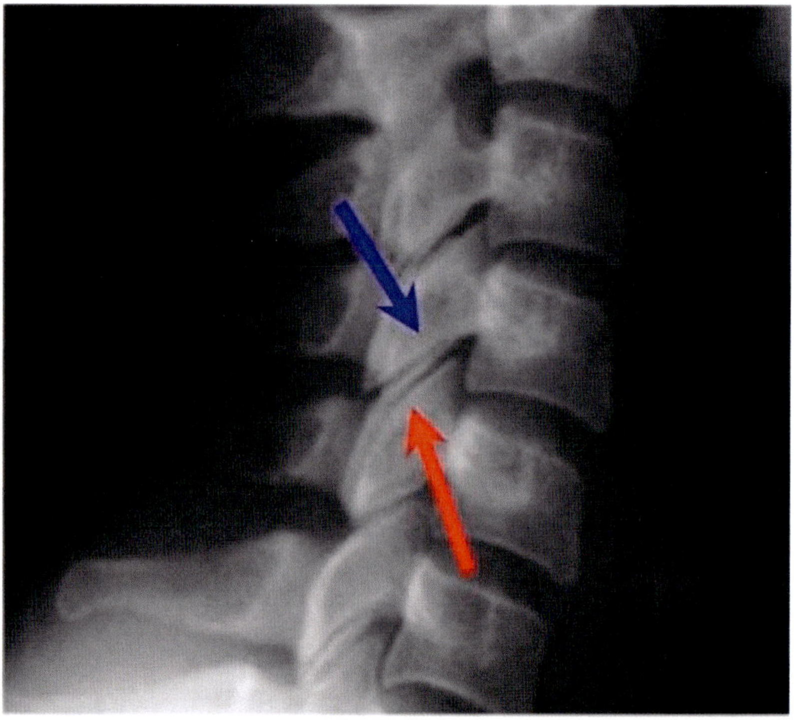

Widely spread, are the instruments that affect the organism with electric signals of a certain form, length and power. However most of them proved to be not very effective due to the lack of monitoring the organism's reaction to electrical stimulation.

By existence of "a dialogue" between the body and the device itself (literally bio-feedback) the SCENAR is referred to as peculiar device, namely an electro-neuro-regulator, which generates every new stimulating pulse according to the body's response to the previous one. This stimulates the body's maximum responsive reaction, which very often cannot be achieved by the other customary and widespread electro stimulators.

The latest achievements in biophysics, physiology and reflexotherapy have assisted in developing new original energy-neuro-adaptive-receptor therapy (SCENAR) devices used for body's pathology diagnostics, physiotherapeutical treatment and rehabilitation.

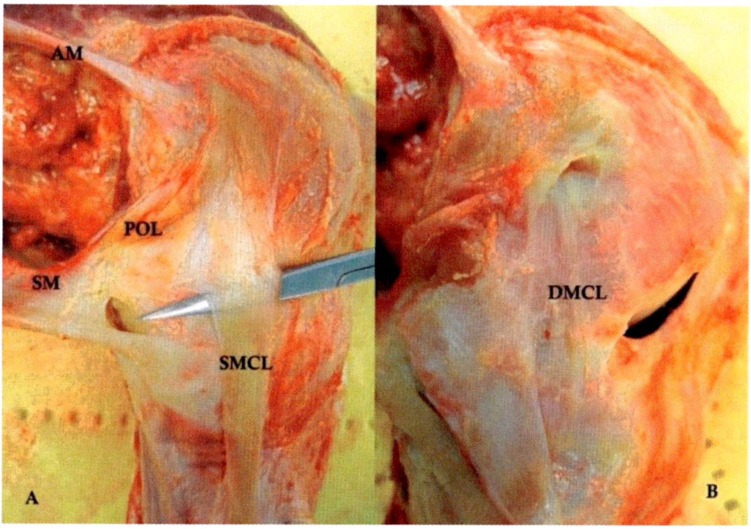
AM
POL
SM
SMCL
A
DMCL
B

All the body's organs and systems are known to be a single whole. Neither organ nor system is functioning in an isolated manner. By virtue of "native-to-the body language”, i.e., neuro-type endogenous impulse, the device forms up a “body-device” stage within the dynamic system. Thus, it becomes possible to create the body’s multilevel and multicomponent feedback loop to correct its adaptation capabilities. It gives an opportunity for very fast and maximally qualitative correction of various pathological states of an organism. The organism, beginning with a cell (nucleolus, mitochondrion, cell membrane, etc.) and ending with organs and systems, represents the most complex set of membranes vibrating in a certain mode. If there is a pathological focus (functional or organic disorder of a tissue structure), the vibration mode changes and becomes irregular.

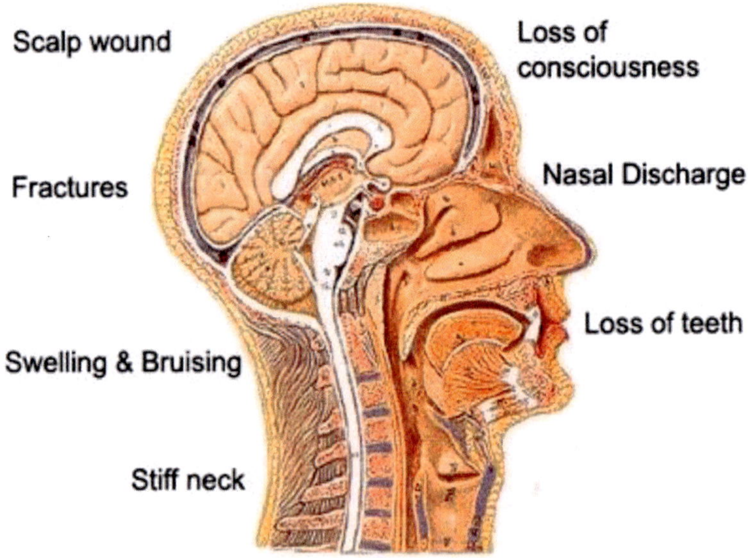
Scalp wound
Loss of consciousness
Fractures
Nasal Discharge
Loss of teeth
Swelling & Bruising
Stiff neck

SCENAR devices act at the cell level and rehabilitate respiratory enzyme chains of the mitochondria (i.e., respiratory ferments structure responsible for cell breathing), cytoplasmic membranes, etc. And so, they recover homeostasis of the cell media (its internal invariability). Generally, the cellular reactions help restore respiratory capacity in tissues and organs, lower concentration of hydrogen ions in tissues, restore or improve utilization of free oxygen by the cell (depending on how far gone is the pathological process), and restore and improve metabolic processes in the body.

Taking into consideration the “affinity” of some electrical currents to the ones of living matter, medicine uses that energy for prophylaxis and treatment of various diseases. From the biophysical point of view, homeostasis is the state in which all the processes responsible for energy transformations in the organism (temperature, acid-base equilibrium, etc.) are dynamically balanced and stable despite environmental changes. The skin plays an essential role in this process. Nerve endings on the skin continually inform the brain of any changes in the body, both inside and outside. Any changes on the skin surface can characterize the body’s condition.

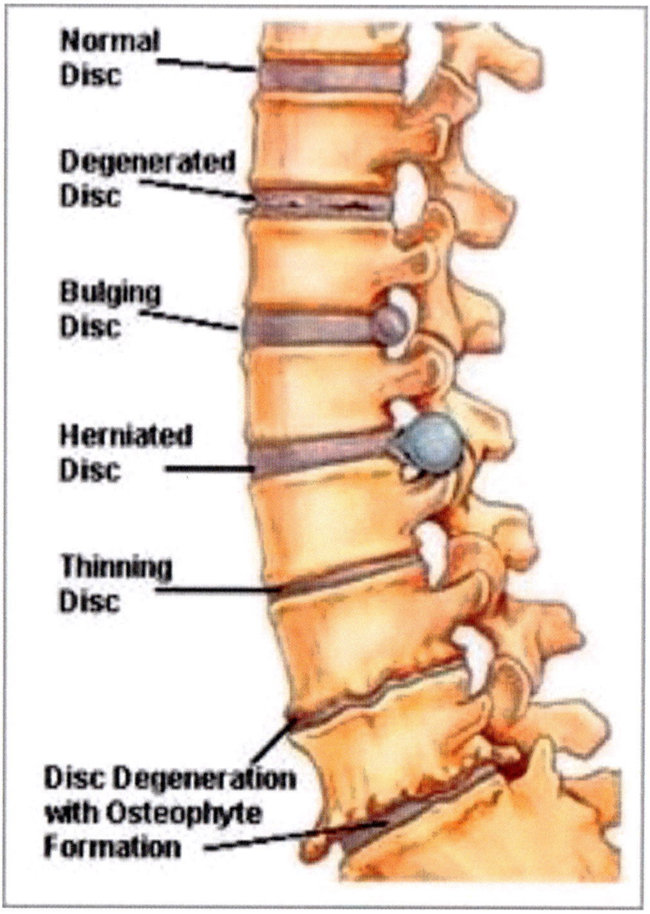
Normal
Disc
Degenerated
Disc
Bulging
Disc
Herniated
Disc
Thinning
Disc
Disc Degeneration
with Osteophyte
Formation

By affecting certain parts of the skin, the SCENAR devices activate practically all the organs and systems of the body. Great numbers of skin receptors help obtain unique healing effects for a wide variety of disease conditions.

Since the brain controls the tissues and organs with electric pulses, it is natural that the device-generated pulses can transdermally influence the internal organs and systems through a "feedback" from the body.

Scenar-devices generate electric pulses which are similar by their form to the brain's neuropulses. Since these pulses "operate" within the physiological parameters and are accordingly transformed in the body in the process of their activity, they are not "alien" and therefore cause no side effects.

SCENAR therapy is regarded as an "intermediate link" between orthodox and traditional eastern medicine. The principals and methodology of SCENAR therapy bring together orthodox and traditional eastern medicine, in particular, acupuncture and its various modifications.

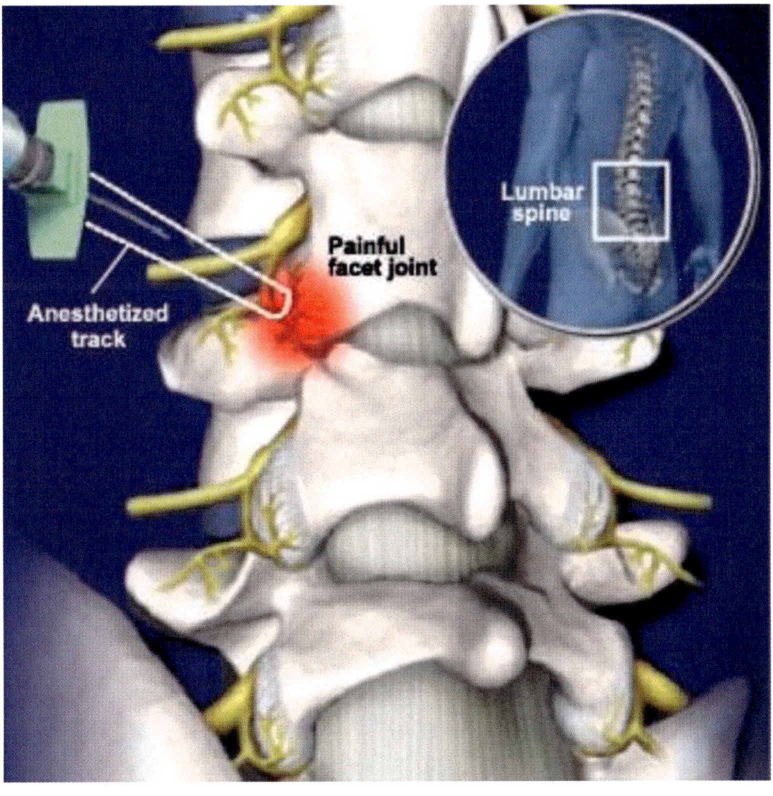
Lumbar spine
Painful facet joint
Anesthetized track

SCENAR sets up a constant 'dialogue' with the organism based on biofeedback. This makes it stand out from other physiotherapeutic devices. It is unique in being a device that uses an individually measured and specifically directed action to achieve its effects.

In SCENAR therapy we talk about pathological systems that occur when a normal functional system becomes disordered in some way and is not corrected by the organism for whatever reason. The SCENAR influences this pathological system and changes it to a functional pathological system, a situation in which the organism itself recognizes that there is a problem and takes the necessary action to re-establish a functional system. The SCENAR thus allows the maturation and completion of these cycles.

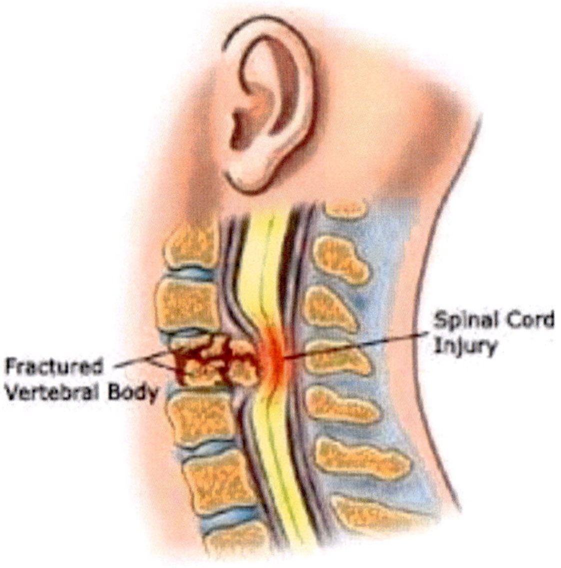
Spinal Cord
Injury
Fractured
Vertebral Body

The RITM SCENAR featuring Interactive Neuro-Stimulation Technology is effective in managing pain associated with soft tissue dysfunction and in controlling chronic, severe pain. It is appropriate for the treatment of both acute and chronic conditions and focuses on decreasing pain and restoring function.

The RITM SCENAR is marketed for the following indications:

Symptomatic relief and management of chronic intractable pain.

Acute and chronic pain relief and the resulting increase in range of motion.

Adjunctive treatment in the management of post surgical and post traumatic pain.

Muscle relaxation, reducing muscle cramps and spasms.

Enhancing neuromuscular re-education.

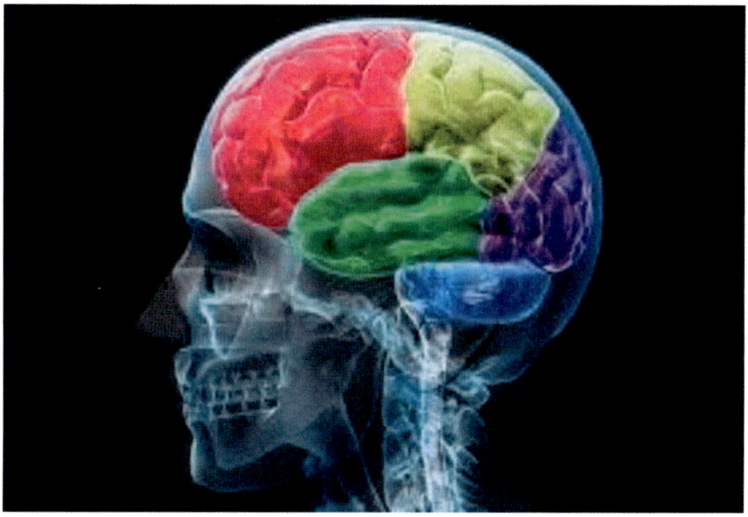

The SCENAR is a unique Neurostimulation device. All cells and tissues in the body function within a normal range of electrical activity. The skin has also presented fascinating electrophysiological behaviors. Extensive work has been done to map the electrical conductivity characteristics of the skin relative to internal functions. Both somatic and visceral dysfunctions are reliably projected into the skin. These projections are detectable by significant changes in the electrical conductivity of the skin. As long as the stressful stimulus remains in place, the patterns of altered conductivity can persist for weeks, months and longer, creating the chronic pain pattern.

The SCENAR is designed to sense this activity and, through a process of interactive feedback, to assist the tissue in its self-regulating processes.

The outcome of the interactive neurostimulation is that it affects the area of pathological activity locally through an increased blood circulation, neuropeptides release, stimulation of the lymph flow, muscle relaxation and centrally, by affecting the CNS, in particular, the autonomic nervous system.

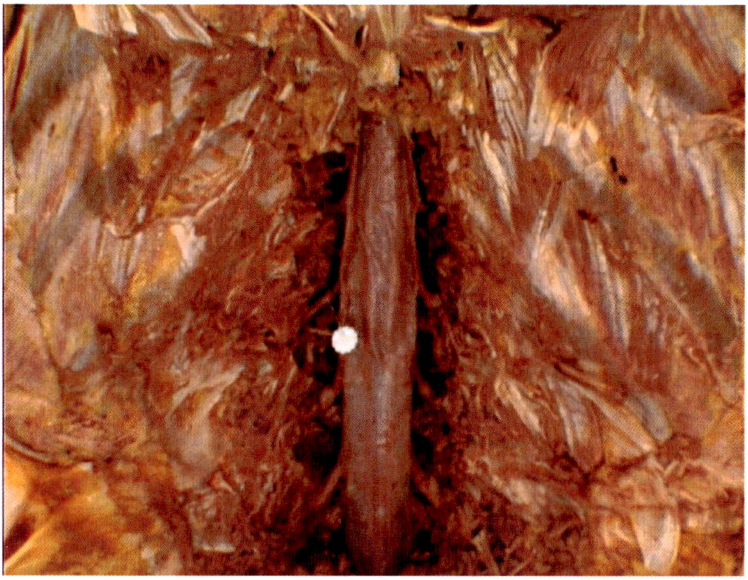

The operator of the SCENAR has the choice of a variety of modes when using the device. If desired it is possible to view aspects of this interaction on screen through sets of numbers and symbols. The device is capable of signaling to the operator when specific results have been achieved. All reactions are real-time and continuously changing according to the body's responses to the impulse. It is also possible to work more freely without attention to the screen and assess the results through easy to recognize signs in the tissue response itself.

The basic mode of operation of a typical Scenar device is to deliver a "dosage" of electrical stimulation impulses to the body via an in-built and/or remote electrodes in direct contact with the skin surface. **These impulses have been tailored to mimic the electrical discharges of the nervous system,** in order to elicit the organism's response with optimum efficiency and minimum disruption to cell function, depending upon the unique requirements of the presenting pain disease dynamics (or lack of same). The action is aimed at both the "fast" pain blocking A-fibres and the "slow" pain producing and peptide generating C-fibres.

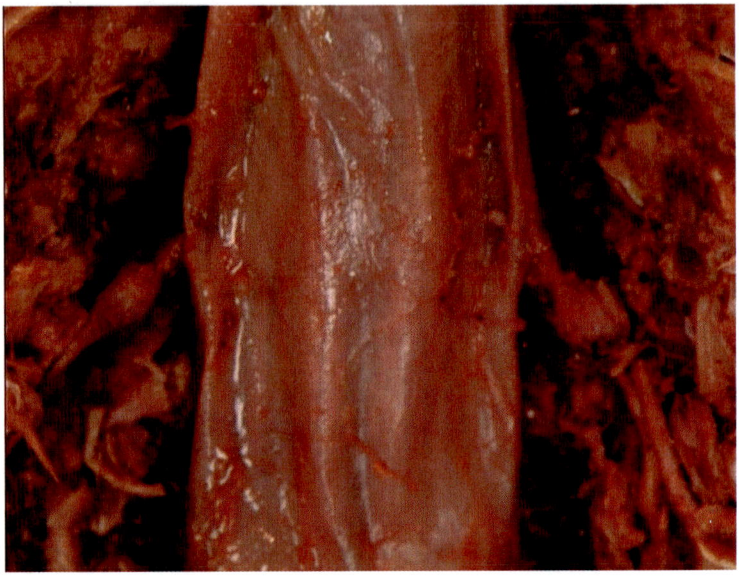

The signal stream, comprising waveform, signal strength (voltage and current) and frequency, can be varied in a number of ways, either by pre-section by the operator or automatically by the control circuitry of the device. The "dosage" can be delivered automatically or overridden at the discretion of the operator, with guidance from visual indicators.

Due to a "feedback" (device-organism-device), SCENAR devices respond to any change in the skin impedance. Any energetic change in the electric pulse of the device stimulates maximum response from the body. Therefore, there is neither discontinued orientation response form the body nor its adaptation to device treatment. Also, there is no decrease in the threshold sensation to a monotonous irritant, as against other electrostimulators. The impulse stimulates cells, tissues and organs and is transformed there into a signal containing information about certain pathology in the body. This information is further transferred to the central nervous system. And so, there is a formed functional system: the cerebrum receives this information, processes it, selects the proper systems of the body to be applied to for the express return to norm and orders them “to start acting”. It activates all the recovery mechanisms in the body, including the energy transfer mechanism, initiating gradual, step-by-step, transition of the body’s functions from pathology to norm.

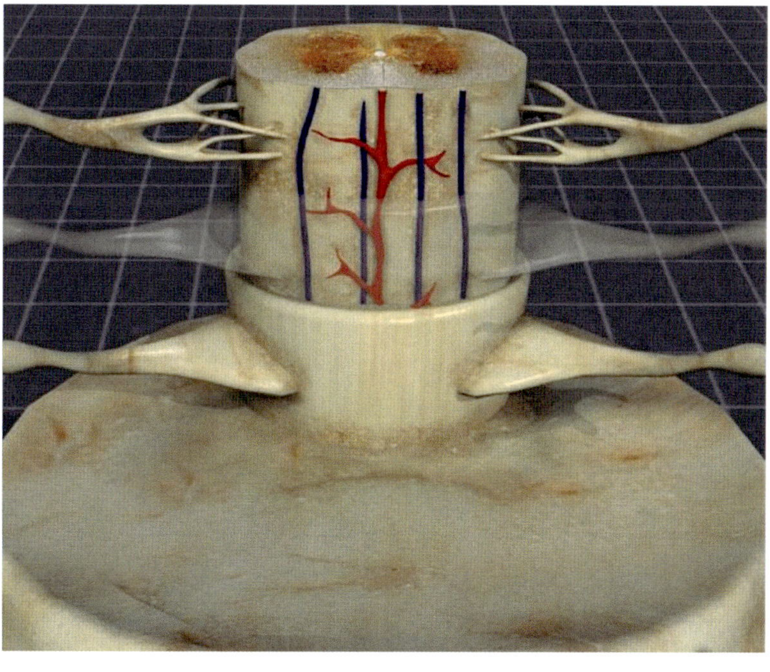

What does SCENAR do to the body? How does it affect the body’s physiology?

This will be a brief answer to a rather in-depth topic and requires a good understanding of the body's physiology to truly understand. We cover this topic extensively in mentoring and training.

In answering the question consider that SCENAR therapy functions on two physiological principles, that our bodies have their own healing capabilities and are continually employing processes of self-regulation to maintain our health.

The SCENAR delivers computer modulated therapeutic electro-stimulation via your skin. The SCENAR treatment produces local effects (i.e., stimulates the skin and blood vessels) as well as a general influence, by affecting neural and hormonal regulation systems.

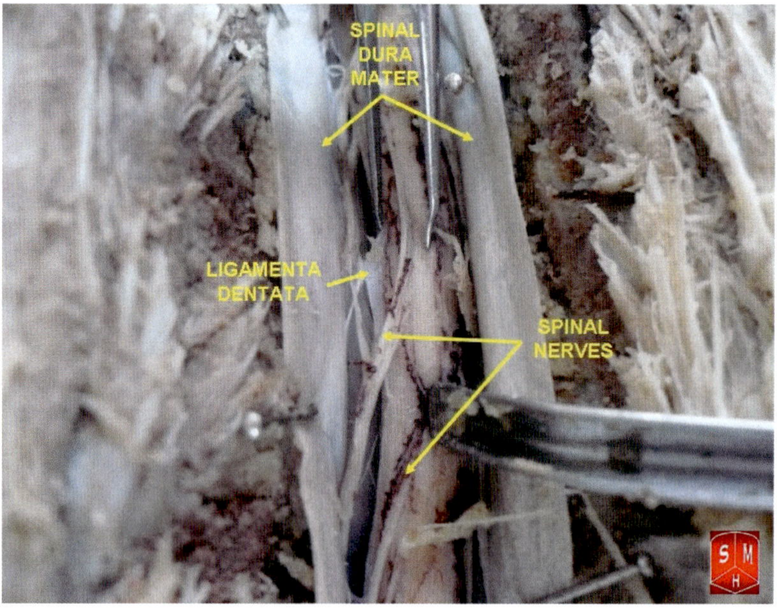
SPINAL
DURA
MATER
LIGAMENTA
DENTATA
SPINAL
NERVES

Due to its high amplitude, small unmyelinated **"C" fibers** are stimulated to a higher degree than with other forms of electrotherapy. Thus, when sufficiently stimulated these **"C" fibers** then trigger neuro and regulative-peptide release in your body. It is the release of these peptides that generates pain relief and effects healing processes in your body. The SCENAR impulse is carried via afferent nerve fibers to the regulatory centers in the brain which in turn respond via efferent nerve fibers. The SCENAR interprets the response and via computer modulation, results in its next impulse being modified accordingly which further provides information back to the brain to either amplify or dampen the pathological signals initiating pain, ultimately leading to homeostasis or stable equilibrium.

The practice of influencing skin nerve endings in particular points to control processes in the organs and systems is called reflex therapy. Various traditional healing methods, like acupuncture, acupressure and moxibustion by millennia of observation and trial discovered a system of specifically active points that can influence the internal organs, taking advantage of the unique relationship between skin and the internal workings of the entire body. Later, as the electric nature of nervous processes was discovered, electric stimulation of the skin entered practice, and the latest step in this development is the SCENAR therapy.

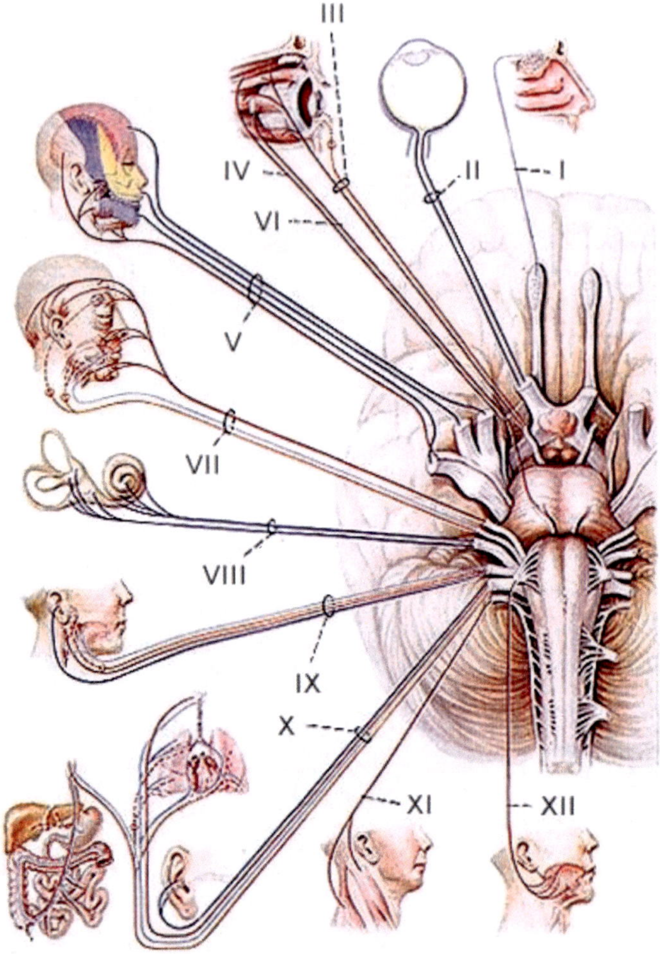
III
IV
VI
II
I
V
VII
VIII
IX
X
XI
XII

The active points on the skin are stimulated by electric impulses patterned after the natural discharges of the nervous system and adaptively controlled by feedback. This produces a unique effect, stimulating and optimizing the regulatory abilities of the nervous system for restoring health and protecting well-being.

The first thing to know is that SCENAR is actually an abbreviation for "self-controlled energo-neuro-adaptive regulator." It is a handheld regenerative electro-therapeutic medical device developed in Russia. In the U.S. market it is classified as a Class II Medical Device and it is available to patients by prescription. SCENAR was actually invented and developed in Russia nearly 20 years ago for the Russian cosmonauts in their Space Research Program. The Russians were proactively thinking about and taking care of the problem of health care and medicine for the cosmonauts just like NASA does for our astronauts. There are "professional" model SCENAR devices and simpler home unit devices for patients.

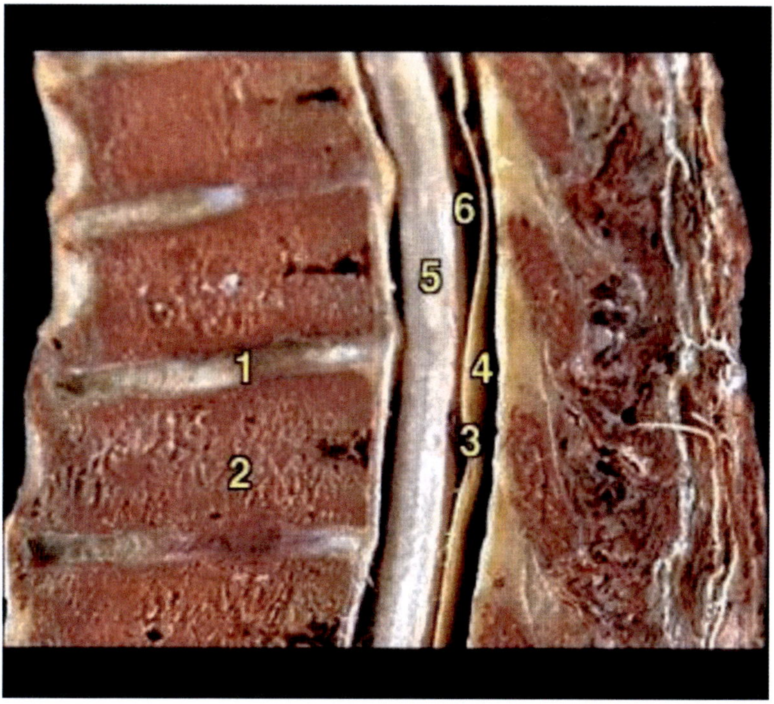
6
5
1
4
3
2

This will be a brief answer to a rather in-depth topic and requires a good understanding of the body's physiology to truly understand. We cover this topic extensively in mentoring and training.

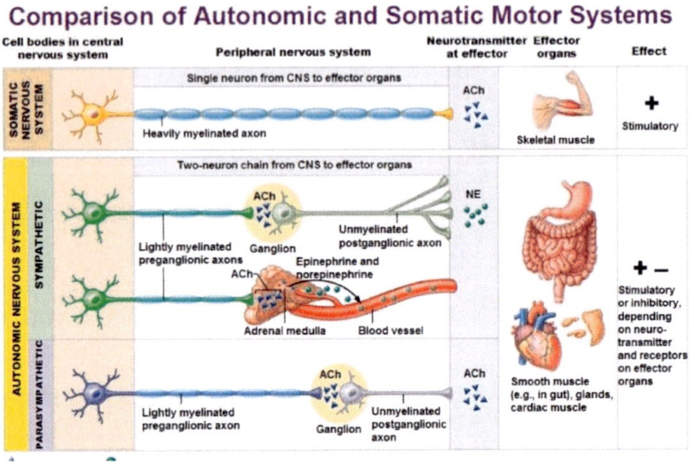
Comparison of Autonomic and Somatic Motor Systems
Cell bodies in central nervous system
Peripheral nervous system
Neurotransmitter at effector
Effector organs
Effect
SOMATIC NERVOUS SYSTEM
Single neuron from CNS to effector organs
ACh
Heavily myelinated axon
Skeletal muscle
+
Stimulatory
AUTONOMIC NERVOUS SYSTEM
SYMPATHETIC
Two-neuron chain from CNS to effector organs
ACh
NE
Unmyelinated postganglionic axon
Lightly myelinated preganglionic axons
Ganglion
Epinephrine and norepinephrine
ACh
Adrenal medulla
Blood vessel
+ –
Stimulatory or inhibitory, depending on neuro-transmitter and receptors on effector organs
PARASYMPATHETIC
ACh
ACh
Smooth muscle (e.g., in gut), glands, cardiac muscle
Lightly myelinated preganglionic axon
Ganglion
Unmyelinated postganglionic axon

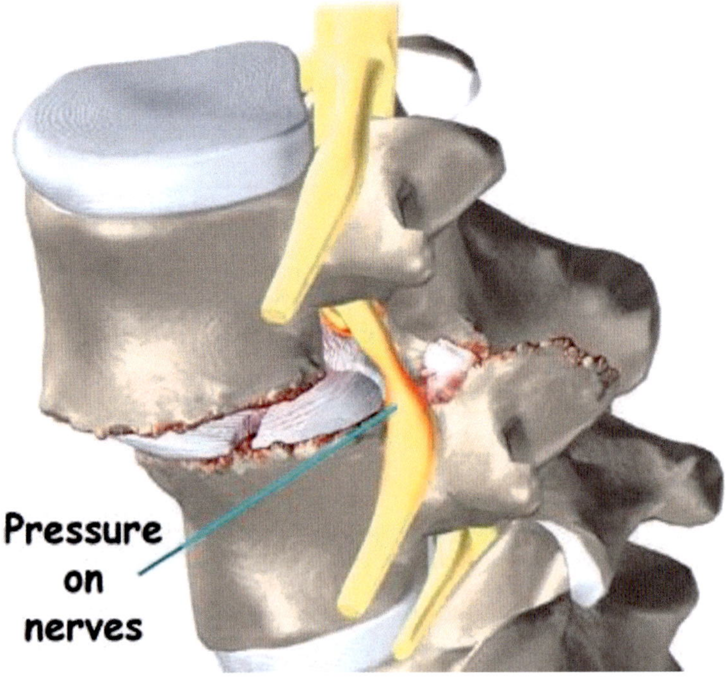
Pressure on nerves

How does Scenar Work?

The SCENAR is operated by placing the device directly onto the skin, where it collects electromagnetic signals, records the skin response and uses its sophisticated software to return a freshly modulated and modified signal back to the body.

In an area of pathological focus, the first sign is usually increased pain sensitivity to pressure; secondly, there is a marked decrease in electrical skin resistance. By sending endogenous biofeedback impulses toward the area of the pathological focus, the SCENAR device can also help the body to identify, “reconnect and recognize” the pathological area. This allows the person’s own body to release certain chemical substances (regulative peptides) which in turn help to regenerate the damaged cells or to restore the disturbed function.

Every event in the body, either normal or pathological produces electrical changes and alterations of the magnetic fields surrounding the body The electric fields produced during muscle movements are widely considered to provide the information that directs the activities of 'generative' cells such as osteoblasts, myoblasts, perivascular cells, fibroblasts and others that lay down or resorb collagen, thereby 'reforming' tissues so that they can adapt to the way the body is used. (Oschman, 1996).

The SCENAR delivers a "dosage" in the form of bi-polar electrical impulses to stimulate the body via built-in or attached electrodes in direct contact with the skin surface, and in accordance with electro-dermal impedance. These impulses have been tailored to mimic the electrical discharges of the nervous system in order to elicit the person's response with optimum efficiency and minimum disruption to cell function. The impulses act on the central nervous system via the ascending pathways of the spinal cord to the cortex of the brain which then conveys impulses to trigger responses in organs corresponding to the area of skin being treated. Additionally, it acts on the peripheral nervous system via the cytoplasm matrix and meridians. The SCENAR impulse by its nature also acts upon the segmental or dermatomal mechanism to act upon spinal reflexes.

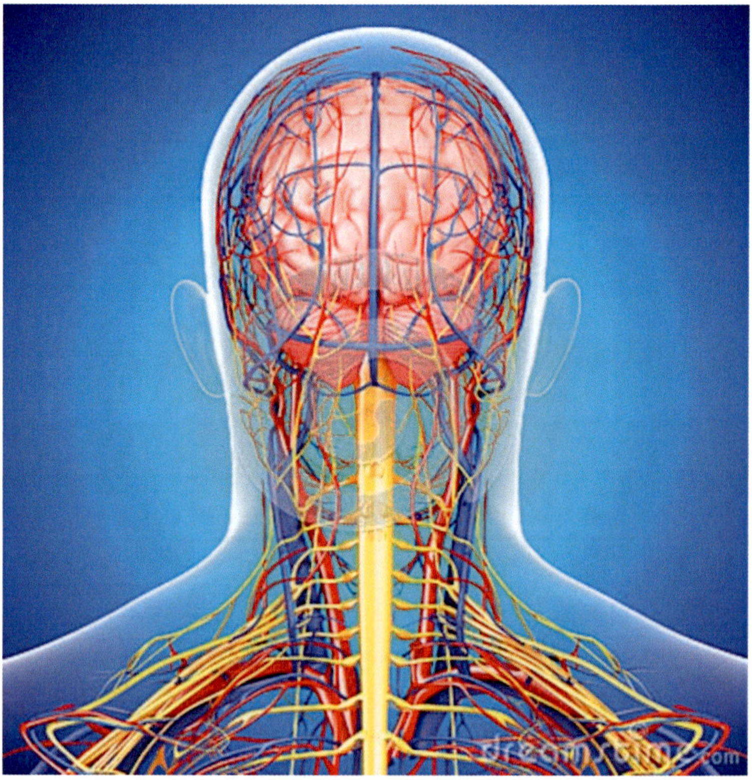

In response to the SCENAR impulse, regulative neuropeptides (chemicals released by nerves) are released in cascade, thus instigating a 'whole body' effect - it operates on both mind and body. It is the biofeedback function of the **SCENAR that provides an individual 'dosing' action** via the skin that promotes restoration of the body's disturbed (or lost) function. The "dosage" can be delivered automatically or over-ridden at the discretion of the therapist with guidance from visual, audio and tactile indicators plus digital diagnostic and treatment protocols.

The practitioner determines where to apply the device by looking for anomalies on the skin surface. These anomalies are indicated by redness, numbness, 'stickiness' (a magnetic-like drag as the device is moved across the skin) or a change in sound emitted from the device. Experience indicates that the body's natural healing process is commenced by treating these "asymmetries".

SCENAR impulses applied to the paravertebral zones, reduce the activity of the Renshaw cells (inhibitory interneurons that are innervated by collaterals from motorneurons and in turn form synapses with the same and adjacent motorneurons to exert inhibition) and therefore, restores the ability of the nervous system to damp down the transmission of pain impulses.

In conventional medicine, the adaptive reaction of the organism to a change in its external environment is called a "disease" and the approach is to "fight" with them in order to expel them from the organism. However, an adaptive reaction is not a disease. There seems to be little real sense in fighting these adaptive reactions: it appears to be more constructive to support the natural response of the organism. This is exactly what the SCENAR aims to do. **Its impulses aim to strengthen the integrity and natural balance of the organism as a whole by stimulating the nervous system to produce neuropeptides.** Neuropeptides are chemicals produced by the nerves, that keep the body balanced and reestablishes the body's natural physiological state in which healing is achieved. Without these regulatory neuropeptides, the body adapts and becomes "stuck" in "disease states" and portions of the body are blocked from communicating with the energetic system that keeps it in balance. **The SCENAR begins a dialogue with these blocked areas by providing a new stream of information.** Once the lines of communication have been reestablished, the information-starved areas keep on "talking".

Chapter 18.
Soft Tissue Injury and Neurological Case Studies

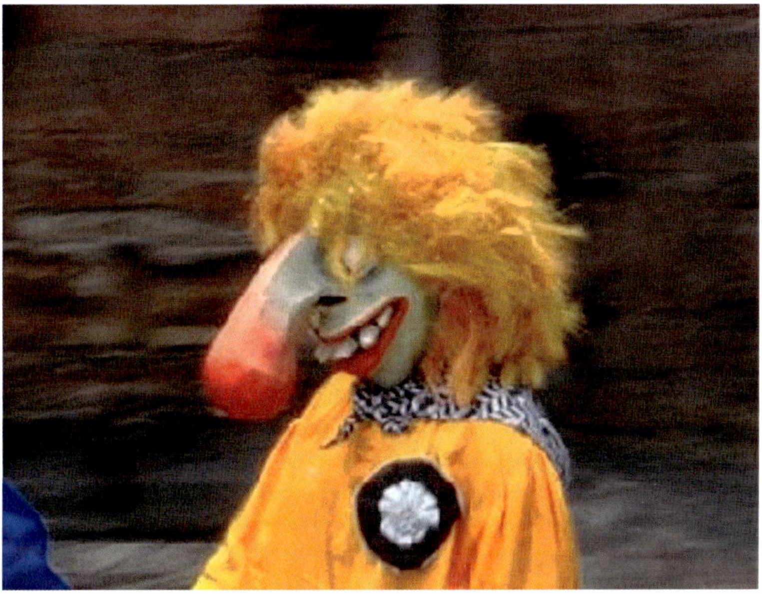

B.H., a thirty five year old businessman presented with an eighteen year old **rotator cuff injury** to his left shoulder. His range of motion was limited to fifty percent of normal with pain. He was treated five times using microcurrent electrical stimulation over a period of one week. His range of motion was increased and his pain was reduced after the first treatment. After the week he was pain free with full range of motion using ten pound weights.

C.B., a seventeen year old girl presented 24 hours after a car accident on the freeway where she suffered a **left-right, front to back and transverse whiplash.** At the time she presented she had no range of motion in her neck and severe pain. She reported that she had not had any medical care. She was treated three times over a five day period of time using microcurrent electrical stimulation. The first treatment reduced her pain by 80% and increased her range of motion by 50%. After the third treatment she reported being fully recovered.

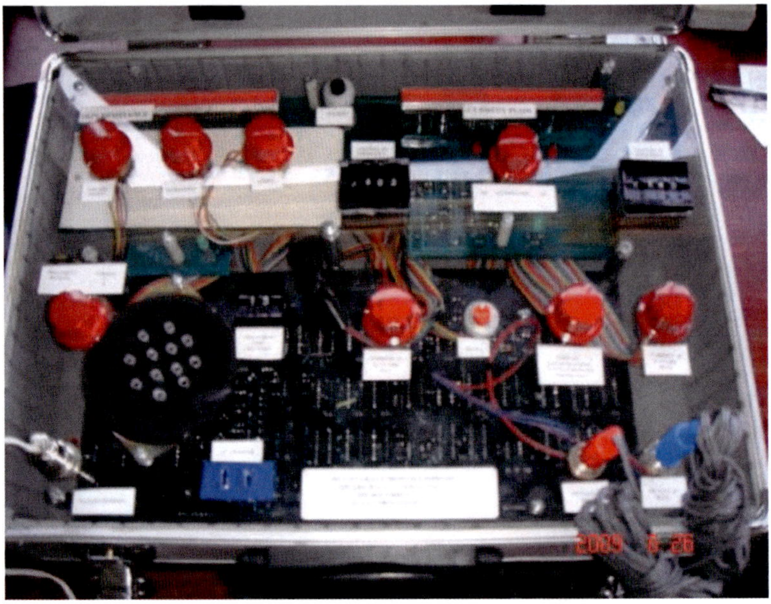
2009 8 26

D.B., a fifty year old female presented with two issues – TMJ and a **chronic injury to her right shoulder** with decreased range of motion and pain. Her TMJ was caused by trauma she sustained at the age of sixteen. She reported constant pain and restricted movement in her jaw with bruxism. Both conditions were treatment using microcurrent electrical stimulation. She had a series of eight treatments over three weeks. She was discharged with both conditions fully resolved. Weeks later she is saying “I don’t have TMJ anymore!”

H.H. presented with chronic **lumbar sacral strain** as a result of long hours of sitting at a computer. She was treated three times per week for two weeks using a combination of electro-therapy devices. She was discharged pain free with full range of motion. She was evaluated a week later with no return of symptoms.

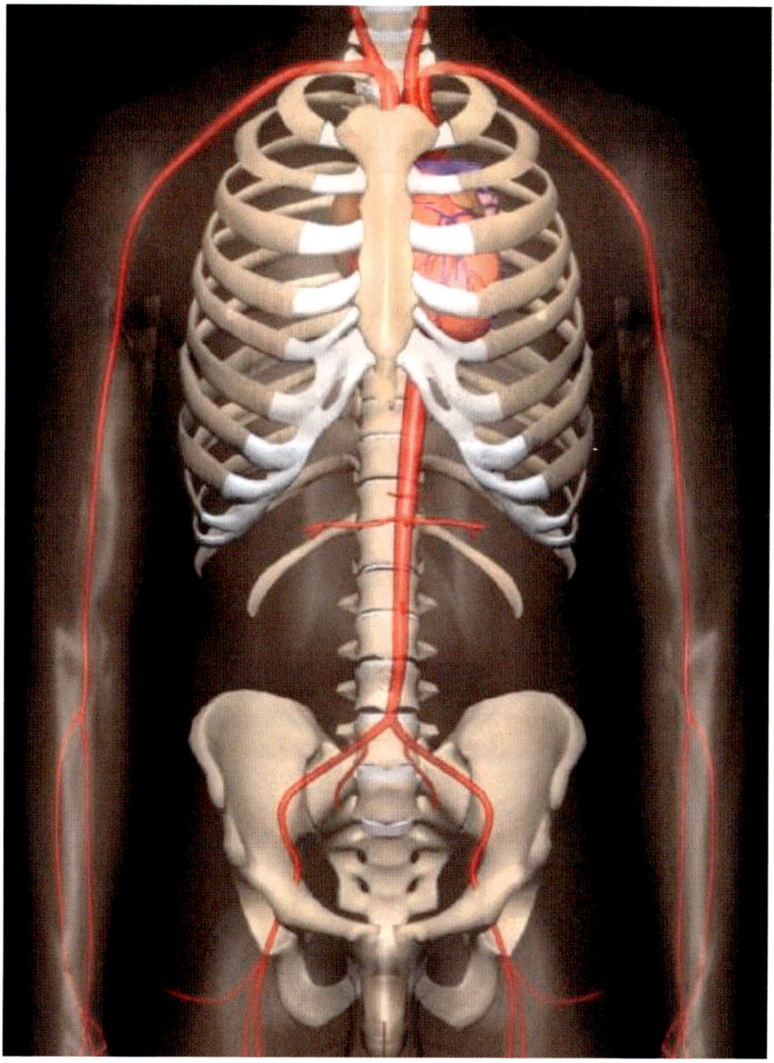

M.K., a Pilate's instructor, presented with **severe pain in her right foot.** She was treated seven times over a period of two weeks using microcurrent electrical stimulation on her foot and ankle. She was discharged as fully recovered.

F.D. presented with **chronic lumbar sacral pain with sciatica** resulting from heavy lifting in her job as a mail carrier. She was treated eight times over a three week period using a combination of electrical stimulation. Patient reported a consistent decrease in her pain and sciatica while at work. She was discharged as fully recovered.

G.H., a carpet cleaner, presented with pain from **lateral epicondylitis of his right elbow** resulting from his work. He was treated five times over 2 weeks using microcurrent stimulation with progressive results. He was discharged pain free and returned to work.

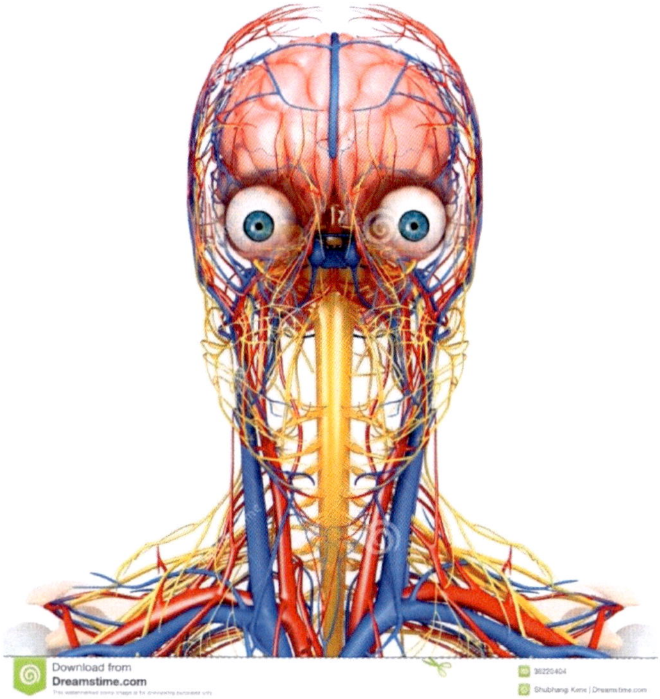
Download from
Dreamstime.com

L.H., a 77 year-old male, presented on March 1, 2007 complaining of **severe chronic pain over the entire surface of the right side of his face**. He stated he had this pain for 20 years and that it prevented him from eating and shaving among other activities. His face was somewhat contorted and his right eye and mouth drooped. He suffered from **Trigeminal Neuralgia**.

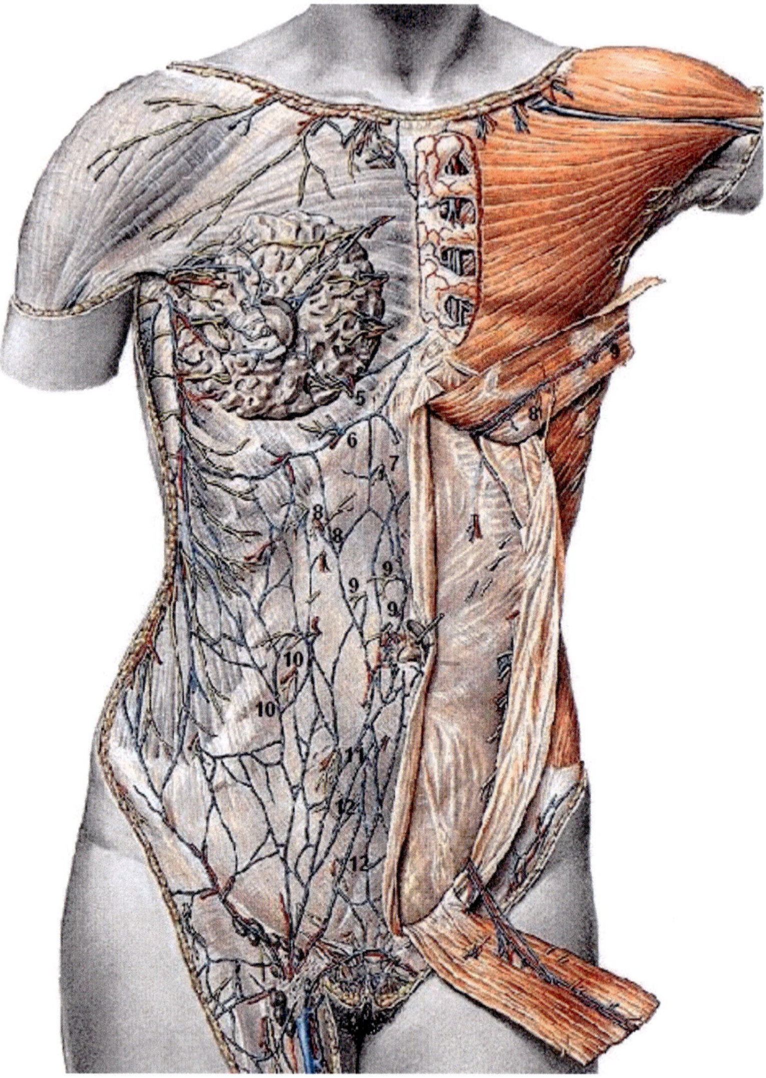
5
6
7
8
8
9
9
9
8
10
10
11
12
12

TN (Trigeminal Neuralgia) is a disorder of the fifth cranial (trigeminal) nerve that causes episodes of intense, stabbing, electric shock-like pain in the areas of the face where the branches of the nerve are distributed - lips, eyes, nose, scalp, forehead, upper jaw, and lower jaw. L.H. was taking three different types of medications including anti-convulsants, anti-spasmodics, and pain medication for the entire 20 years of his disease as prescribed by his doctors. At one point during this period, he had surgery on his face to deaden one of his facial nerves. The surgery had no lasting effect.

He was treated four times per week with the SCENAR electro-medicine treatment device for four weeks in the office. As a result, as of March 30, 2007, **his face is symmetrical, he has no pain and he is off of his medications. His personality, which was for 20 years depressed and morose due to the pain and the drug side effects, is now happy and lively. He is going out socially with his wife, dancing, brushing his teeth, eating and shaving with no pain.**

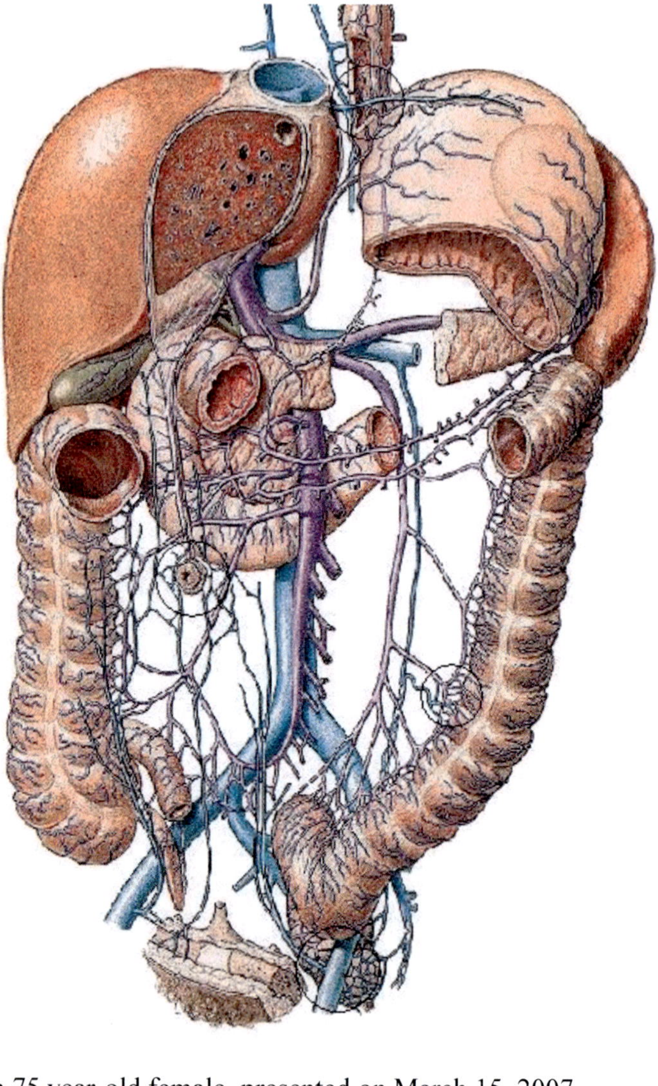

J.C., a 75 year-old female, presented on March 15, 2007 complaining of pain in her hands as the result of the onset of **Rheumatoid Arthritis**. She also complained of the severe stiffening of her two middle fingers as in a spasm on a regular basis. She was not on pain medication and her health was otherwise good.

She was treated with a Microcurrent electro-medicine treatment device and then the SCENAR treatment device three times per week for 3 weeks. Currently, she is reporting no pain and stiffness and no spasm. She shows off now by snapping her fingers for anyone who will watch. I feel we can prevent her arthritis from progressing by occasional treatment.

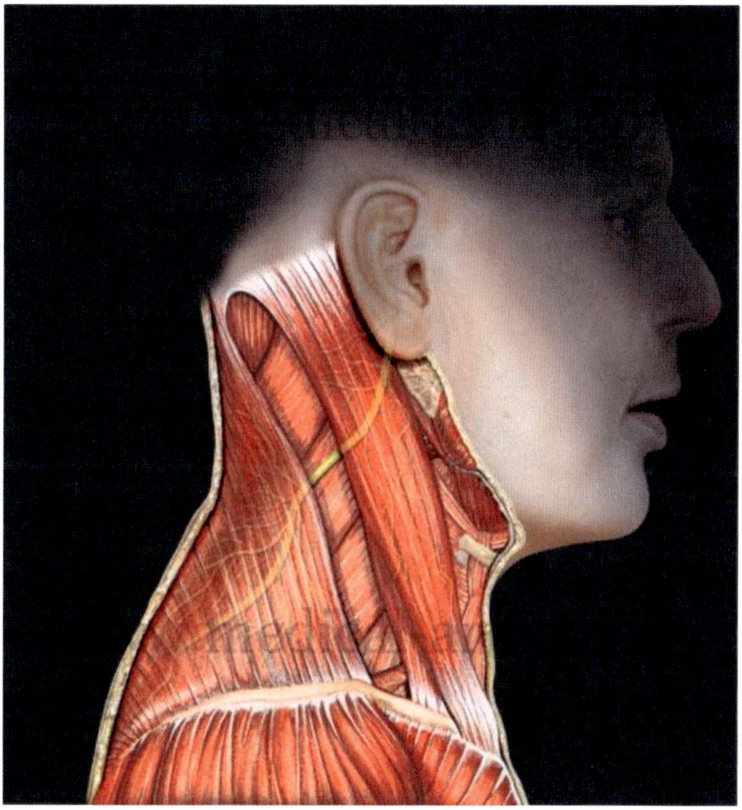

Case studies for spinal cord repair post trauma resulting in partial or complete severing at the cervical or upper thoracic level.

Darren, a 23 year-old male, presented with a total perseveration of his cervical spine as the result of a car accident wherein he exited the vehicle upon collision at high speed resulting in complete severing of his spinal cord at the C-3 4 level. This resulted in total disability of movement and bladder and bowel function, a quadriplegic. Therapy consisted of 14 months treatment including 3 forms of electro-therapy, exercise and visualization training by me.

As Darren progressed, he became able to eat, brush his teeth and hair, then move his pelvis, stand with assistance, learn to use a self propelled wheelchair and finally stand and walk unassisted after 14 months of therapy and daily exercise. He has since moved to Hawaii to pursue his work as an artist painter. Yes, he paints with his hand.

Leslie, a 32 year-old woman, presented with complete perseveration of the spinal cord at T- Level as the result of a car accident. This left her a paraplegic with no use of her legs. She was wheelchair bound. Therapy consisted of 9 months of treatment including 3 forms of electro-therapy, exercise and visualization training by myself. As a result, she was able to abandon the wheelchair and walk either with a walker, a cane, and sometimes unassisted. I will have to say that if she had continued therapy for 4 more months, she would have progressed further.

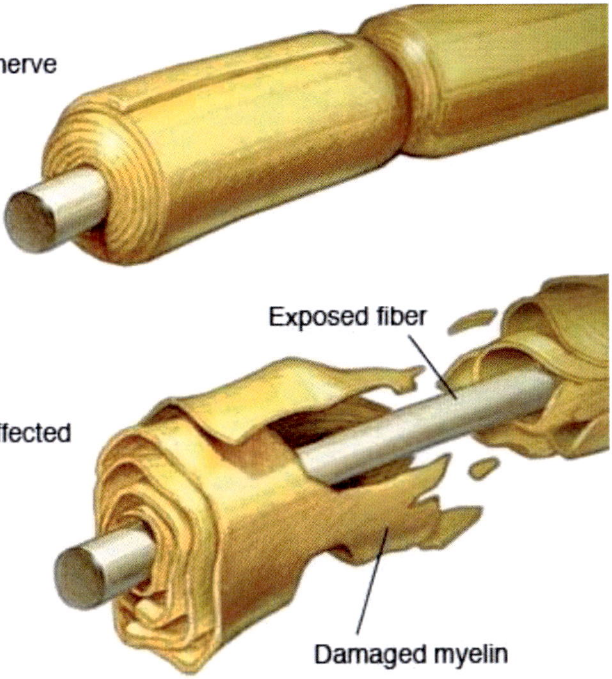
Normal nerve
Exposed fiber
Nerve affected by MS
Damaged myelin

© MAYO FOUNDATION FOR MEDICAL EDUCATION AND RESEARCH. ALL RIGHTS RESERVED.

John, a 46 year-old male, presented with a fractured back and severed spinal cord at T-8 9, the result of a fall off a mountain cliff. As a result, he was wheelchair bound and unable to walk. Therapy consisted of 8 months of treatment including three forms of electro-therapy, exercise and visualization training by me. As time progressed, he became able to leave his wheelchair, move his pelvis, and walk with a walker, then a cane and finally unassisted.

Lenore, a 37 year-old female, presented with partial persevereation of her spinal cord at C – 5 6 Level, resulting very limited use of her arms and hands and no use of her legs. Therapy consisted of 12 months of treatment including 3 forms of electro-therapy, exercise and visualization training by me. As the therapy progressed, she became able to use her Hands and arms. During the last four months of therapy she was able leave her wheelchair and begin to walk, first with assistance and then without.

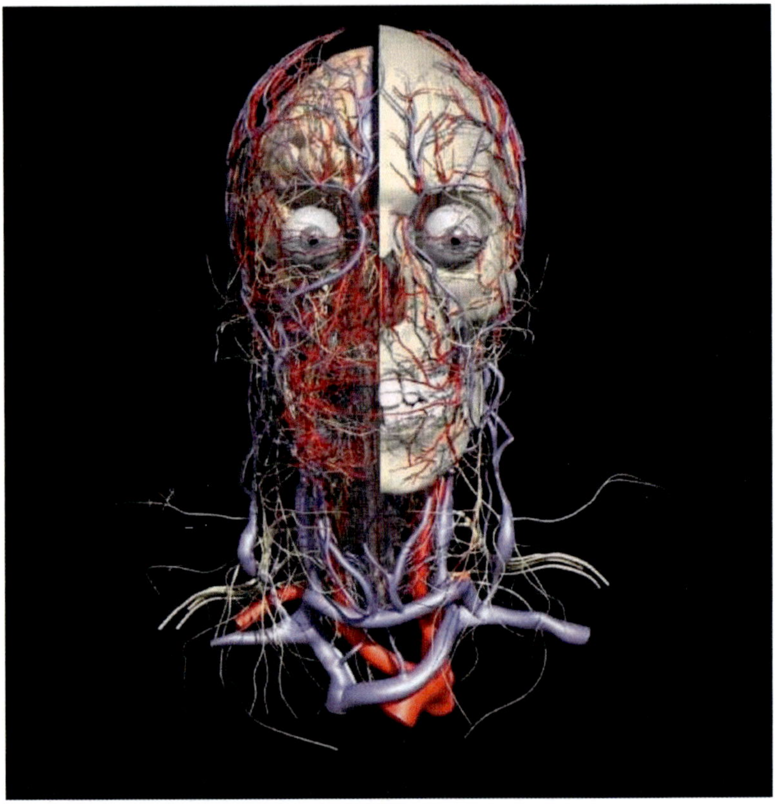

Greg is 28 year-old male who suffered a compression fracture of his neck with compression of his spinal cord at C- 4 5. As a result, he was rendered a complete quadriplegic. He had no use of his arms, hands, fingers, legs, feet, bowel or bladder. Therapy consisted of 7 months of treatment including three forms of electro-therapy, exercise and visualization training by me.

He has some use of his right arm and hand and he is able to leave his fully automated wheelchair and use a manual one to wheel himself around. He has bladder and bowel control and is able to have sex with his wife on a regular basis. He is still in therapy, and will be for about eight more months. He is right on schedule in progress, with the 21 other patients I have worked with.

So these are five typical cases from 20 years of work with Quadriplegics and paraplegics. Their progress is consistent, seems to be on the same schedule and always works. The only soft factor in all of this is: How much time and effort the patient is willing to put into their rehabilitation. This is not just my work. The patient has to commit to several hours a day for a year or more, to make it work.

Index

Made in the USA
Middletown, DE
10 November 2024

64228846R00261